Stanley Stephens.

Jan '83

Rehabilitation of the Neurological Patient

REHABILITATION OF THE NEUROLOGICAL PATIENT

L. S. ILLIS
MD, BSc, FRCP
Consultant Neurologist
Wessex Neurological Centre
Clinical Senior Lecturer in Neurology
University of Southampton Medical School

E. M. SEDGWICK
BSc, MD
Consultant in Clinical Neurophysiology
Wessex Neurological Centre
Senior Lecturer in Clinical Neurophysiology
University of Southampton Medical School

H. J. GLANVILLE
FRCP, DPhyMed
Emeritus Foundation Professor
Europe Chair of Rehabilitation
University of Southampton Medical School

With a Foreword by
Baroness Masham of Ilton

BLACKWELL SCIENTIFIC PUBLICATIONS
OXFORD LONDON EDINBURGH
BOSTON MELBOURNE

DISTRIBUTORS

USA
  Blackwell Mosby Book Distributors
  11830 Westline Industrial Drive
  St. Louis, Missouri 63141

Canada
  Blackwell Mosby Book Distributors
  120 Melford Drive, Scarborough
  Ontario M1B 2X4

Australia
  Blackwell Scientific Book Distributors
  214 Berkely Street, Carlton
  Victoria 3053

British Library
  Cataloguing in Publication Data

Illis, L. S.
  Rehabilitation of the neurological patient.
  1. Nervous system—Diseases
  2. Rehabilitation
  I. Title   II. Sedgwick, E. M.   III. Glanville,
H. J.
  362.1′968   RC350.4

ISBN 0-632-00595-5

Contents

List of Contributors

P. BACH-Y-RITA, Veterans Administration Hospital, Martinez, California, and Departments of Physical Medicine and Rehabilitation and Human Physiology, University of California, Davis, USA.

M. DEVOR, Life Sciences Institute, The Hebrew University of Jerusalem, Israel.

C. D. EVANS, Purley, Surrey, UK. Formerly Consultant in Rheumatology and Rehabilitation to the Oxford Area Health Authority (Teaching).

R. C. L. FENELEY, Department of Urology, Southmead Hospital, Bristol, UK.

H. L. FRANKEL, National Spinal Injuries Centre, Stoke Mandeville Hospital, Aylesbury, Bucks, UK.

H. J. GLANVILLE, Emeritus Foundation Professor, Europe Chair of Rehabilitation, University of Southampton Medical School, Southampton, UK.

L. S. ILLIS, Wessex Neurological Centre, Southampton General Hospital, and University of Southampton Medical School, Southampton, UK.

R. LANGTON HEWER, Department of Neurology, Frenchay Hospital, Bristol, UK.

D. M. LONG, Department of Neurological Surgery, The Johns Hopkins Hospital, Baltimore, Maryland, USA.

The late P. J. R. NICHOLS, formerly of Mary Marlborough Lodge, Nuffield Orthopaedic Centre, Headington, Oxford, UK.

J. M. NIGHTINGALE, Departments of Electrical Engineering and Electronics, University of Southampton, Southampton, UK.

E. M. SEDGWICK, Wessex Neurological Centre, Southampton General Hospital, and University of Southampton Medical School, Southampton, UK.

M. J. TORRENS, Department of Neurosurgery, Frenchay Hospital, Bristol, UK.

R. O. WELLER, Department of Neuropathology, Southampton General Hospital, and University of Southampton Medical School, Southampton, UK.

C. B. WYNN PARRY, Royal National Orthopaedic Hospital, London, UK.

OBITUARY—PHILLIP NICHOLS

PHILLIP NICHOLS died suddenly, after a short illness, before he was able to revise his manuscript for this publication. The editors have revised the manuscript and we think that Phillip would have approved this published form.

Phillip Nichols had a distinguished career in rehabilitation in the Royal Air Force and subsequently made an outstanding contribution to rehabilitation of the severely disabled at Mary Marlborough Lodge, Oxford. Until his death he was adviser in rehabilitation to the Department of Health and Social Security.

He will be sadly missed by his many friends and by his patients.

Hugh Glanville, L. S. Illis, E. M. Sedgwick

Foreword

It is with great pleasure that I congratulate Dr L. S. Illis, Dr E. M. Sedgwick and Professor Hugh Glanville on producing this book. They are experts in their fields of medicine. Sometimes the most difficult aspects of life are swept under the carpet. For a long time there has been a need to bring to the fore the rehabilitation of the neurological patient.

Over the past fifteen years or so there has been an increasing interest in the nature of neurological deficit following experimental lesions of the nervous system, and the nature of recovery as the nervous system adapts. More recently, there has been a great stimulus to investigating the problems of neurologically disabled people. This stimulus has come from workers as diverse as neuropathologists, experimental neurophysiologists and engineers. Although it is unrealistic to look towards a cure for neurological disability, as for example in spinal cord injury, one can undoubtedly look towards considerable improvement in neurological function by the application of known techniques and by the cooperation of rehabilitation doctors, neurologists, neurophysiologists and engineers. The so-called basic sciences of anatomy and physiology are particularly relevant to neurological disablement and the principles of neurological rehabilitation. There is, however, no single textbook on neurological rehabilitation which brings together the basic sciences, rehabilitation principles and research in rehabilitation.

This book has been compiled with that particular facet in mind. The three parts of this book indicate firstly the changes which occur as a result of a lesion in the adult central nervous system and indicate the capacities which exist within the central nervous system for change at structural and functional level. In a sense, this part of the book outlines the basic science of rehabilitation on which assessment and treatment programmes must be based. Secondly, the major part of the book deals with specific neurological problems outlined by authors who are eminent in their particular fields and who are all engaged in running a clinical service. Thirdly, the final chapters review some new approaches to rehabilitation. This section deals not so much with established procedures, but is an indication of future possibilities based on existing research in engineering, in the use of alternative sensory channels and in the use of repetitive stimulation to possibly modify the function of the nervous system.

In a book of this scope there are bound to be many omissions, both intentional and unintentional. For example, it is impossible in a book of this type to give practical details of physiotherapeutic procedures which may be used in neurological rehabilitation. In due time much of this book will become out of date and doctors and patients will welcome the advances that make it out of date. In the meantime, it serves its intended function as a much needed review of this new, cooperative, field of functional neurological and neurophysiological medicine.

I hope this book will help the readers to understand more fully the concept of neurological disablement and to help them to be more aware of the need for comprehensive rehabilitation.

Susan Masham
January 1982

Preface

It has been stated that an improvement in rehabilitation standards could mean more to millions of people than almost any other medical advance (Secretary of State for the Social Services, UK, 1973). For years specialists in various fields have been exhorted to carry out the rehabilitation of patients within their own speciality. At the same time the general field of rehabilitation has tended to lack intellectual excitement and fulfilment, and has failed to capture the imagination of medical students.

This volume represents the attempt of specialists in Neurology, Neurophysiology and Rehabilitation to indicate the possibilities for rehabilitation of the neurological patient. The book is not intended as a handbook of techniques, although many techniques are described. There are three main sections in the book: the first section deals with basic sciences, that is, the altered anatomy and physiology as a result of a lesion in the central nervous system, and indicates the way this knowledge may shape rehabilitation techniques and the great importance of applying neurophysiological methods in the assessment and management of patients with chronic neurological deficit. In the second section the problems of patients with specific disorders are dealt with by experts in their fields. The third section of the book is the most controversial, and indicates some possibilities for the future. These possibilities may never be realized, but they indicate ways in which neurological rehabilitation may grow. There are many other prospects for the future, for example the possibility of encouraging regeneration in the central nervous system. This is something which one would hardly have dared talk about ten or fifteen years ago, but in recent years there has been an upsurge of interest in this possibility.

Perhaps the most encouraging aspect of the book is the way in which specialists from disparate fields come together with a common aim. For too long the field of rehabilitation has been neglected by specialists such as neurologists, neurophysiologists and urologists. Perhaps the time has come for an enlightened Government to establish small but active Neurological Rehabilitation Research Units, where teams such as indicated in this book could work on the common problems involving neurological deficit and pain.

ACKNOWLEDGEMENTS

It is a pleasure to acknowledge the immense help we have received from Dr Ray Tallis of the Wessex Neurological Centre.

Without the hours of patient and painstaking secretarial work of Miss Gillian Green the editors' task would have been impossible and we gratefully record our appreciation.

The Muscular Dystrophy Group of Great Britain have kindly permitted us to use material from one of their publications in Chapter 11.

Chapter 1
What is Rehabilitation?

Sommerville (1975) suggested that rehabilitation was first used in common English parlance in the meaning of 'making able' and 'making able again' to denote readoption of denominational dress by transgressors who had been temporarily denied the privilege of wearing it.

Rehabilitation is a word which is used increasingly in different contexts, it therefore suggests different things and there is no specific acceptance of its meaning. To some it means reinstatement, or even instatement for the first time in the physical sense, others will interpret it as applying to the reinstatement of offenders, addicts and people suffering from psychiatric disorders. It is within the definition formulated in the Mair Report (1972), *Medical Rehabilitation: the Pattern for the Future*, that the meaning is taken for this book: 'Rehabilitation implies the restoration of patients to their fullest physical, mental and social capability'; and one might add 'in the shortest possible time'.

When we relate this concept to the problem of neurological disability, which is often progressive, which usually affects many rather than single functions, which usually excludes cure as a possible outcome of rehabilitation, the objective will be to help the patient to achieve the best possible quality of life in the circumstances. The patient cannot be considered singly; for example, a wheel-chair existence directly affects everyone with whom the sufferer is associated, including family, people at work, and many others in society whom he regularly meets. In his book, Cooper (1976) introduces the concept of the Fourth World of handicapped people who are with us and need the support of family and friends. These people are not two entities, but one organism irretrievably locked together and bound 'by a combination of concern, love, despair, frustration and feelings of guilt'. Parents and loved ones, too, are in a sense citizens of this Fourth World because they are drawn into it. Doctors and others, whose role it is to help disabled people, must learn to understand these human and social relationships in order to develop the knowledge to counsel and to help them wisely. Cooper rightly points out that the rule for survival has always been 'adapt or perish', and emphasizes that our contribution must be to help victims and their relatives to accept what is inevitable, to correct what is correctable and to build new lives by adapting to new circumstances.

The report on specific technical matters from the 29th World Health Assembly

1

(World Health Organization, 1976) states that rehabilitation is usually defined as the third phase of medicine, prevention being the first and curative care the second. Throughout the report the term is used, as here, to define interactions which in general aim to provide treatment and services to patients who are already disabled or at risk due to an interference with function. In 1969, the WHO expert committee (World Health Organization, 1969) defined rehabilitation as follows: 'the combined and coordinated use of medical, social, educational and vocational measures for training or retraining the individual to the highest possible level of functional ability'. This definition relates mainly to intervention aimed at the individual with less emphasis upon altering the factors in immediate surroundings or in society which all bear heavily upon the problem.

An understanding of the word rehabilitation by no means eliminates the confusion surrounding the use of common terms such an *impairment, functional limitation, handicap* and *disability*.

DEFINITIONS

Impairment, for practical purposes, means 'a missing or defective part, tissue, organ or mechanism of the body . . .' (World Health Organization, 1969).

Functional limitation may or may not result from impairment, as defined above, and such limitations may be regressive or progressive depending upon the cause.

Handicap 'reflects the value attached to an individual's status when it departs from the norm. In the context of health care handicap is the disadvantage that is consequent upon impairment and disability . . .' (Wood, 1975).

Disability '. . . describes a functional departure from the norm and as such it mediates between impairment and handicap. In the context of health care disability is the loss or reduction of functional ability and activity that is consequent upon impairment' (Wood, 1975).

Obviously impairment, for example the loss of a leg, will be a disadvantage and therefore a handicap to a rock climber. On the other hand, such loss will little affect a sedentary worker's efficiency at work. Disability consequent upon the same cause will be variously reflected in different individuals consequent upon their attitudes, social status, occupation and so on.

The International Classification of Diseases (ICD) deals with diagnoses but not with their outcome. At the Conference for the Ninth Revision of the ICD, 1975, a resolution recommended a tentative draft classification of impairments and handicaps for trial purposes and the work was undertaken by P. H. N. Wood, ARC Epidemiological Research Unit, Manchester. It is an important step because at present there is no standard accepted classification of impairment and handicap, and consequently no common scientific classification of impairment and handicap such as would provide a base line for research and evaluation by ensuring that 'like' is being compared with 'like'.

Other workers have contributed to this problem, for example Agerholm (1975) and Taylor (1977) who draw attention to the inter-relationship of physical impairment, functional limitation, disability and social handicap. These attempts at clarification of terms and of coding are particularly important in the field of neurological rehabilitation which needs a common language as a prerequisite for the measurement of the many factors which, for need of a better word, we describe as function.

WHO has many important functions in relation to rehabilitation. For example, there are probably 380 000 000 disabled people in the world (World Health Organization, 1976), but where do priorities lie for prevention and intervention? With limited resources where can they be best used? Would it be by providing protein and vitamins for the third world or are there some areas in which finance should be applied to aid research into neurological disorders, for example, which are responsible for the most severely handicapped people amongst us? For the first time in decades there is real evidence that such people can begin to hope for a better future through new approaches.

POTENTIAL FOR IMPROVEMENT

The Sherrington concept of neurophysiology no longer explains observed facts. It does not, for example, explain how a man whose sensory apparatus had been destroyed by neurovirus was totally dependent when admitted to our unit and subsequently 'recovered'. The main features were complete absence of proprioception and patchy loss of cutaneous sensation. Eventually he became totally independent and returned to gainful employment although at that point routine neurological examination revealed no objective deviation from the pre-recovery state. Similarly, it is usual that following acute cord or brain damage, stabilization occurs after a period of two or more years, but we have no evidence that upper neurons regenerate although they seem to attempt to do so by inexpedient sprouting. What then happens? Illis (1973) has postulated how alternative connections would be possible between cell stations. He shows how such interconnections could prevent the total failure of a system if one station were destroyed. On the other hand, failure would follow if alternative pathways did not exist. In this book, Devor states the paradox in recovery of the central nervous system. He puts his finger on the point in the statement that 'among the so called "plastic" changes the physical basis of rehabilitation will be found'.

We do not know enough about the presence or connections of alternative pathways, about how to recruit them or how to influence the 'plastic' changes which undeniably happen. It is interesting to draw an analogy with Victorian engineers (Rolt, 1970) who found solutions to practical problems before they understood the scientific basis for them, and doctors who observe the complexity of hand function for example and understand the implications of the mechanisms that provide it but not all their details. Control engineers view hand function as a challenge to be reproduced by electronic circuitry and mechanical hardware (Glanville, 1976). Their exciting progress was partly determined by ingenuity in devising sensors and circuitry to perform some of the functions of the interneurone system, so that simple commands would evoke an element of automatic function that is inherent but elusive in our comprehension of the human mechanism.

Comparison of the performance of biomechanical and electronic mechanisms leads, not surprisingly, to the observation of differences between them and for example, how biological sensors are capable of both coarse and very fine responses according to the requirements of a given movement. Other instances illustrate how normal physiology has been better understood through the need to develop devices to carry out similar functions. For example, computers, calculators and memory banks can carry out, or could be programmed to accomplish, some functions of which the brain is capable. How far the mechanisms are or are not electronically similar is open to conjecture. We do know, however, a good deal about neurophysiological responses in the brain and computer science now suggests how the brain might handle certain tasks. In another instance it was commonly observed that weak muscles from poliomyelitis could be strengthened by exercise. It seemed that perseverance by the rehabilitation team and the patient were of prime importance. If improvement did occur it tended to continue for about two years. When electromyography was used to study action potentials in these patients recovery seemed to correspond with the appearance of 'giant potentials'. The reason for their appearance and their association with recovery was later explained by the discovery of peripheral sprouting of motor units to innervate adjacent denervated muscle fibres—a hitherto unknown phenomenon. It follows that the organized study of recovery and deterioration of function by qualified personnel at all levels, against the background knowledge of the normal central nervous system, must be rewarding. Imagination as well as the means to develop new diagnostic tools will play an important part.

Our problem is to unravel the complex circuitry of the central nervous system because until we can do so a specific approach to its rehabilitation is impossible.

The regenerative powers of the peripheral nervous system, improved techniques in nerve and tendon surgery, and better orthotic devices have greatly improved the outlook in plexus and peripheral nerve lesions. Wynn Parry (1966) points out here and elsewhere that recovery can be accelerated by good aftercare and re-education. He demonstrates through careful serial assessments how motor as well as sensory function can be re-educated in the hand more quickly and completely through training than by a passive approach. He describes, too, how transcutaneous electrical stimulation has proved useful in a number of painful peripheral nerve disorders. His work is supported by carefully compiled evidence which justifies the therapy advised even if the physiological reasons for the observed effects are not always fully understood. Similarly Illis and Sedgwick in this book have studied in depth and longitudinally a few patients undergoing spinal cord stimulation and their work points to the effects that can be expected or at least hoped for. In practice this means that careful observation makes it possible to advise patients what improvement they could expect and what are the attendant risks. The mechanisms underlying improvement are not known, but Cook's observation that his patients treated for intractable pain by cord stimulation suffering from concurrent multiple sclerosis showed functional improvement has been confirmed by other workers and the amount, duration and quality of improvement are being verified so that cord stimulation in selected cases has passed beyond the stage of 'experimental therapy'.

Unfortunately, in the past, failure to carry out scientific evaluation of outcome to support clinical impression has caused good, or at least useful, forms of intervention to fall into disrepute and useless interventions to be perpetuated. Thus electrical stimulation fell into disrepute and almost total rejection in the United Kingdom during the three decades after the Second World War on the grounds that it represented a form of passive treatment whilst active treatment, i.e. 'doing exercises', would always achieve a better result. Electrical stimulation, nevertheless, had a few protagonists, some of whom would hold one form of faradic stimulator to be 'better than' another. Certainly output parameters of faradic stimulators varied wildly, and possibly therefore some did give better results than others, but claims were not supported by real evidence and it was not until the appearance of square wave stimulators with good output control that serious interest was aroused again. Now electrical stimulation has many uses which include functional electronic stimulation (Dimitrijevic *et al.*, 1968; Glanville, 1972) in which functional motor effects as well as inhibitory effects upon the spastic calf, in hemiplegia, are described.

MEASUREMENT OF FUNCTION

To measure function accurately, repeatably and objectively is exceedingly difficult because function is compounded of an immense multitude of factors which are as difficult to identify, isolate and measure. The need to measure in order to compare and to assess the outcome of intervention is not in doubt, and whilst many workers are continuously trying to devise and improve methods the clinician will often have to innovate and compromise in choices to suit his need to test the value and cost effectiveness of alternative therapies.

The UK armed forces adopted a rough classification for troops in order to measure their suitability for service. During the Second World War a system called PULHEEMS was introduced which was designed to provide a profile of the individual. Each initial represents a capability which is classified from 1 (perfect) to 8 (nil) for each individual:

P   Physical capacity
U   Upper limbs
L   Lower limbs
H   Hearing
E   Eyesight L
E   Eyesight R
M   Mental capacity
S   Stability (emotional)

It now becomes simple to match the capability of an individual for specific jobs in the services. The score under each heading also gives a rough profile of capability. Obviously a low scorer under H would be a bad choice for a radio operator—motivation however, does sometimes produce extraordinary exceptions! (e.g. a double lower limb amputee who continued a distinguished career as an operational pilot during the Second World War). The system does not give the detail needed for most scientific evaluation, but it probably did influence thinking about scoring systems in common use in *daily living departments* of rehabilitation units where it is necessary to assess the individual as to ability in independence etc. Most units tend to invent their own systems for this purpose, based upon ability of the individual to carry out essential tasks for independent living without assistance, with aids or with assistance. Some include a time factor because obviously to be able to dress without help is valueless if it takes all day! A seminar at the Northwick Park Hospital dealt with these complex problems (Yates, 1976) including the quality of life (and how to measure it), and amongst other contributions there is a useful description of a move by the British Association of Occupational Therapists to standardize Activities of Daily Living assessment (Jay, 1976). Nichols (1976), however, questioned whether Activities of Daily Living indices were of any value on the grounds that they are subjective and therefore not reliable or repeatable, for a whole variety of reasons. Whiting and Lincoln (1980) discuss an Activities of Daily Living assessment for stroke patients. Evans in this book describes a practical system for the evaluation of progress in brain-damaged patients. The system identifies the point at which improvement stops and therefore when emphasis should change from active to supportive programmes. The decision is always a difficult one for the clinician to make, but clear guidelines are helpful in indicating when to conserve rather than to misapply scarce resources. Lynn and co-workers (1977) describe how a programmed signal can produce a spot tracing or 'target' on a cathode ray screen. The signal can be followed by a patient using a manual device to manipulate in order to maintain a circular marker around the target. Accuracy in following the target can be estimated by scanning and it then becomes possible to show the degree of error expressed numerically during the task. Although the actual activity is valueless in terms of usefulness in the life situation, it is nevertheless a valuable measure in assessing accuracy in performing the task, which requires manipulative skill, coordination and response in tracking the target.

Again, Miller and co-workers (1978) demonstrated the EMG patterns of arm movement and muscle activity in 20 subjects whilst turning a cranked wheel. This activity involves the patterns of muscle activity common to the reaching and retrieving movements of daily living. It was possible to define normals and recognize the effects of learning the task and the abnormalities introduced by spasticity.

There are many complex and sophisticated approaches to the problem of measuring locomotion, for example walkways with multi-channel EMG record-ing, cine photography in several planes, pressure plate studies and so on, but the case for simple feedback systems is valid both to measure function and as an aid to re-educative procedures. Calibration of such apparatus is a problem and digital displays are helpful in the clinical use of feedback apparatus. More rational and better therapy will be possible as better techniques for measuring are developed. Sophisticated apparatus in main research centres does not replace the need for the simpler inexpensive tools for making objective measurements in small clinical departments where much of the remedial work is done.

COMMUNICATIONS

Failure to exchange knowledge and experience is an important cause of failure to provide services that could be available for patients. Thus research teaching and services need to be integrated between main centres and peripheral units for the benefit of both. Special Interest Groups have been set up in the Wessex Region in the UK, largely with the problem of communications in mind. Their functions are:

1. to evaluate, measure and create standards in rehabilitation practice
2. to improve services through greater efficiency
3. to promote research where it is seen to be needed
4. to improve education in rehabilitation, and
5. to share information arising from clinical work.

The model which has been adopted shows signs of success in practice and it lends itself particularly well to neurological disability which poses severe prob-lems in rehabilitation whose solution does not rest in the hands of any single individual. Such a group must be multi-disciplinary, consisting of physicians, surgeons, therapists, ergonomists, psychologists, engineers, to mention only a few. It must be headed by a coordinator who is someone with sufficient grasp of the whole field to plan and conduct meetings of good academic and practical standard. The group also requires secretarial support. In practice the groups in Wessex consist of about 80 regular attenders who represent all the district hospitals in the region. Essentially they are working groups and therefore define needs and allocate tasks, and meetings take place when members of the group have produced something to discuss rather than at regular intervals. In practice meetings take place two or three times a year. The activities of groups are part research, part teaching and learning, and part related to the improvement of practice. The outcome is a general improvement of standards and a means for quick dissemination of new knowledge, for introducing new principles in care and, above all, for evaluating the outcome of rehabilitation activities. There would be other ways of tackling the same problems and the exact organization of any schemes would depend upon local resources, personalities and geography. The objective, however, would remain the same, namely to improve practice based on scientific studies rather than by reliance on custom or empiricism and to generate new knowledge. Groups may not carry full competence in all aspects within their membership; therefore access to university departments and faculties is of great value. The support of libraries, teaching media, statistics, ergonomics, mathematics and engineering are needed and are forthcoming from an academic source.

Of great value, too, at an international level are complementary programmes between main centres. Meetings supported by charity have brought workers together from all parts of the world in order to share experience and to effect exchanges of scientific and medical staff.

It is not the purpose of this chapter to describe the organization of rehabilitation units or services. They are described elsewhere (Glanville, 1976; Cochrane & Glanville, 1975; Glanville, 1956; Nichols, 1980). An important need today is to ensure that new knowledge about neurological disability is communicated to providers of services so that good developments can be incorporated into practice. Unfortunately much that could be done for patients is not available to them, often through poor communication and lack of awareness rather than from lack of resources by the providers of services.

COORDINATION

Much good would come from a policy to develop research teaching and services in a few main centres designed to combine both the acute and rehabilitative phases of care for patients with neurological disorders. Too often key people in the neurological team are denied the experience of involvement during rehabilitation which is essential to research and to the growth of knowledge for the reasons indicated earlier. The study of improvement and the reasons for its taking place have received too little attention but do require increasing study. Academic posts in neurological rehabilitation should be set up to bridge the gap between the acute and restorative phases of care and to ensure that appropriate emphasis is given to the task of harnessing data to increase knowledge and how to use and teach it wisely. The contribution of the paramedical professions to improving the lot of the neurologically disabled is inestimable. These professions require good post-graduate experience and it will be best provided for them in comprehensive centres of the kind envisaged. Centres could not work realistically in isolation for they must stimulate and help to develop community, social and voluntary services as well as public awareness of the needs of disabled people. So long as professionals consider only their own limited roles in relation to neuropathology and disability resulting from it there will be little progress. Whilst resources remain a major obstacle, enthusiastic leadership and the adjustment of attitudes costs nothing. Not least important for the future is an urgent need, namely to include in undergraduate medical curricula a realistic exposure to the problems of disability and to restorative medicine.

REFERENCES

AGERHOLM M. (1975) Handicap and the handicapped. A nomenclature of classification of intrinsic handicaps. *Royal Society of Health Journal*, **1**, 3–8.

COCHRANE G. & GLANVILLE H.J. (1975) Rehabilitation today. *Update*, **10**, 1357–72.

COOPER I.S. (1976) *Living with Chronic Neurological Disease*, pp. 11–21. W. W. Norton & Co., New York.

DIMITRIJEVIC M.R., GRACANIN F., PREVEC T. & TRONTELJ J. (1968) Electronic control of paralysed extremities. *Biomedical Engineering*, **3**, 8–14.

GANDY M., LYNN P.A., MILLER S. & REED G.A.L. (1978) Quantitative assessment of patterns of muscle activity in the arm. *International Journal of Rehabilitation Research*, **1**, 356.

GLANVILLE H.J. (1956) A unit for early rehabilitation in a general hospital. *Annals of Physical Medicine*, **3**, 101–2.

GLANVILLE H.J. (1972) Electronic control of paralysis. *Proceedings of the Royal Society of Medicine*, **65**, 233–5.

GLANVILLE H.J. (1976) An inaugural lecture. *What is Rehabilitation?*, p. 13. University of Southampton.

ILLIS L.S. (1973) Experimental model of regeneration in the central nervous system—I. Synaptic. *Brain*, **96**, 47–60.

JAY P. (1976) How association sought a standard way to record assessment. *Occupational Therapy*, **39**, 299–300.

LYNN P., REED G.A.L., PARKER W.R. & LANGTON HEWER R. (1977) Some applications of human-operator research to the assessment of disability in stroke. *Medical and Biological Engineering and Computing*, **15**, 184–8.

MAIR REPORT (1972) *Medical Rehabilitation: the Pattern for the Future*. Scottish Home and Health Department, Social Health Services Council. HMSO, London.

NICHOLS P.J.R. (1976) ADL Indices of any value. *Occupational Therapy*, **39**, 160–3.

NICHOLS P.J.R. (1980) *Rehabilitation Medicine: the Management of Physical Disabilities*, 2e, Chapter 1. Butterworths, London.

PARRY C.B. WYNN (1966) *Rehabilitation of the Hand*, 2e. Butterworths, London.

ROLT L.J.C. (1970) *Victorian Engineering*. Penguin Press, Allen Lane.

SOMMERVILLE J.D. (1975) *Workshop on Disablement and Rehabilitation in Developing Countries*, 7–18, p. 11. Department of Social Studies, Selly Oak College, Birmingham, United Kingdom.

TAYLOR D.G. (1977) Physical impairment social handicap. *Office of Health Care Economics*, **60**, 6–7.

WHITING S. & LINCOLN N. (1980) An ADL assessment for stroke patients. *Occupational Therapy*, **43**, 44–6.

Wood P.H.N. (1975) Classification of impairments and handicaps. Doc. No. WHO 1 CD/9 Rev. Conf/7515, p. 2. Geneva.

World Health Organization (1969) Technical Report, No. 419, p. 13. 1.4.1.

World Health Organization (1969) Technical Report, No. 419, p. 7. 1.2(1).

World Health Organization (1976) 29th World Assembly. A20 Inf. Doc. 1, p. 13. 1.4.1.

World Health Organization (1976) A29. Inf. Doc/1, p. 17, Table 1.

Yates E. (1976) Measuring the quality of life. *Occupational Therapy*, **39,** 299.

PART I
ALTERED STRUCTURE
AND FUNCTION

Although there is no nerve cell division in the adult CNS the capacity for change exists and is manifest after a lesion.

Part I of this book describes these changes and indicates rules which they follow, both at a structural and functional level. This is the science of rehabilitation on which assessment and treatment programmes must be based. An understanding of pathology and altered physiology is even more important in rehabilitative neurology than in diagnostic neurology.

Chapter 2

Damage to
the Nervous System

Recovery of function following a partial lesion in the central nervous system (CNS) remains one of the major problems in neurology. Gradual and progressive recovery of function may occur in some patients but not in others and this has never been adequately explained. The standard procedures used to promote recovery (for example, rehabilitation techniques and the use of drugs) have little effect on recovery of integrated function as opposed to preventing the development of secondary complications. In succeeding chapters the natural history of various neurological lesions is described and the methods of aiding the process of recovery are discussed. This chapter is concerned with the nature of the lesions, the pathological processes at work, the effect of such lesions in producing the abnormal clinical picture, and indications of how recovery may perhaps be aided using the knowledge gained from neuropathology and experimental neurology. The way in which plasticity has been explored in the mammalian nervous system and its importance with reference to human pathology is discussed fully by Dr Devor in Chapter 3.

ORGANIZATION OF CENTRAL AND PERIPHERAL NERVOUS SYSTEMS

Although neuronal cell bodies may be localized in specific regions of the brain, spinal cord, sensory ganglia and autonomic ganglia, their dendritic ramifications and axonal processes are often widely spread. The active metabolism of neurons is reflected in their large nuclei and prominent nucleoli; abundant rough surfaced endoplasmic reticulum and polyribosomes forming Nissl granules within the neuronal cell bodies are also an indication of their high level of protein production (Peters *et al.*, 1976). Numerous mitochondria are dispersed throughout the cell soma and within dendrites and axons. Various substances and cell organelles are transported by axoplasmic and dendritic flow both away from (orthograde transport) and towards (retrograde transport) the neuronal cell body (Olsson & Kristensson, 1979). The fast phase of axoplasmic flow at 400–450 mm/day occurs through the cisternae or smooth endoplasmic reticulum (Droz *et al.*, 1975) and is concerned with the transport of neurotransmitters and enzymes from the neuron cell body along the axon, and with the transport of material for the renewal of axonal and synaptic vesicle membrane. A similar system of smooth endoplasmic reticulum is involved in the retrograde axoplasmic flow material from the periphery to the cell body; viruses (Kristensson, 1978) and tetanus toxins (Price *et al.*, 1975) are transported in this way. The slow phase of axoplasmic flow is concerned with the transport of axonal proteins at a rate of a few millimetres a day. Although the exact mechanism of the slow phase of axoplasmic flow is not clear, it may be associated with the longitudinally orientated microtubules and neurofilaments which are so prominent in axons and dendrites (Peters *et al.*, 1976).

Much of the surface of the dendrites and cell bodies of neurons within the central nervous system is covered by boutons terminaux forming synaptic connections from afferent neurons. Similar but modified synaptic connections are also seen in the periphery at muscle endplates and at autonomic nerve endings. The larger axons in both the central and peripheral nervous system are myelinated and nerve impulses are transmitted by saltatory conduction. Myelin in the central nervous system is formed by compaction of cell membranes derived from oligodendroglial cells (Warwick & Williams, 1973; Peters *et al.*, 1976); each cell myelinates several axons (Fig. 2.1). Schwann cells form myelin in the peripheral nervous system, but each Schwann cell only myelinates one segment of one axon (Weller & Cervós-Navarro, 1977).

Virtually the whole of the central nervous system is maintained in a special environment by the blood–brain barrier (Bradbury, 1979). Proteins, protein-bound moieties and other substances which penetrate many organs throughout the body are denied entry to the major portion of the central nervous system by the blood–brain barrier maintained by capillary endothelia (Brightman *et al.*, 1970). Astrocytes closely invest capillaries throughout the central nervous system and may well play an important role in maintaining the optimum milieu for neuronal function. A similar barrier exists in the main trunks of peripheral nerves (Ahmed & Weller, 1979), but there is no such blood–nerve barrier within dorsal root ganglia and autonomic ganglia where proteins and other substances pass more readily from the blood into the interstitial spaces (Jacobs *et al.*, 1976). Peripheral nerves are also surrounded by a multilayered perineurial sheath (Fig. 2.1) which exerts a barrier function upon substances diffusing into the nerve and surrounding tissue (Olsson & Kristensson, 1973; Ahmed & Weller, 1979).

PATHOLOGICAL REACTIONS IN THE NERVOUS SYSTEM

Neurons do not divide in postnatal life so that if a neuron dies following an insult it is not replaced and its connections are lost. The nervous system, and neurons in particular, are very sensitive to hypoxia, ischaemia and hypoglycaemia (Brierley, 1976). Toxic damage to the central nervous system from heavy metals (Cavanagh, 1979) and from a wide variety of organic compounds (Spencer &

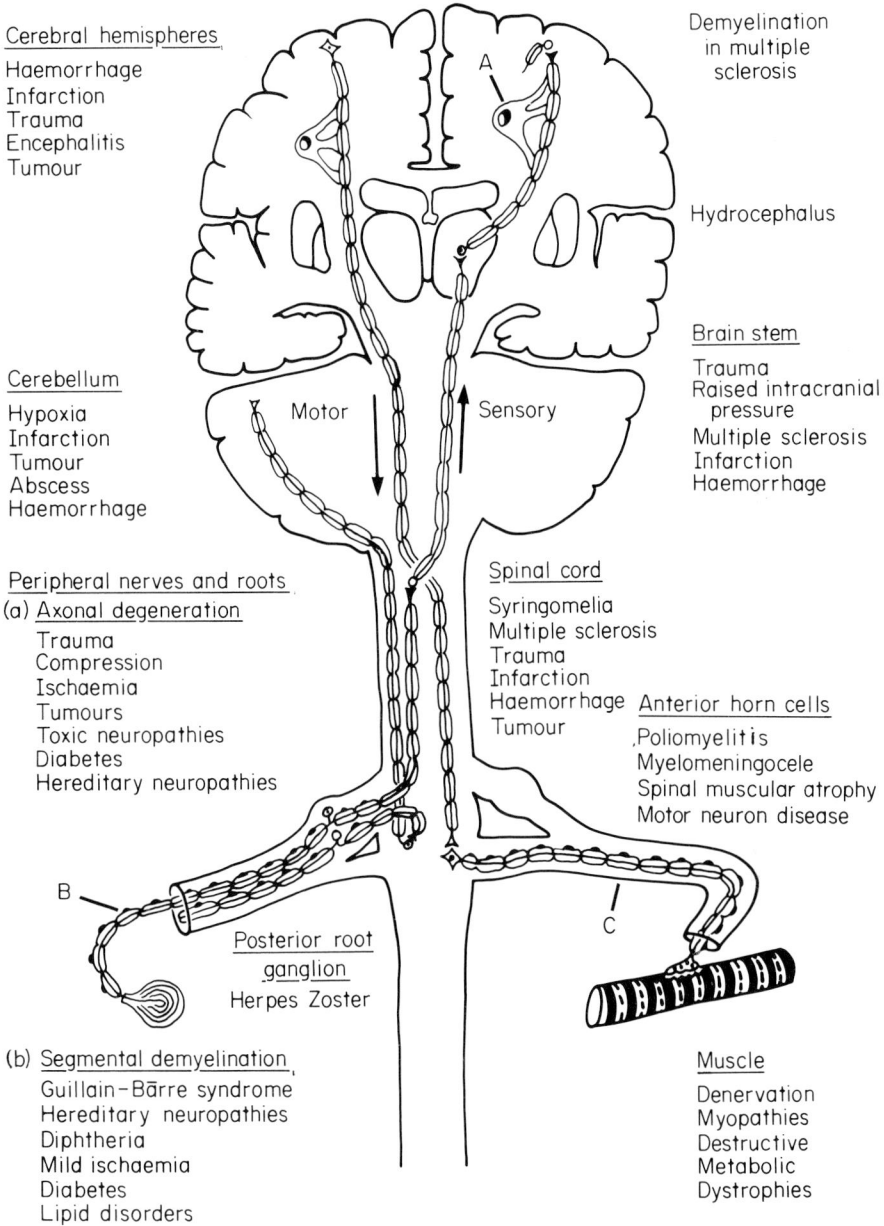

Cerebral hemispheres

Haemorrhage
Infarction
Trauma
Encephalitis
Tumour

Demyelination
in multiple
sclerosis

Hydrocephalus

Brain stem

Trauma
Raised intracranial
   pressure
Multiple sclerosis
Infarction
Haemorrhage

Cerebellum

Hypoxia
Infarction
Tumour
Abscess
Haemorrhage

Motor   Sensory

Peripheral nerves and roots

(a) Axonal degeneration

   Trauma
   Compression
   Ischaemia
   Tumours
   Toxic neuropathies
   Diabetes
   Hereditary neuropathies

Spinal cord

Syringomelia
Multiple sclerosis
Trauma
Infarction
Haemorrhage
Tumour

Anterior horn cells

Poliomyelitis
Myelomeningocele
Spinal muscular atrophy
Motor neuron disease

Posterior root
   ganglion
Herpes Zoster

(b) Segmental demyelination

   Guillain–Bārre syndrome
   Hereditary neuropathies
   Diphtheria
   Mild ischaemia
   Diabetes
   Lipid disorders

Muscle

Denervation
Myopathies
Destructive
Metabolic
Dystrophies

Fig. 2.1 Diagram to show the site and nature of major neuropathological lesions. Oligodendroglial cells (A) are shown myelinating several segments of an axon in the central nervous system whereas Schwann cells (B) only myelinate one segment of one axon. Peripheral nerves are surrounded by a multilayered cellular perineurial sheath (C).

Schaumburg, 1980) may result in the death of neurons. Similarly, certain viruses such as polio virus, Herpes simplex, and rabies may specifically infect neurons and cause their destruction (Adams, 1976). Not all neurons are equally sensitive to pathological insults; in general, the phylogenetically newer parts of the nervous system such as the cerebral cortex and neocerebellum are more vulnerable to damage by hypoxia, ischaemia and hypoglycaemia. Neurons in the brain stem and spinal cord, on the other hand, are less sensitive to such insults, but the reasons for this pattern of differential sensitivity are not fully understood. Some areas of the brain are particularly prone to damage from ischaemia, especially in boundary zones between regions of arterial supply when there is loss of auto-regulation of cerebral blood flow under conditions of hypotension and poor perfusion (Brierley, 1976).

Axons in the central nervous system may be damaged as a result of trauma, intracerebral haemorrhage, infarction, the actions of toxins or by tumour invasion. Motor or sensory tracts are particularly concentrated in the internal capsules, cerebral peduncles, pons, medulla and spinal cord, so that even small pathological lesions in these regions of the central nervous system may produce severe neurological deficit. Alternatively, the very widespread axonal damage which can occur in cerebral trauma may result in extensive neurological defects. When an axon is damaged or severed, orthograde and retrograde axoplasmic flow continues so that axonal swellings form on either side of the point of axonal division. Thus damaged tracts can often be identified in the early stages following a head injury by the presence of such axon balloons (Strich, 1961). The distal ends of severed axons start to degenerate soon after the injury and after a few days the fragmented axon and myelin is phagocytosed by activated microglia and macrophages derived from blood monocytes. Degenerating axons may be traced through their distal pathways by staining sections of the tissue for myelin breakdown products which appear as neutral lipid droplets of cholesterol ester some three to six weeks after axonal damage.

Early regeneration end bulbs or axon balloons at the ends of the proximal axonal stumps are seen as large oval swellings approximately 50 μm and approximately 20 μm in diameter; it is from these swellings, full of mitochondria, neurotubules and neurofilaments, that regenerating axon sprouts emerge. During the phase of regeneration, the neuronal cell body may undergo the changes of chromatolysis. The cell body of the neuron swells and becomes spherical in shape; the nucelus adopts an eccentric position within the cell and the nucleolus enlarges. Discrete Nissl granules of rough surface endoplasmic reticulum disappear and the cellular RNA becomes dispersed throughout the cytoplasm. Originally, chromatolysis was considered to be a degenerative phenomenon, but it is now known that it represents a stage of increased protein synthesis associated with axonal regeneration (Kreutzberg, 1972; Torvik, 1976). Chromatolysis is most marked when the axon is severed near its origin from the cell body and may be seen in the first weeks after injury. Despite the active axonal regeneration in the early stages this phenomenon is short lived in the central nervous system in virtually all pathways (Berry, 1979). Regeneration in the peripheral nervous system, on the other hand, is much more successful, especially if the main trunk of the nerve is preserved free from scar tissue (Sunderland, 1968).

Myelin sheaths are selectively destroyed in demyelinating diseases and the axons are preserved, at least, in the initial stages of the disease. Conduction of impulses across the demyelinated segments of axon is considerably reduced and may fail altogether. Destruction of myelin may be due to death of the myelin-supporting cells and/or due to direct attack upon the myelin sheath itself (Lampert, 1978). In multiple sclerosis, there is loss of oligodendroglial cells from the demyelinated plaques and very little remyelination occurs. Eventually the plaques become gliotic and the axons degenerate (Lumsden, 1970; Oppenheimer, 1976). Demyelination also occurs in the peripheral nervous system in a number of neuropathies, e.g. post-infectious polyneuropathy (Guillain-Barré syndrome) (Prineas, 1972), diphtheritic neuropathy and, to a greater or lesser extent, in ischaemic and compressive neuropathies (Weller & Cervós-Navarro, 1977). There is a similar slowing of nerve conduction across the affected segments, but in contrast to the central nervous system, remyelination within the peripheral nervous system occurs rapidly and, in the absence of axonal damage, recovery from the neuropathy may be complete. Some chronic neuropathies exhibit features which suggest that there is repeated demyelination and remyelination within the nerve. The result is the formation of a typical histological picture of onion-bulb whorls and the clinical finding of hypertrophic nerves.

THE EFFECTS OF DAMAGE TO BRAIN TISSUE

If a few widely spaced neurons are damaged by an insult such as hypoxia they may die and be ingested by microglial cells and there may be little scarring of the brain tissue. In larger lesions, however, neuronal death and damage to astrocytes, vessels and oligodendroglial cells within the tissue induces an acute inflammatory response with exudation of oedema fluid and polymorphonuclear leucocytes in the ensuing few hours. Alteration of the blood–brain barrier allows protein-rich fluid to enter the damaged area and the surrounding brain, and cerebral oedema develops (Klatzo, 1979). In the cortex, the oedema fluid accumulates within astrocytes, but in the white matter oedema fluid spreads readily between nerve fibre elements and may lead to extensive brain swelling. Investigative procedures such as Technetium-isotope brain scans and computerized axial tomography with Conray (meglumine iothalamate) enhancement demonstrate well the breakdown of the blood–brain barrier in areas of brain damage.

Within the first 12–24 hours following an injury to brain tissue, microglia surrounding the area of damage become activated and over the subsequent few days these cells, together with more numerous macrophages derived from blood monocytes, invade the necrotic area. When the brain damage is due to a virus infection, lymphocytes will also be prominent in the cellular exudate, whereas polymorphonuclear leucocytes accompany bacterial infections. The ultimate outcome of the lesion will depend upon its size, and upon whether all the tissue elements in the area of damage have been destroyed. Large infarcts may remain as areas of softening within the brain for many months or years; eventually the necrotic material is removed by macrophages and a cyst forms surrounded by glial scar tissue formed from reactive astrocytes. Necrotic tissue is more rapidly removed from very small areas of brain damage and after a few weeks only a few reactive astrocytes may remain in the damaged area. Tracts containing the axons arising from the damaged neurons degenerate and eventually become shrunken and gliotic.

In multiple sclerosis, the axons are initially preserved and only the oligodendroglia and myelin sheaths are destroyed. Chronic multiple sclerosis plaques, however, contain few axons and are seen as firm sclerotic grey plaques of gliosis within the grey and white matter.

BRAIN DAMAGE IN NEUROLOGICAL DISEASE

There are a variety of pathological lesions where significant damage to the nervous system occurs and the neurological defects are disabling for the patient. In the context of rehabilitation, it may be important to emphasize the non-progressive lesion, but the pathology of tumours should also be discussed especially where they are benign in character and the progression of neurological damage may be arrested by treatment. Special attention, however, is paid to lesions resulting from cerebrovascular disease, trauma, virus infections, and multiple sclerosis.

Cerebrovascular Disease

Intracerebral haemorrhage associated with hypertension most commonly occurs in the region of the basal ganglia (Russell, 1954; Yates, 1976). Its disruptive effects commonly involve the internal capsule and blood may burst through into the ventricular system. Haemorrhage into the brain stem and cerebellum is less common than intracerebral haemorrhage but has a similar disruptive effect upon surrounding tissues. In addition to direct damage to adjacent nerve fibres and neurons, haemorrhage into the brain substance may cause the problems associated with space-occupying lesions (see below).

Although rupture of a berry aneurysm frequently results in a subarachnoid haemorrhage, intracerebral haemorrhage may occur if the aneurysm is deep within the lateral fissure. In such cases, the pressure from an arterial haemorrhage is sufficient to form a large haematoma in the inferior regions of the frontal lobe or within the temporal lobe adjacent to the aneurysm. Another important complication of a ruptured berry aneurysm which occurs in the early stages is

infarction of cerebral tissue. Spasm of cerebral arteries is induced by the presence of blood within the subarachnoid space (Owman *et al.*, 1979) and may cause extensive infarction (Heros *et al.*, 1976) of territory supplied by the anterior or middle cerebral arteries.

Infarction with irreparable destruction of brain tissue may affect any part of the central nervous system, including the cerebral hemispheres, brain stem, cerebellum or spinal cord. Thrombotic occlusion of atherosclerotic carotid, vertebral or cerebral arteries may result in infarction in their areas of supply. Occlusion of intracranial arteries by emboli arising from atherosclerotic plaques in the larger vessels in the neck or from mural thrombi in an infarcted left ventricle or a fibrillating left atrium may also produce large and small infarcts. Showers of emboli may cause multiple small infarcts throughout the brain with less noticeable focal neurological deficits but with a devastating effect on intellectual function.

Trauma

A severe head injury may damage the brain in several ways; a proportion of injuries are fatal, but other patients survive with widespread brain damage and complicated neurological defects. Fractures of the skull which involve branches of the middle meningeal arteries or disrupt lateral venous sinuses in the posterior fossa may produce extradural haemorrhages which, unless treated, may cause the death of the patient from brain compression and displacement. Tearing of the cortical veins as they enter the superior sagittal sinus may result from a head injury and brain compression or displacement may ensue from a subdural haematoma.

The direct effects of trauma upon the brain include contusion or bruising at the site of impact of the head injury and as a similar, often a more severe, *contre-coup* injury. Such contusions involve the surface of the brain and are most frequently seen in the frontal and temporal lobes. Severe brain damage also occurs due to shearing lesions within the brain substance itself. During the trauma, swirling movements develop within the brain so that long tracts like the fornix, and commissural tracts such as the anterior commissure and corpus callosum, may be torn. Similarly, throughout the white matter, axons within fibre tracts are disrupted, most especially around small blood vessels. The extent of the shearing lesions may be seen macroscopically as petechial haemorrhages in patients dying soon after brain injury. More commonly, however, they are only detected by microscopic examination of the brain where axonal swellings representing abortive attempts at regeneration are seen within the damaged tracts (Strich, 1961). Shearing damage may also affect the brain stem, especially the midbrain and the superior cerebellar peduncles. There are two main effects of the shearing lesions; fibres within the affected tracts are actually divided and, as they do not effectively regenerate, the patient loses valuable intracerebral connections. The second major effect is that the widespread brain damage induces an inflammatory reaction within the brain and massive cerebral oedema may ensue.

A further important complication of head injuries must be mentioned. Obstruction of the airway in an unconscious patient may result in severe hypoxic damage to the brain, especially to the cerebral cortex, hippocampus and cerebellum. Similarly, patients who are shocked for a prolonged period from loss of blood may suffer cerebral ischaemia, particularly if they are trapped in an upright position following the trauma. Cerebral infarction in hypotension may involve large areas of the cerebral cortex or may be confined to boundary zones between areas of major cerebral artery supply (see page 16).

Virus Infections

Damage to the nervous system may result from direct invasion by a virus or from an allergic post-infectious encephalomyelitis (Croft, 1969). Direct invasion of the nervous system may cause not only death of the infected neurons but also considerable tissue oedema. Herpes simplex encephalitis is frequently complicated by extensive necrosis and oedema of the temporal lobes; if the patient survives, the severe memory loss from temporal lobe damage may be accompanied by neurological defects resulting from the effects of the cerebral oedema (see below). Polio virus infection may cause widespread destruction of anterior horn cells and neurons in cranial nerve nuclei so that the post-encephalomyelitic neurological disabilities in this disease are largely the result of muscle denervation.

Multiple Sclerosis

Multiple sclerosis is a primary demyelinating disease of the central nervous system in which the myelin is selectively destroyed but the axons are largely preserved in the early stages. Post-mortem studies of the brain and spinal cord of patients who have survived with the disease for many years have shown that numerous plaques of demyelination may be present throughout the nervous system. They range from a few millimetres in diameter to a centimetre or more. The plaques are not in fact flat, they have volume although they appear as plaques in sections of brain. No part of the central nervous system seems to be exempt from involvement by multiple sclerosis although there may be more plaques in the spinal cord in some patients, whereas in others brain lesions are more numerous. There are certain sites in the brain which appear to be most frequently involved. The optic nerves commonly contain plaques; large demyelinated plaques in the cerebral hemispheres are most frequently found in the periventricular white matter and small plaques are often at the periphery of cerebral gyri, either contiguous with the cortex or wholly involving the cortex. Although the small plaques are widely distributed throughout multiple sclerotic brains, Lumsden did find a distinct predilection for the superior frontal gyrus; however, no relationship to arterial supply was found. In the 36 brains examined by Lumsden (1970), 8% had 100–465 small gyral plaques in the brain whereas 16% of cases had less than 3 plaques. Approximately 80% of small 1–10 mm plaques in a series of 10 multiple sclerosis brains were in the cerebral hemispheres and 20% in the brain stem and cerebellum.

Multiple sclerosis plaques which have been present for many years appear as firm (sclerotic) grey, sharply defined areas of gliosis devoid of myelin and virtually devoid of axons. They probably take many months or years to reach this form. In the acute stages of a multiple sclerosis lesion, the plaque is soft and granular. Histologically, there is perivascular accumulation of lymphocytes, invasion of the area by macrophages and destruction of myelin. Although some axonal degeneration is seen, axons are usually well preserved in the early stages. A striking loss of oligodendroglial cells from multiple sclerosis plaques may be observed and there is little, if any, remyelination. Reactive astrocytes increase in numbers within the plaque during the stage of myelin breakdown and, as the debris is removed, gliotic scar tissue composed of astrocyte processes remains.

The precise cause of multiple sclerosis is at present unknown, but the presence of large numbers of lymphocytes in early plaques suggests that a delayed hypersensitivity reaction to a virus or another antigen may play a role in demyelination. Furthermore, raised levels of immunoglobulins with an oligoclonal pattern in the CSF (Siden & Kjellin, 1978) and antibodies to oligodendroglia (Abramsky *et al.*, 1977) in these patients suggests that humoral immunological factors also play a role in the disease. The significance of raised virus antibodies, particularly to measles, in the CSF of multiple sclerosis patients is uncertain.

Antel *et al.* (1979) observed a reduction in suppressor T-lymphocyte activity during exacerbations in multiple sclerosis with a rise to levels above normal during remission. It is possible that the balance between helper and suppressor T-cells is disturbed and thus the regulation of immunocompetent cells in multiple sclerosis may be deficient. The restriction of multiple sclerosis to certain geographical areas (Acheson, 1977), and the recently reported association between HLA and multiple sclerosis, suggest that a genetically determined defect in immunological response may play a role in the pathogenesis of the disease (Batchelor *et al.*, 1978).

Secondary Effects of Space-occupying Lesions and Cerebral Oedema

In addition to their primary destructive effects, cerebral lesions may induce secondary complications due to their space-occupying nature (Fig. 2.2). A rapid increase in the volume of the intracranial contents occurs with an intracerebral haemorrhage and following subdural or extradural haemorrhage. Similar, but

Falx
cerebri

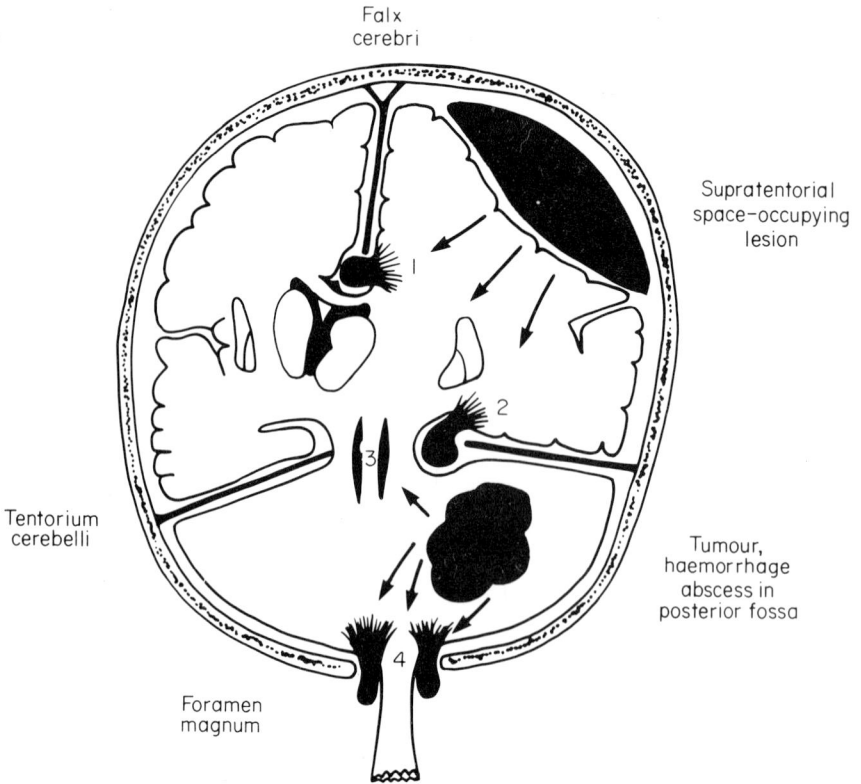

Supratentorial
space-occupying
lesion

Tentorium
cerebelli

Tumour,
haemorrhage
abscess in
posterior fossa

Foramen
magnum

Fig. 2.2   Diagram to summarize the major effects of supra and infratentorial space-occupying lesions:
1.   herniation of the cingulate gyrus under the falx
2.   herniation of the uncus and parahippocampal gyrus through the tentorial incisure; branches of the posterior cerebral artery become compressed by the free edge of the tentorium
3.   brain stem compression and haemorrhage accompanying herniation of the para-hippocampal gyrus
4.   herniation of the cerebellar tonsils through the foramen magnum with compression of the medulla.

often a less rapid increase in brain volume may accompany the cerebral oedema induced by trauma, cerebral infarction or by a cerebral abscess. Raised intra-cranial pressure associated with gliomas and meningiomas may have a slow onset, but infarction or haemorrhage within a glioma may induce a very rapid increase in intracranial pressure. There is a limited amount of cerebrospinal fluid which can be displaced from the cranial cavity by an enlarging space-occupying lesion; when this reserve capacity is exhausted, displacement of the brain occurs. An expanding lesion in one hemisphere or a localized subdural or extradural haemorrhage displaces the brain towards the opposite side. In addition, brain tissue may be forced to herniate through narrow openings between dural compartments (Fig. 2.2). Probably the most important of these openings is the incisura in the tentorium cerebelli, through which the brain stem and posterior cerebral arteries pass from the posterior into the middle cranial fossa. With an enlarging unilateral supratentorial lesion, the brain stem may be compressed from side to side and depressed towards the posterior fossa; in addition, the most medial portion of the temporal lobe on the affected side, i.e. the uncus and the parahippocampal gyrus, may be forced down between the free edge of the tentorium and midbrain. The uncal and parahippocampal gyral herniation has three main effects. First, compression of the brain stem is often accompanied by haemorrhage into midbrain and pons. Midbrain damage of this type may be responsible for the patient's altered level of consciousness and is frequently fatal. There may be severe neurological defects in those who survive. Cerebrospinal fluid flow through the aqueduct may also be impaired by midbrain compression with resultant obstructive hydrocephalus. Another important complication of parahippocampal gyral herniation is occlusion of branches of the posterior cerebral artery on the affected side with consequent infarction of the visual cortex and of the inferior aspect of the temporal lobe. Patients recovering with this lesion will have visual field defects. The third main effect of herniation at the tentorial incisura is compression of the oculomotor nerve with the consequent effects upon pupillary and eye movements.

Expanding supratentorial lesions may also cause herniation of the cingulate gyrus under the falx cerebri and, if severe, the gyrus may become infarcted. Space-occupying lesions in the posterior fossa, either in the cerebellum, brain stem, fourth ventricle or in the cerebellopontine angles, cause herniation of the cerebellar tonsils through the foramen magnum resulting in compression of the medulla and impairment of CSF flow through the foramen magnum.

Hydrocephalus

Hydrocephalus results from blockage of the CSF pathways either within the ventricles, aqueduct or subarachnoid space. Tumours or haemorrhage within the ventricular system are potent causes of hydrocephalus. More insidious impedance to cerebrospinal fluid flow may occur with occlusion of the subarachnoid space following haemorrhage from a birth injury or a ruptured berry aneurysm and subsequent fibrosis of the subarachnoid space. Similarly, meningeal fibrosis may follow meningitis, particularly tuberculous meningitis. As the normal cerebrospinal fluid circulation is prevented, the ventricles enlarge, fluid is forced into the periventricular white matter and is probably drained into the blood through the periventricular blood vessels (Lorenzo, *et al.*, 1970). Pathological studies of hydrocephalic brains both in man and in experimental animals suggest that the major damage to the brain occurs in the periventricular white matter and this may be the main cause of lasting neurological defects especially in hydrocephalic children (Weller & Shulman, 1972; Weller & Mitchell, 1980).

Damage to the Spinal Cord

Direct penetrating injuries, fracture dislocations of the spine, prolapsed inter-vertebral discs or, more rarely, spinal extradural haematomas may cause severe local damage to the spinal cord either from compression, shearing or from interference with the blood supply and subsequent infarction (Hughes, 1977). Meningiomas, Schwannomas, metastatic tumour or infective bone lesions can also result in cord compression. Infarction of the spinal cord may be a compli-cation of a dissecting aneurysm of the aorta or follow occlusion of the spinal arteries. Intramedullary gliomas and vascular malformations also damage the spinal cord as they grow or bleed.

Although a destructive lesion could be limited to a few segments of the cord, the effects are usually more widespread due to degeneration of the long ascending and descending tracts passing through the damaged area. Some recovery of function may occur within the first weeks following a non-progressive destructive spinal cord lesion and is probably due to the subsidence of oedema. As in the rest of the central nervous system, however, there is little, if any, effective regeneration of transected axons in the long tracts of the spinal cord.

A degenerative cyst forms at the site of a destructive lesion and the cord becomes softened as the damaged tissue is moved by macrophages. Astrocytes proliferate around the edge of the damaged area and form a glial scar. If the glial limiting membrane of the spinal cord is broken, axons may regenerate from the dorsal roots into the damaged segment of the cord and invade the glial scar (Blakemore, 1976). These neurites are usually myelinated by Schwann cells and they do not extend far into the spinal cord.

Spinal cord damage in syringomyelia differs in character and timing from that seen with trauma. As the syrinx expands within the centre of the cord its main effect is initially upon the spinothalamic tracts, causing dissociated sensory loss. Anterior horn cell destruction over several segments may occur and, as the syrinx is most often found in the cervical region of the cord, there is wasting of the muscles in the arms. Signs of long tract damage are relatively late in their appearance.

Multiple sclerosis may involve the spinal cord at any level, but lesions in the cervical cord are about twice as common as those elsewhere in the cord (Oppen-heimer, 1978). The plaques may be roughly circular in outline, but in the cervical cord they are often fan-shaped and involve the lateral columns of white matter. Large plaques of demyelination may extend over the whole cross-section of the cord producing a transverse myelitis. Histologically the cord plaques are similar to the cerebral lesions; initially the axons are preserved, but as the plaques become older and more gliotic, axons are lost, resulting in degeneration and atrophy of long tracts (Oppenheimer, 1976).

REGENERATION AND RECOVERY IN THE CENTRAL NERVOUS SYSTEM

When either the brain or spinal cord is damaged by haemorrhage, infarction, hypoxia or trauma, there is an inflammatory reaction which is accompanied by alteration in the blood–brain barrier and subsequent tissue oedema. From experimental studies it is known that the exudation of fluid starts soon after the insult and oedema develops within the next 24 hours (Klatzo, 1979; Bradbury, 1979). Thereafter, the blood–brain barrier is progressively restored and, in small lesions, it may be intact after two or three weeks (Mitchell *et al.*, 1979). Recovery of function in the early stages after an insult is probably due mainly to the subsidence of oedema in the surrounding structurally intact neural tissue. Despite early axonal sprouting and regeneration in the central nervous system, growth in the majority of axons ceases after about two weeks (Cajal, 1928). True regeneration does, however, occur in monoaminergic fibres (Bjorklund *et al.*, 1975), in non-myelinated cholinergic axons and in neurosecretory fibres (Berry, 1979) (Fig. 2.3). Why axonal regeneration is for the most part abortive in the central nervous system still remains a problem. The presence of scar tissue at the site of injury may inhibit regeneration, but although there is little regeneration across the tissue in the adult or fetal central nervous system, uninjured fetal axons do grow through damaged areas (Berry, 1979). It appears, therefore, that scar tissue and degenerate nervous tissue may not necessarily prevent axonal growth. It is possible that the lack of appropriate nerve growth factors in the adult brain may inhibit regeneration. Growth of selected neurons is stimulated by nerve growth factor (NGF) for a limited period during development of the mammalian nervous system, but NGF has no effect in the adult (Varon, 1975). As yet no pharmacological agent has been shown to stimulate significant regeneration in the central nervous system, although the pentapeptides, which include the morphine agonist, encephalin, may possess some axon growth-promoting properties (Martin, *et al.*, 1975).

Numerous collateral axon sprouts are formed during the early phases of regeneration and one factor which may inhibit axon growth is the formation of synapses in adjacent tracts proximal to the site of injury. Such synapses may be formed by the regenerating axons or their collaterals in the injured rat spinal cord and their establishment may suppress further regeneration (Bernstein & Bernstein, 1971; Berry, 1979).

The lack of regeneration in the central nervous system is in sharp contrast to the regenerative capacity of the peripheral nervous system. It is possible that the satellite cells play a role in regeneration and that whereas Schwann cells have

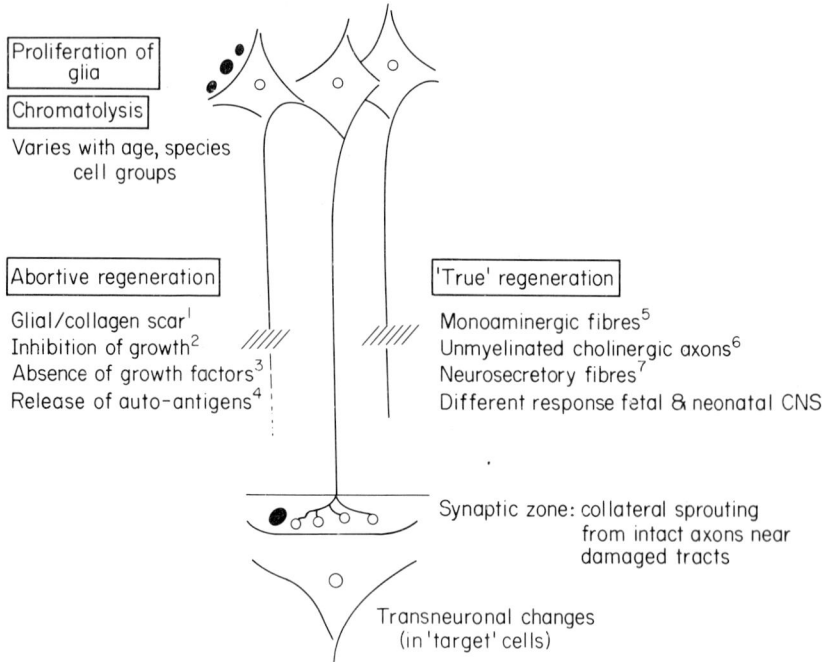

Fig. 2.3 Summary of the problem of CNS regeneration:

1. The barrier hypothesis: the glial/collagen scar forms a dense barrier through which no regenerating axons can penetrate. There are many inconsistencies in this hypothesis and it is doubtful if this is now tenable.

2. Aberrant synaptic contacts: possibly the physical barrier of the glial and fibroblast scar deflects growing axons into adjacent tissue where the axons then form synaptic contacts with other axons and dendrites. Bernstein and Bernstein (1969) suggest that CNS neurons are inhibited from further growth after forming such synaptic connections.

3. Absence of growth factors: Kiernan (1978) suggests that all central axons would regenerate if they had available to them their specific growth-promoting factor.

4. Injury may release substances from the CNS to the blood or vice versa. Antibodies, reacting with CNS antigens, may be taken up by growing axons and transported to the parent cell body and inhibit protein synthesis and axon growth (Berry & Riches, 1974).

5. Monoaminergic fibres may regenerate across CNS lesions and this has never been fully explained. Possibly they have a faster rate of growth which enables them to pass the barrier site before the scar is organized or they may release specific enzymes.

6. Central cholinergic fibres have been shown to regenerate if the tissue contains a peripheral cholinergic and noradrenergic supply, but heavily myelinated fibres do not regenerate.

7. Complete transection of pituitary stalk leads to regeneration of neurosecretory fibres into the neurohypophysis, but neurosecretory axons will not regenerate into pieces of cerebral cortex. Apparently neurosecretory axons are only able to regenerate in the presence of pituicytes. Berry & Riches (1974) suggest that these unmyelinated neurosecretory fibres are outside the blood–brain barrier and their constituent proteins are not therefore sequestered antigens like those in most other central fibres.

the capacity to stimulate and regulate growth; oligodendrocytes appear to lack such a property. Regenerating axons from damaged dorsal roots do not penetrate the spinal cord unless they are accompanied by Schwann cells; even then they do not penetrate very far.

In spite of the lack of anatomical and physiological evidence of regeneration in the injured central nervous system, recovery of function does occur.

THE NATURE OF RECOVERY

There are many ways of looking at the nature of recovery of function in the CNS and most of them are not mutually exclusive. Von Monakow's concept of 'diaschisis' (1902) was first suggested as the explanation for long delayed spontaneous recovery after a lesion in the CNS.

Von Monakow suggested that if a part of the CNS is destroyed, the distant part with which it was in neuronal contact may stop functioning. After some period of time the so-called 'depressed' area recovers its ability to function. However, Von Monakow was unable to explain the mechanism of recovery although it was clear that recovery of function would be due to removal of 'depression' with no real reorganization of the CNS taking place. The second major opinion as to the nature of recovery involves plasticity of the nervous system, so that recovery of function is consequent upon reorganization of the nervous system directed towards the re-establishment of the structural basis of the function originally lost. In this way, one could describe recovery of function as following Le Chatelier's principle: if a system is in equilibrium and one of the conditions of the system is altered, it will adjust itself in such a way as partially to neutralize the change of condition.

If the nature of recovery is obscure, even more so is the mechanism by which it is produced. Recovery of function may be due to an opening up of paths not normally or previously used by the organism, as is suggested by Pavlovian physiology and by more recent anatomical and physiological studies, or it may be due to a reorganization of the structurally undamaged central nervous system after a lesion has occurred. Probably it is a combination of both. Spinal shock serves as an interesting illustration of the effect of a lesion and the possible nature of recovery.

Spinal Shock

The term 'spinal shock' was introduced by Marshall Hall (1850), though the actual phenomena were described earlier by Hall in 1833 and Whytt in 1750. Spinal shock signifies the effect of sudden injury or transection of the spinal cord. It is characterized by sensory and motor paralysis and then, later, by gradual recovery of reflexes. Nobody has ever given a totally convincing explanation of the recovery of reflexes following their complete abolition.

Spinal shock occurs at any level of transection below the mid-pons. Above this level a transection produces decerebrate rigidity. Following transection below the pons, nerve cells in the spinal cord are suddenly cut off from all descending influences and undergo a dramatic change in their capacity to react. There is no consistent uniformity of opinion with regard to the importance of different pathways in producing spinal shock. However, in lower animals the important descending influences are probably reticulospinal and vestibulo-spinal, whereas in higher animals, including man, corticospinal connections are probably more important. It is usually assumed that the importance of the pathways in producing spinal shock is a reflection of their specificity. However, it may equally be argued that the importance lies in their relative contribution to the total spinal cord input. The fact that the depression of spinal shock is much more severe when transection is below the pons does not necessarily mean that there is some particularly important aborally directed control arising in pontine nuclei, since it could equally mean that the difference in transection above and below the pons is due to the relative contribution to the descending pathways made by different levels of the neuraxis. That is, the greater the number of descending pathways interrupted, the more likely that shock will ensue because the more severely disorganized will be the area upon which these descending pathways converge. A higher contribution of inputs from a particular centre does, of course, confer some specificity, but it is not necessary to assign the capacity for production of spinal shock on to the centre or its pathway.

It is usually considered that the shock is due to some withdrawal of impulses flowing down the spinal cord from higher levels although another possible view is that the failure of neuronal function is due to inhibition. It is worth noting, and may be of importance in attempting to review the causation and recovery in spinal shock, to realize that headward of the transection there is also a change in the reflex response (Creed *et al.*, 1932).

Of particular interest in spinal shock are the experiments of Teasdell and Stavraky (1953), in which one limb of the cat was deafferented by section of the posterior roots; electrical stimulation of the basis pedunculi produced no response in the corresponding limb, but 5–47 days later responses were evoked more readily in the denervated than in the normal limb. This is a similar, but reversed, state of affairs to that pertaining in spinal shock.

From this brief account of spinal shock two facts emerge: in the 60 odd years since Sherrington summarized spinal shock as a withdrawal of synaptic transmission, neurophysiology has had very little to add. More surprisingly, nobody had ever looked at the spinal cord to see what was actually happening until the late 1950s and early 1960s (Liu & Chambers, 1958; Illis, 1963).

The 'target area' of nerve fibres in any part of the nervous system is the neuronal surface where connections are made. Wyckoff and Young (1956) were the first to focus attention on the motoneuron surface as a whole and subsequently many workers have demonstrated that the motoneuron surface of an anterior horn cell in the cat spinal cord, for example, has up to 30 000 synaptic endings on its surface (Aitken & Bridger, 1961; Illis, 1964a; Young, 1964). These endings occupy at least 70% of the cell and dendrite surface and clothe the cell surface like a mosaic, the constituent parts of which are separated by a small space occupied by glial cells and processes. There are, therefore, units in the central nervous system which have up to 30 000 or more inputs from diverse sources and one output ending in many places. Probably within the area encompassed by one glial cell and its process there are inputs from different sources since it is known that the boutons of any incoming fibres are widely scattered over the cell surface. This zone, consisting of boutons terminaux, post-synaptic thickenings, glial cells and their processes may be called the 'synaptic zone'. It is the only part of the nervous system where information from one unit is accessible to another unit and the only place where one part of the nervous system can influence another part. It is the basis of both the reflex and the 'higher' behaviour of the animal. It has been studied in great detail from the point of view of the effect of partial lesions, sprouting of new terminals, the reaction of glial cells, the effect of toxins and the effect of repetitive stimulation (Illis, 1964b; 1973a, b; 1969; Illis *et al.*, 1966; Illis & Mitchell, 1970). Prior to this time the nerve cell surface was thought to be the site of a few hundred synaptic endings. With particular regard to spinal shock, it has been shown that the period of temporary absence of reflexes in spinal shock, and the period during which Teasdell and Stavraky failed to evoke a response in a deafferented limb by stimulation of the basis pedunculi, coincide reasonably well with the phase of apparent widespread anatomical disruption of the synaptic zone following partial denervation (Illis, 1963). In experimental studies if one follows the reactions of the synaptic zone, there is a stage of more or less stable equilibrium reached which has been termed the stage of functional reorganization and it is suggested that possibly neurological function returns at this stage. The reflexes return in an altered form because the organization of the synaptic zone is altered. Although it is difficult to compare accurately the anatomical changes with the phases of spinal shock because the synaptic zone shows a progressive change which may well begin before 24 hours, and because the exact time sequence of the return of reflexes following cord transection is difficult to determine from the literature, it is quite clear that following cord section in the cat, reflexes below the lesion are obtainable after about one hour. However, not all reflexes are so readily obtainable and over a long period of time reflexes are returning and still changing in their nature. They come back in the order: knee jerk, crossed extensor and extensor thrust. The last to appear is the scratch reflex and Sherrington (1910) observed that the scratch reflex six weeks after cord section was still irregular, feeble and easily fatigued.

It is thus suggested that the synaptic zone may be profoundly altered by the denervation of a critical number of boutons terminaux with the consequences not only of degeneration of these boutons but disorganization of the whole synaptic zone, resulting in depression of activity of a nerve cell. With time the deafferented boutons would degenerate, but those with intact fibres would reorganize to reform the partial mosaic that is seen at the stage of functional reorganization.

Spinal shock, however, is not a static phenomenon with a beginning and an end. There is a traumatic beginning, but the return of function is an evolving process and investigation of the nature of this return must include investigation of the capacity of the nervous system to learn, and the capacity of the central nervous system to regenerate.

Multiplication of nerve cells ceases at or soon after birth and is followed by nerve cell death which continues throughout the life of all mammals. This means that development of central nervous system function must depend on organization rather than on the mere number of nerve cells, and suggests that it is the *type* of connection between nerve cells that is important rather than the *fact* of connection. That is, it is the relative importance or density of endings which any neural connection supplies to its target synaptic zone which is important in determining the function of that particular set of pathways.

Biological Models

It is helpful, when considering how the nervous system reacts to a lesion and the importance this may have in terms of recovery, to consider biological models of nervous integration. There are two main types of such models—those with a random or diffuse structure, and those with a well-localized or specific structure. A rapid association of sensory information coming from widely differing sources and of differing modalities obviously requires a richly cross-connected nerve network. The importance of cross connectivity in producing flexibility is indicated in Fig. 2.4.

The existence of highly specific inborn circuits in the CNS implies the genetic determination of synaptic connections and reduces to a minor role the effect of use and disuse on connectivity. However, complete randomness of connection is contrary to known anatomical facts, but genetically rigid connection could not possibly subserve the multitude of genetically unpredictable activities which occur during the lifetime of an organism. In the random type of model, nonspecificity of organization produces stability against disturbance. There is, however, a sharp transition from stability to instability as the connectance reaches a critical level (Gardner & Ashby, 1970; May, 1972). This is probably a general system property since it is so widespread in a variety of systems (Ashby, 1968). It appears that the larger and more complex a system becomes, the more a change in condition either produces no effect at all or a sudden and large consequence at one critical level. In the CNS this instability is guarded against, since any specific circuits would reduce the randomness of the structure. If

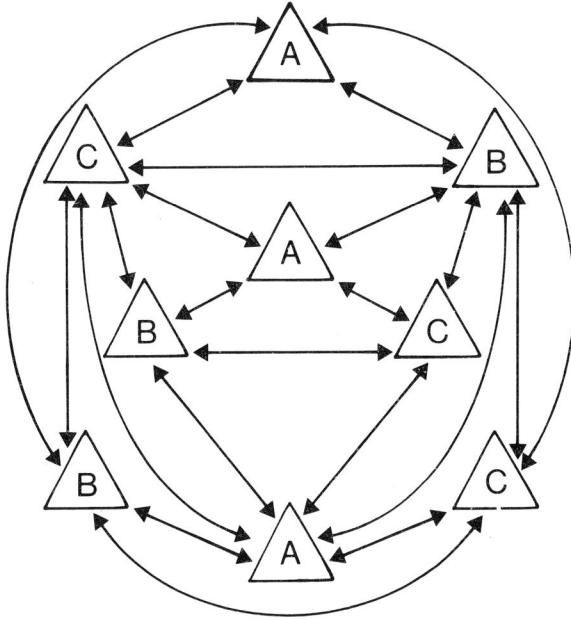

Fig. 2.4 Schematic diagram indicating the connections of nine cells of three types, A, B and C (the lines indicate connectivity and not actual axons). Because of the random connectivity it is possible to have a firing sequence A, B, C, B, A, utilizing any of 99 different pathways. A specific pathway would greatly reduce flexibility.

specific circuits only are present then stability does not exist in the presence of perturbation (see Fig. 2.5).

The simplest form of the diffusely structured nervous system is where the probability of any one unit of the system being connected to any other unit is equal. Assuming the property of synaptic facilitation, such a structure could be altered as a result of a sensory input and perform a variety of learned tasks (Harth & Edgar, 1967). Some specificity would be established as a result of repetitive stimulation, since the effect of such stimulation is to produce a demonstrable structural change in appropriate synapses (Bazanova *et al.*, 1965; Darinskii & Korneeva, 1969; Illis, 1969).

The acceptance of this type of random-specific model as a means of studying the functioning of the CNS assumes the relative unimportance of connections, and indeed of the nerve cells themselves, as regards integration at least, and throws into prominence the areas of connectivity or areas of discontinuity of the nervous system. The relative contribution of a pathway to the synaptic zone is not rigid but can be altered by use, by disuse, by degeneration and regeneration and by the effect of toxins. (The concept of relative contribution and the consequent plastic properties of the synaptic zone are illustrated in Chapter 3.)

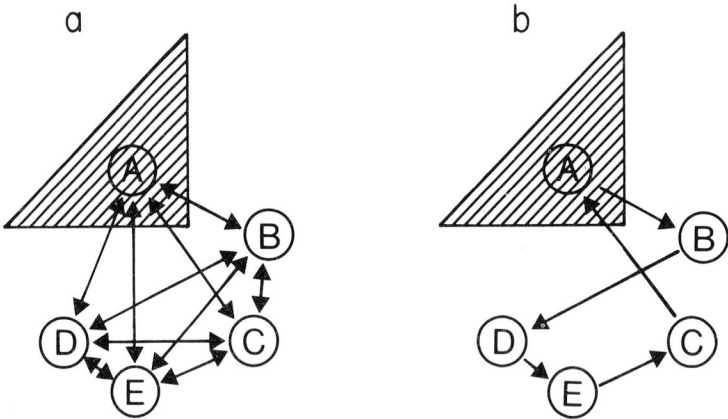

Fig. 2.5a Model of the CNS with random connectivity. A lesion at A does not produce catastrophic effects (unless it is very large) as regards the functioning of the net. For the net to continue functioning, existing pathways are used although some of these may have been little used previously. (The arrows do not represent actual connections but indicate that the chance of any one unit being connected to any other unit is equal.)

Fig. 2.5b Model with a specific structure. A lesion at A now produces complete disruption. For the net to continue functioning completely new connections would have to be established. (Reproduced *Lancet*, Illis, 1973.)

The Effect of a Partial Lesion

The normal clinical neurological state in an organism with an anatomically intact nervous system is a function of the complex and dynamic pattern of impulses arriving at all levels of the nervous system (Fig. 2.6). Changes in the environment are signalled by alteration in the spatial and temporal pattern of discharges and in the rate, amplitude and shape of the signals. These factors are, in turn, altered by and, at the same time, make up the 'central excitatory state' — a somewhat loose concept which refers to the level of excitability of the CNS and embraces sensory information from the environment, sensory information generated by motor activity and information from within the CNS. Minor changes in the micro-environment of nerve cells and their processes may produce marked functional changes; for example, a rise in temperature may produce conduction block; lowering the concentration of calcium ions may theoretically alter conduction velocity (Schauf & Davis 1974).

The effect of a lesion includes not only specific neurological deficits due to loss of the functions subserved by the damaged structures, but also to more wide-spread and less understood effects (Fig. 2.7), which may be of great importance.

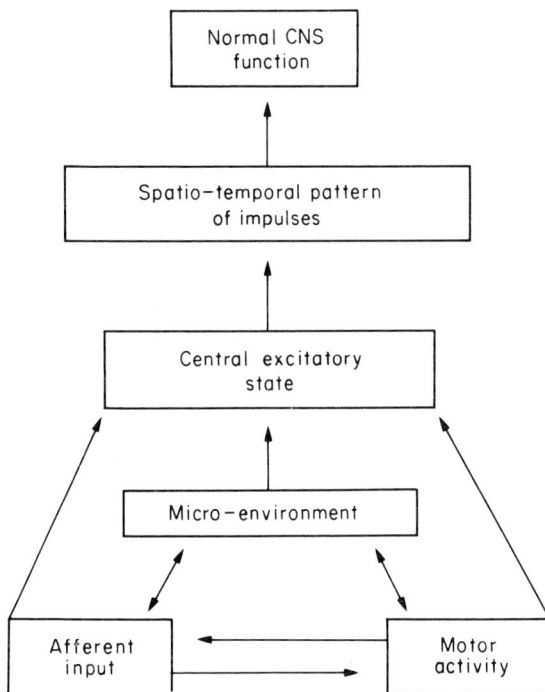

Fig. 2.6 Schematic diagram indicating the functional factors which determine the normal clinical state.

Most of the early work on regeneration in the CNS was limited to nerve cells or axons, and this restriction was responsible for the failure of regeneration studies to offer any explanation of recovery of function after a lesion involving the CNS in the mammal, or any hope of clinical application. In the peripheral nervous system, partial denervation of a muscle results eventually in sprouting from terminal fibres to reinnervate previously denervated motor end plates. In an analogous way, sprouting has been demonstrated in mammalian spinal cord and in the brain. It would appear that the CNS may respond to a lesion by active reorganization involving mechanisms which are known to be operative in neurogenesis and in the maintenance of function in the face of a naturally occurring loss of neurons. There is evidence that neurons can support a larger terminal arborization than they usually do. Not only can an increase in terminal innervation (sprouting) occur, but changes in the structure of undamaged synapses and an increase in the territory of functional axon terminals indicate that connectivity can itself be altered by environmental change (Blakemore, 1977). There is improved connectivity in the fibres which have the heaviest input—a fact from which the concept of synaptic competition has been derived.

In summary, the effect of a lesion is not only to produce specific deficits. In

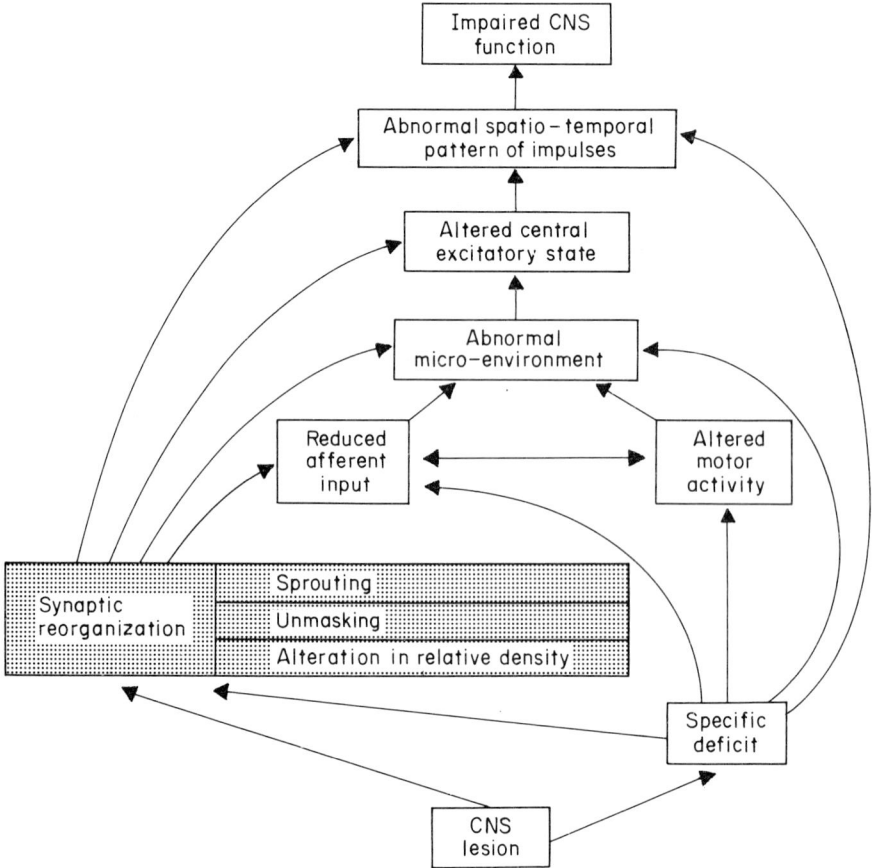

Fig. 2.7 Schematic diagram indicating the functional factors resulting from a partial lesion emphasizing the role of the intact nervous system in producing neurological deficit.

addition, the lesion triggers off a sequence of events, including sprouting of intact terminals, and in this way produces altered connectivity within the intact central nervous system. Destruction of a major input to a neuron or neuron pool will not only have a negative effect; it will also have a positive effect of making previously minor inputs relatively more important and thus alter the relative density of endings in any particular neuron or neuron pool. This by itself would have a far-reaching effect on neuronal functioning.

Although sprouting produces a reorganization at synaptic level, it is not necessary for a structural lesion to occur. An alteration of neural activity may produce a marked change in reorganization. Deafferentation may also 'unmask' a pre-existing but relatively insignificant neural pathway (see Chapter 3).

Conclusion

The intact nervous system reacts in response to a lesion. It is possible to produce structural changes in the central nervous system by environmental changes and it appears that previously unused, or little used, pathways may become effective following degeneration of major connections, or by altering neural activity. This not only provides a theoretical basis for attempting to improve neuronal function in patients who have a partial lesion of the central nervous system but suggests that the problem of rehabilitation of such patients should be via active procedures aimed at the intact, but poorly functioning, central nervous system.

DAMAGE TO THE PERIPHERAL NERVOUS SYSTEM

There are two major responses to peripheral nerve damage, viz. axonal degeneration and segmental demyelination (Weller & Cervós-Navarro, 1977), and provided that neuronal cell bodies, Schwann cells and major nerve trunks remain intact, the peripheral nervous system exhibits a far greater capacity for regeneration than the central nervous system.

Following axonal damage, the distal end of a nerve degenerates, but within 48 hours the proximal axon swells at its terminal end and forms a regenerating end-bulb. After some six days, several small axon sprouts grow from each end-bulb into the distal stump of the nerve along bands of proliferating Schwann cells. The regenerating axons grow into the distal part of the nerve in clusters and after seven to ten days individual axons are invaginated into Schwann cells and myelinated. Regenerating axons grow distally at 2–5 mm per day depending upon the species and upon whether distal connections can be established.

The other major response to nerve damage is segmental demyelination where the myelin sheath is stripped off the axon over one or several segments along the nerve; the axon remains intact. There is slowing of nerve conduction across the demyelinated segment, but remyelination is often very rapid starting within a few days and leading to return of normal conduction velocities and recovery of function within two to three weeks (Bradley, 1975).

Chronic disablement of patients due to peripheral nerve disease occurs when the anterior horn cells or dorsal root ganglion cells are destroyed, or when effective regeneration of damaged axons is prevented either by physical barriers or by metabolic disorders. Segmental demyelination may be recurrent due to repeated immunological attack or due to metabolic and genetic abnormalities within the remyelinating Schwann cells.

Destruction of Motoneurons

Patients with myelomeningocoeles may suffer considerable damage to neurons in the spinal cord so that there is denervation of the bladder and muscles in the lower limbs. Compression of the spinal cord and syringomelia may also cause local destruction of anterior horn cells. Motoneuron loss occurs in virus diseases, particularly poliomyelitis, and loss of these cells is also a feature of motor neuron disease and spinal muscular atrophies. Inherited or sporadic disorders such as Friedreich's ataxia and hereditary sensory neuropathies exhibit extensive loss of dorsal root ganglion cells with degeneration of large myelinated fibres within sensory nerves and degeneration in the posterior columns of the spinal cord.

Failure of Axonal Regeneration in Peripheral Nerves

Axons may fail to regenerate or make contact with their end organs following trauma, especially if there is extensive scar tissue within the injured nerve or if the distance for regeneration is very great (Sunderland, 1968; Asbury & Johnson, 1978). Traumatic or amputation neuromas may form at the severed end of a nerve or even at the site of a nerve crush where continuity of the nerve is preserved (Weller & Cervós-Navarro, 1977), but it is not known why some neuromas are painful whereas others are not. A tangle of nerve fibres and Schwann cells in small fascicles surrounded by perineurium may be seen in a traumatic neuroma a few months after the injury, but later, fibrous tissue may predominate. Repeated damage to peripheral nerves may inhibit regeneration as in entrapment neuropathies or when there is persistent ischaemia.

Toxic neuropathies occur following exposure to a variety of drugs or industrial chemicals (Schaumburg & Spencer, 1979; Spencer & Schaumburg, 1980) and they are usually due to axonal degeneration involving the distal ends of long sensory and motor axons. The distal ends of long tracts in the spinal cord are also affected so that axonal degeneration is seen in the gracile, spinocerebellar and corticospinal tracts. Axons in the peripheral nerves may take many months or years to regenerate following withdrawal from exposure to the toxin. Central nervous system axons do not regenerate so residual signs may be predominantly ataxia and spasticity due to long tract damage.

Axonal degeneration also occurs in endocrine neuropathies, uraemia, amyloid and diabetic neuropathy; regeneration may depend upon adequate treatment of the primary disorder.

Disorders of Remyelination

Segmental demylination occurs in acute post-infectious polyneuritis (Guillain-Barré syndrome); in many cases remyelination is rapid and recovery is virtually complete. Relapsing forms do occur, however, where there is repeated segmental demyelination and remyelination, and further loss of neurological function will accompany each episode. Some hereditary neuropathies including certain types of Charcot-Marie-Tooth disease and Dejerine-Sottas disease appear to be due to a failure of Schwann cells to appropriately remyelinate demyelinating axons (Aguayo, 1978). The repeated segmental demyelination and remyelination are associated with extensive Schwann cell proliferation and formation of the 'onion-bulb' whorls and thickened nerves of hypertrophic neuropathy. Disorders of lipid metabolism such as metachromatic leukodystrophy and Refsum's disease also result in disordered myelination.

PROGRESSIVE MUSCLE DISEASE

Disordered muscle function may result from the loss of nerve supply to muscle groups as in motor neuron disease, acute and chronic peripheral neuropathies, and in spinal muscular atrophy; muscles waste and become weak. Reinnervation by collateral sprouts from preserved nerves frequently occurs in the early stages of chronic disorders such as spinal muscular atrophy, but progressive loss of motoneurons eventually leads to extensive denervation and muscle atrophy.

Primary muscle diseases (myopathies) may be due to destruction of muscle fibres or due to metabolic disorders involving the whole patient or just the muscle cells themselves. Inflammatory disorders such as sarcoidosis or parasitic infections may also affect muscles. Polymyositis is characterized by the destruction and regeneration of muscle fibres; it may be acute, subacute or chronic in its course and may be associated with other diseases including polyarteritis nodosa, rheumatoid arthritis, lupus erythematosis and with carcinomas. There are therapeutic measures which can be taken to treat polymyositis and arrest the progress of muscle destruction. Such treatment is not effective in muscular dystrophies, which are progressive destructive disorders of muscle usually with an hereditary basis. Dystrophies are characterized by a cycle of muscle cell degeneration and regeneration which is particularly prominent in the Duchenne dystrophy; eventually there is extensive loss of muscle tissue and replacement by fibro-fatty tissue. In other dystrophies, including limb-girdle, facioscapulohumeral and myotonic dystrophies, the muscle cell destruction is less marked and the disease may be only slowly progressive.

Many of the congenital myopathies and metabolic myopathies due to mitochondrial abnormalities or disorders of glycogen metabolism may show little destruction of muscle fibres, but muscle function may be defective.

Biopsy in the Diagnosis and Assessment of Neuromuscular Disease

When taken in conjunction with clinical and electrophysiological data, the histological features of a biopsy from the sural or another sensory nerve are often valuable in assessing the pathology and progress of a neuropathy or peripheral nerve lesion. Axonal degeneration can be assessed from the loss of large and small myelinated fibres and the cause of the neuropathy may be evident; for example, vasculitis may be present in biopsies from patients with rheumatoid arthritis and polyarteritis nodosa, or amyloid deposition may be seen in the vessel walls in amyloidosis. Regenerating axons form clusters of small-diameter fibres and their presence is a useful guide to the potential for recovery in traumatic and vascular nerve lesions.

Segmental demyelination occurs not only in the Guillain-Barré syndrome, where it often affects only nerve roots, but also in diphtheritic neuropathy, to a variable extent in diabetes, and in less severe compressive and vascular neuropathies. Demyelinated and remyelinating nerve fibres can be detected in teased-fibre preparations and in transverse sections of nerve biopsies. The appearance and size of 'onion-bulb' whorls in the nerves of patients with recurrent demyelinating neuropathies and in chronic hereditary hypertrophic neuropathies, e.g. Charcot-Marie-Tooth and Dejerine-Sottas disease, is often valuable in establishing a diagnosis and in assessing progression of the disease (Weller & Cervós-Navarro, 1977). Lipid disorders including sulphatide lipidosis (metachromatic leukodystrophy) are associated with segmental demyelination in peripheral nerves where the abnormal lipid accumulates in Schwann cells and macrophages. Diagnosis and characterization of the enzyme defect, however, is usually from cultures of the patient's fibroblasts.

The introduction of enzyme histochemical techniques has greatly extended the use of muscle biopsy in the diagnosis and assessment of muscle disease. As with peripheral nerve lesions, biopsies of muscle can usually only be fully assessed when adequate clinical data are available. Atrophy of small or large groups or muscle fibres is seen in biopsies of those muscles affected by motor nerve lesions. In spinal muscular atrophy and motor neuron disease, the denervation is usually accompanied in the early stages by reinnervation from collateral sprouts of surviving nerves. Such reinnervation can be detected by enzyme histochemistry (Dubowitz & Brooke, 1973).

Histological methods are often useful in assessing the degree of muscle destruction and regeneration in myopathies and dystrophies. Differentiation of muscle fibres within the biopsy by histochemical techniques is, however, usually essential for firm categorization of muscle diseases (Dubowitz & Brooke, 1973). By these techniques, Duchenne and Becker dystrophies can be distinguished from each other as can limb-girdle, facioscapulohumeral and myotonic dystrophies. Furthermore, the Type 2 fibre atrophy of polymyalgia rheumatica can only be reliably detected histochemically. Enzyme defects in some glycogen storage diseases are also detectable by histochemistry whereas the characterization of abnormalities in mitochondria and other cell organelles in congenital myopathies may require electron microscopy in addition to histochemistry.

VALIDITY OF PROJECTION FROM EXPERIMENTAL ANIMALS TO MAN

Man is very different from other animals, particularly in the anatomy and physiology of his nervous system, in his bipedal locomotion and in his social organization. Such differences cast doubt upon the validity of animal experiments and their relevance to human disease. There are, however, large areas where the same biological principles obtain for man and other animals. This applies to many tissues including the nervous system where, for example, fundamental principles of axonal degeneration and regeneration broadly correspond as do the properties of the blood–brain barrier and other basic biological functions. Thus, although problems which involve the unique anatomy and physiological nature of the human nervous system are often difficult to investigate in a meaningful way, it is often possible to dissect a problem and to investigate certain facets in experimental animals. In this way, a picture of pathological events may be built up by combining the results of animal studies with observations in man. Accurate clinical observations are often very valuable in localizing a lesion and monitoring its progress but may give little indication of the pathological process involved. Post-mortem studies, on the other hand, are static and tissue is frequently too poorly preserved for detailed pathological investigation. Nevertheless, sufficient indication of the pathological process may be attained to allow various aspects to be investigated in experimental animals and a complete picture of events to be established. Experimental studies often offer a wide scope for the elucidation of basic pathological problems and for preliminary investigations of therapeutic procedure.

FUTURE POSSIBILITIES FOR RESEARCH

Scope for research to improve rehabilitation of the neurological patient lies in two main fields, viz. prevention of tissue damage during the acute stages of a disease and the promotion of regeneration during the recovery phases.

It is becoming increasingly clear that immunological mechanisms are involved in the destruction of myelin in multiple sclerosis. Characterization of the immunological processes and their prevention or moderation by immunosuppression could lead to a reduction of neurological damage. Similarly, the role of oedema in causing or ameliorating tissue damage is unclear and still requires elucidation. Promotion of regeneration is perhaps the most difficult aspect to investigate unless the relevant pharmacological agents become available. Many of the future advances in recovery of neurological function may lie in an increased understanding of plasticity of the nervous system and promotion of this phenomenon during rehabilitation.

REFERENCES

ABRAMSKY O., LISAK R.P., SILBERBERG D.H. & PLEASURE D.E. (1977) Antibodies to oligodendroglia in patients with multiple sclerosis. *New England Journal of Medicine*, **297**, 1207–11.

ACHESON E.D. (1977) Epidemiology of multiple sclerosis. *British Medical Bulletin*, **33**, 9–14.

ADAMS J.H. (1976) Virus diseases of the nervous system. In *Greenfield's Neuropathology* (Eds. Blackwood W. & Corsellis J.A.N.), 3e, pp. 292–326. Edward Arnold, London.

AGUAYO A.J. (1978) Biological behaviour of Schwann cells: inherited neuropathies. *Journal of Neuropathology and Experimental Neurology*, **37**, 569.

AHMED A.M. & WELLER R.O. (1979) The blood-nerve barrier and reconstitution of the perineurium following nerve grafting. *Neuropathology and Applied Neurobiology*, **5**, 469–84.

AITKEN J.T. & BRIDGER J.E. (1961) Neuron size and neuron population density in the lumbo-sacral region of the cat's spinal cord. *Journal of Anatomy*, **95**, 38–53.

ANTEL J.P., ARNASON B.W.G. & MEDOF M.E. (1979) Suppressor cell function in multiple sclerosis: correlation with clinical disease activity. *Annals of Neurology*, **5**, 338–42.

ASBURY A.K. & JOHNSON P.C. (1978) *Pathology of Peripheral Nerve*. W. B. Saunders Company, Philadelphia, London.

ASHBY W.R. (1968) The contribution of information theory to pathological mechanisms in psychiatry. *British Journal of Psychiatry*, **114**, 1485–98.

BATCHELOR J.R., COMPSTON A. & McDONALD W.I. (1978) The significance of the association between HLA and multiple sclerosis. *British Medical Bulletin*, **34**, 279–84.

BAZANOVA I.S., EVDOKIMOV S.A., MAIROV V.N., MERKULOVA O.S. & CHERNIGOVSKII V.N. (1965) Morphological and electrical changes in interneuronal synapses during passage of rhythmic impulses. In *Federation Proceedings*, 1966, **25**, T187–90.

BERNSTEIN J.J. & BERNSTEIN M.E. (1969) Ultrastructure of normal regeneration and loss of regenerative capacity following teflon blockage in goldfish spinal cord. *Experimental Neurology*, **24**, 538–57.

BERNSTEIN J.J. & BERNSTEIN M.E. (1971) Axon regeneration and formation of synapses proximal to the site of lesion following hemisection of the rat spinal cord. *Experimental Neurology*, **30**, 336–51.

BERRY M. (1979) Regeneration in the central nervous system. In *Recent Advances in Neuropathology*, Vol. I (Eds. Smith W.T. & Cavanagh J.B.), pp. 67–111. Churchill Livingstone, Edinburgh.

BERRY M. & RICHES A.C. (1974) An immunological approach to regeneration in the central nervous system. *British Medical Bulletin*, **30**, 135–40.

BJÖRKLUND A., JOHANSSON B., STEVENI U. & SVENDGAARD N-A. (1975) Re-establishment of functional connections by regenerating central adrenergic and cholinergic axons. *Nature, London*, **523**, 446–8.

BLAKEMORE C. (1977) Genetic instructions and development of plasticity in the kitten's visual cortex. *Philosophical Transactions Royal Society London*, B278, 425–34.

BLAKEMORE W.F. (1976) Invasion of Schwann cells into the spinal cord of the rat following local injections of lysolecithin. *Neuropathology and Applied Neurobiology*, **2**, 21–39.

BRADBURY M.W. (1979) *The Concept of a Blood–Brain Barrier*. John Wiley & Sons, Chichester and New York.

BRADLEY W.G. (1975) *Disorders of Peripheral Nerves*. Blackwell Scientific Publications, Oxford.

BRIERLY J.B. (1976) Cerebral hypoxia. In *Greenfield's Neuropathology* (Eds. Blackwood W. & Corsellis J.A.N.), 3e, pp. 43–85. Edward Arnold, London.

BRIGHTMAN M.W., KLATZO I., OLSSON Y., REESE T.S. (1970) The blood–brain barrier to proteins under normal and pathological conditions. *Journal of the Neurological Sciences*, **10**, 215–39.

CAJAL S.R.y. (1928) *Degeneration and Regeneration in the Nervous System*. Oxford University Press, London.

CAVANAGH J.B. (1978) Metallic toxicity and the nervous system. In *Recent Advances in Neuropathology*, Vol I, (Eds. Smith W. Thomas & Cavanagh J.B.), pp. 247–75. Churchill Livingstone, Edinburgh.

CREED R.S., DENNY-BROWN D., ECCLES J.C., LIDDELL E.G.T. & SHERRINGTON C.S. (1932) *Reflex Activity of the Spinal Cord.* Oxford University Press, London.

CROFT P.B. (1969) Para-infectious and post-vaccinial encephalomyelitis. *Postgraduate Medical Journal*, **45**, 392–400.

DARINSKII Y.A. & KORNEEVA T.E. (1969) Change in number and size of synapses on motoneurones of frog spinal cord with prolonged stimulation of posterior roots. In *International Abstracts of Biological Sciences 1971*, **60**, 80.

DROZ B., RAMBOURG A. & KOENIG H.L. (1975) The smooth endoplasmic reticulum: structure and role in the renewal of axonal membrane and synaptic vesicles by fast axonal transport. *Brain Research*, **93**, 1–13.

DUBOWITZ V. & BROOKE M.H. (1973) *Muscle Biopsy: a Modern Approach.* W. B. Saunders Company, Philadelphia.

GARDNER M.R. & ASHBY W.R. (1970) Connectance of large dynamic (cybernetic) systems: critical values for stability. *Nature. Lond.*, **228**, 784.

HALL M. (1833) On the reflex function of the medulla oblongata and medulla spinalis. *Philosophical Transactions of the Royal Society*, **123**, 635–65.

HALL M. (1850) Quoted by Sherrington (1910).

HARTH E.M. & EDGAR S.L. (1967) Association by synaptic facilitation in highly damped neural nets. *Biophysical Journal*, **7**, 689–717.

HEROS R.C., ZERAS N.T. & NEGORO M. (1976) Cerebral vasospasm. *Surgical Neurology*, **5**, 354–62.

HUGHES J.T. (1977) *Pathology of the Spinal Cord*, 2e. Lloyd-Luke, London.

ILLIS L.S. (1963) Changes in spinal cord synapses and a possible explanation for spinal shock. *Experimental Neurology*, **8**, 328–35.

ILLIS L.S. (1964a) Spinal cord synapses: the normal appearances by the light microscope. *Brain*, **87**, 543–54.

ILLIS L.S. (1964b) Spinal cord synapses in the cat: the reaction of boutons terminaux at the motorneurone surface to experimental denervation. *Brain*, **87**, 555–72.

ILLIS L.S. (1969) Enlargement of spinal cord synapses after repetitive stimulation of a single posterior root. *Nature, London*, **223**, 76–7.

ILLIS L.S. (1973) Regeneration in the central nervous system. *Lancet*, **i**, 1035–7.

ILLIS L.S. (1973a) Experimental model of regeneration in the CNS: I. Synaptic changes. *Brain*, **96**, 47–60.

ILLIS L.S. (1973b) Experimental model of regeneration in the CNS: II. The reaction of glia in the synaptic zone. *Brain*, **96**, 61–8.

ILLIS L.S. & MITCHELL J. (1970) The effect of tetanus toxin on boutons terminaux. *Brain Research*, **18**, 283–95.

ILLIS L.S., PATANGIA G.N. & CAVANAGH J.B. (1966) Boutons terminaux and tri-ortho-cresyl phosphate toxicity. *Experimental Neurology*, **14**, 160–74.

JACOBS J., MACFARLANE R.M. & CAVANAGH J.B. (1977) Vascular leakage in the dorsal root ganglion of the rat, studied with horse-radish peroxidase. *Journal of the Neurological Sciences*, **29**, 95–107.

KIERNAN J.A. (1978) An explanation of axonal regeneration in peripheral nerves and its failure in the central nervous system. *Medical Hypotheses*, **4**, 15–26.

KLATZO I. (1979) Cerebral oedema and ischaemia. In *Recent Advances in Neuropathology*, Vol. I (Eds. Smith W. Thomas & Cavanagh J.B.), pp. 27–39. Churchill Livingstone, Edinburgh.

KREUTZBERG G.W. (1972) Neural degeneration and regeneration. In *Pathology of the Nervous System*, Vol. III (Ed. Minkler J.), pp. 2678–87. McGraw-Hill, New York.

KRISTENSSON K. (1978) Retrograde transport of macromolecules in axons. *Annual Review of Pharmacology and Toxicology*, **18**, 97–110.

LAMPERT P.W. (1978) Autoimmune and virus-induced demyelinating diseases. *American Journal of Pathology*, **91**, 176–208.

LIU C.N. & CHAMBERS W.W. (1958) Intraspinal sprouting of dorsal root axons. *Archives Neurology and Psychiatry (Chicago)*, **79**, 46–61.

LORENZO A.V., PAGE L.K., WATTERS G.V. (1970) Relationship between cerebrospinal fluid absorption and pressure in human hydrocephalus. *Brain*, **93**, 679–92.

LUMSDEN C.E. (1970) The neuropathology of multiple sclerosis. In *Handbook of Clinical Neurology*, Vol. 9 (Ed. Vinken P.J. & Bruyn C.W.), Ch. 8, pp. 217–309. North Holland Publishing Company, Amsterdam.

MARTIN J.B., RENAUD L.P. & BRAZEAU P. (1975) Hypothalamic peptides: new evidence for 'peptidergic' pathway in the CNS. *Lancet*, **ii**, 393–5.

MAY R.M. (1972) Will a large complex system be stable? *Nature, London*, **238**, 413–14.

MITCHELL J., WELLER R.O. & EVANS H. (1979) Re-establishment of the blood–brain barrier to peroxidase following cold injury to the mouse cortex. *Acta Neuropathologica*, **46**, 45–9.

MONAKOW C. VON (1902) Quoted by Sherrington (1910).

OLSSON Y. & KRISTENSSON K. (1973) The perineurium as a diffusion barrier to protein tracers following trauma to nerves. *Acta Neuropathologica*, **23**, 105–11.

OLSSON Y. & KRISTENSSON K. (1979) Recent application of tracer techniques to neuropathology, with particular reference to vascular permeability and axonal flow. In *Recent Advances in Neuropathology*, Vol. I (Eds. Smith & Cavanagh J.B.), pp. 1–25. Churchill Livingstone, Edinburgh.

OPPENHEIMER D.R. (1976) Demyelinating diseases. In *Greenfield's Neuropathology* (Eds. Blackwood W. & Corsellis J.A.N.), 3e pp. 470–99. Edward Arnold, London.

OPPENHEIMER D.R. (1978) The cervical cord in multiple sclerosis. *Neuropathology and Applied Neurobiology*, **4**, 151–62.

OWMAN C., EDVINSSON L., ÓLIN T., SAHLIN C. & SVENDGAARD N–A. (1979) Pathophysiology of cerebral vasospasm: transmitter changes in perivascular sympathetic nerves, and increased pial artery sensitivity to norepinephrine and serotonin. In *Cerebrovascular Diseases* (Eds. Price T.R. & Nelson E.), pp. 295–305. Raven Press, New York.

PETERS A., PALAY S., WEBSTER H. DEF. (1976) *The Fine Structure of the Nervous System*. The neurons and supporting cells. W. B. Saunders Company, Philadelphia.

PRICE D.L., GRIFFIN J., YOUNG A., PECK K. & STOCKS A. (1975) Tetanus toxin: direct evidence for retrograde intraaxonal transport. *Science*, **188**, 945–7.

PRINEAS J.W. (1972) Acute idiopathic polyneuritis: an electron microscope study. *Laboratory Investigation*, **26**, 133–47.

RUSSELL D.S. (1954) The pathology of spontaneous intracranial haemorrhage. *Proceedings of the Royal Society of Medicine*, **47**, 689–704.

SCHAUF C.L. & DAVIS F.A. (1974) Impulse conduction in multiple sclerosis: a theoretical basis for modification by temperature and pharmacological agents. *Journal of Neurology, Neurosurgery and Psychiatry*, **37**, 152–61.

SCHAUMBURG H.H. & SPENCER P.S. (1979) Toxic neuropathies. *Neurology*, **29**, 429–30.

SHERRINGTON C.S. (1910) *The Integrative Action of the Nervous System*. Constable, London.

SIDEN A. & KJELLIN K.G. (1978) CSF protein examinations with thin-layer isoelectric focusing in multiple sclerosis. *Journal of Neurological Sciences*, **39**, 131–46.

SPENCER P.S. & SCHAUMBURG H.H. (1980) *Experimental and Clinical Neurotoxicology*. Williams & Wilkins, Baltimore.

STRICH S.J. (1961) Shearing of nerve fibres as a cause of brain damage due to head injury. A pathological study of twenty cases. *Lancet*, **ii**, 443–8.

SUNDERLAND S. (1968) *Nerve and Nerve Injuries*. Williams & Wilkins, Baltimore.

TEASDELL R.D. & STAVRAKY G.W. (1953) Responses of de-afferented spinal neurons to corticospinal impulses. *Journal of Neurophysiology*, **16**, 367–75.

TORVIK A. (1976) Central chromatolysis and the axon reaction: a reappraisal. *Neuropathology and Applied Neurobiology*, **2**, 423–32.

VARON S. (1975) Nerve growth factor and its mode of action. *Experimental Neurology*, **48**, 75–92.

WILLIAMS P.L. & WARWICK R. (Eds.) (1980) *Gray's Anatomy*, 36e. Longman, Edinburgh.

WELLER R.O. & CERVÓS-NAVARRO J. (1977) *Pathology of Peripheral Nerves*. Butterworths, London.

WELLER R.O. & MITCHELL J. (1980) Cerebrospinal fluid oedema and its sequelae in hydrocephalus.

In *Brain Edema: Diagnosis, Pathology and Therapy* (Ed. Cervós-Navarro J.). Raven Press, New York.

WELLER R.O. & SHULMAN K. (1972) Infantile hydrocephalus: clinical, histological and ultrastructural study of brain damage. *Journal of Neurosurgery*, **36,** 255–65.

WHYTT R. (1750) Quoted by Sherrington (1910).

WYCKOFF R.W.G. & YOUNG J.Z. (1956) The motoneuron surface. *Proceedings of the Royal Society*, B144, 440–50.

YATES P.O. (1976) Vascular disease of the central nervous system. In *Greenfield's Neuropathology* (Eds. Blackwood W. & Corsellis J.A.N.), 3e, pp. 86–147. Edward Arnold, London.

YOUNG J.Z. (1964) *A Model of the Brain.* Oxford University Press, London.

Chapter 3
Plasticity in the Adult Nervous System

Recovery of function after nervous system injury remains a paradox. On the one hand, the nervous system of mammals does not heal itself. Except for olfactory receptor cells (Graziadei & Graziadei, 1977), neurons that die are not replaced. On the other hand, as evidenced in many of the chapters in this volume, neural function usually does improve in the weeks and months following injury, sometimes dramatically. Our best lead so far is the accumulating body of evidence that the neuroanatomical and neurophysiological picture after brain damage is not static. It is safe to guess that among the so-called 'plastic' changes that follow injury, the physical basis of rehabilitation will be found. The term 'plasticity' deserves some comment. Plasticity is a loosely defined concept that stands in contrast to elasticity and to brittleness. Following impact an elastic object returns to its original form. A brittle object shatters. A plastic object may survive and continue to function, but it is changed by the experience.

In trying to understand recovery of function, one must know what, in essence, was lost. Consider a hypothetical situation in which a particular group of cells is destroyed and as a result a particular behavioural function, say speech, is lost. It cannot be concluded that the speech 'centre' has been destroyed. The functional loss means only that the rest of the brain cannot perform the function without the contribution normally made by the damaged cells. That contribution might be a minor one, say, setting the level of excitability of some other group of cells. Through many of the mechanisms that will be discussed in this chapter, the excitability of the target cells could be restored and with it behavioural function. Von Monakow (1914) called processes such as this 'diaschisis', i.e. functional loss due to depression of a neural mechanism not itself destroyed.

On the other hand, it is possible that somewhere in the central nervous system (CNS) there is a specific, localized group of cells that organizes the neural impulse sequences of speech. Such a hypothetical cell cluster might properly be called a 'speech centre', and its destruction would also result in the functional deficit. In this case, however, recovery might require massive and perhaps impossible reorganization of remaining neural aggregates. We do not know to what extent brain functions are localized in centres. Indeed, this has long been one of the central debates of neurological science (Teuber, 1974). The matter will probably be resolved only as the details of functional circuitry are eventually

44

worked out. Finally, even if a vital circuit element were destroyed, plastic changes such as the substitution of parallel channels or the mobilization of redundant capacity could still support rehabilitation.

When discussing changes that follow nervous system injury, the term 'sprouting' will be used frequently. It refers to new growth of neural processes by protoplasmic extension from axon terminals, nodes of Ranvier, axon stumps (in the case of regeneration) etc. Sprouting occurs in many circumstances (Fig. 3.2). 'Reactive' sprouting (Cotman & Lynch, 1976) refers to new growth of intact fibres usually as a result of nearby denervation. 'Regenerative' sprouting refers to new growth from near the end of a cut fibre. 'Compensatory' sprouting refers to new growth of one branch of an axonal tree when a distant branch is cut. It is unclear to what extent the mechanism underlying sprouting in these three situations is different (see legend of Fig. 3.2).

This chapter will provide a glimpse at a broad range of plastic changes that may bear on functional restitution following nervous system injury to adult mammals. Where relevant, the reader will be directed to in-depth reviews of particular issues. Early pathophysiological processes such as the decline of oedema and recovery from ion imbalances are specifically excluded (see Chapter 2). So, also, are external interventions such as the use of prostheses or neuroaugmentative devices (see Chapters 12, 13, 14).

PLASTICITY IN THE NEWBORN VERSUS ADULT

Critical Periods of Plasticity

Extensive experimental and clinical observations indicate that in young animals and children there is often a remarkable degree of functional sparing after CNS injuries that are devastating when they occur in adulthood (Kennard, 1940; Eidelberg & Stein, 1974). On the other hand, recovery is minimal after some types of injury (Teuber & Rudel, 1962) and in others it may be at a high cost. The sparing of language after early left hemisphere damage, for example, is accompanied by substantial intellectual and perceptual deficits, not seen after equivalent lesions in adults (Woods & Teuber, 1973; Milner, 1974). Even given such qualifications, however, the relative lability of the newborn brain is impressive. A comparison of adult and neonate may therefore be a good point of departure.

A number of experimental studies have found major quantitative differences in the physical reaction of the adult and newborn brain to traumatic injury, and environmental manipulations. For example, Guillery (1972), Kalil (1973) and Hickey (1975) enucleated one eye in kittens, thus deafferenting the corresponding layers in the lateral geniculate nucleus. Several months later the connections of the remaining eye were studied. There is normally a sharp boundary between the layers receiving input from each of the two eyes. In kittens enucleated before nine days of age, however, the border was breached and sprouts from the intact eye invaded the territory of the enucleated eye. No translaminar spread was detected after enucleation at later stages.

Sprouting of intact fibres into a partially denervated nucleus is a common finding in developing systems. The reader is referred to a number of excellent reviews of this subject (Bernstein & Goodman, 1973; Stein *et al.*, 1974; Eidelberg & Stein, 1974; Vital-Durand & Jeannerod, 1975; Jacobson, 1978; Cotman, 1978). This discussion is restricted to a description of three preparations in which the variable age at the time of injury has been studied specifically.

EXAMPLE 1: THE SUPERIOR COLLICULUS (SC)

Our first case study will be of axonal reorganization in the superior colliculus (SC) of the golden hamster. Most fibres of the left optic nerve cross at the optic chiasm and make synaptic terminals in the right diencephalon. Many of these then continue on and make synaptic terminals in a map-like fashion in the superficial cell strata of the SC. Schneider (1970; 1973; 1976) found that if the superficial SC strata on the right are destroyed at birth, recently arrived and/or newly ingrowing fibres from the left eye react in three ways. They increase their distribution in the right diencephalon, they form synaptic connections in the deep layers of the right SC, and, most surprisingly, they cross the midline and terminate on the medial edge of the left SC. The rest of the left SC, of course, is occupied by the right eye which has been forced to yield only a part of its territory to the invader. If the right eye is also removed, anomalous fibres of the left eye spread out and occupy the whole left SC. The capacity to invade the remainder of the left SC is limited in time. It occurs if competition from the right eye is removed on or before the 10th day postpartum, but it does not occur if one waits until the 14th day (So & Schneider, 1978).

Two other properties of this system stand out. First, the amount of anomalous growth in one location depends on the amount of anomalous growth in others. For example, the more invasion of the left SC, the less sprouting is found in the right diencephalon. Second, sprouts invade not only areas that have been denervated as a result of the SC lesion (e.g. the lateral posterior nucleus of the thalamus), but also areas that have not been denervated (e.g. the contralateral SC and the ipsilateral dorsal terminal nucleus). These data suggested to Schneider (1973) that developing neurons tend to conserve their total axonal arborization. When distal branches are 'pruned' off, increased intrinsic growth pressure causes remaining axonal branches to invade nearby tissue and occupy available terminal space in competition with normal inputs ('compensatory sprouting', Fig. 3.2).

EXAMPLE 2: THE LATERAL OLFACTORY TRACT (LOT)

The lateral olfactory tract (LOT) commences in the olfactory bulb as a tight caudally running bundle, but soon fans out and terminates in a thin sheet in the most superficial cortical layer throughout the pyriform lobe (Heimer, 1968; Devor, 1976a). In contrast to the map-like distribution of the optic tract, the LOT fibres form a widely branched and non-topographic projection. Consider first experiments in which the whole LOT was cut across leaving the (target) cortex distal to the cut intact (Devor, 1976b). When this was done within one day of birth, many fibres simply grew over the slit and continued on their way. These successful fibres were probably newly outgrowing ones that had not actually been severed since fibres no longer crossed the cut when the experiment was repeated on day three, the age at which the last outgrowing fibres cross the level of the cut. Instead, when the LOT was cut on day three there was a tremendous build-up of axonal arbor proximally. This involved both a laminar expansion of the LOT distribution at the expense of intracortical association fibres, and lateral and medial spread beyond the normal cytoarchitectonic borders of olfactory cortex (Fig. 3.1). In addition, LOT fibres in the olfactory tubercle grew laterally opposite to their normal direction, and partially reinnervated the olfactory cortex distal to the cut. By the 7th day reinnervation of the distal cortex ceased, by the 17th day lateral and medial spread ceased and by the 43rd day laminar expansion ceased. No sign of LOT rearrangement was seen after tract section in the adult. The consequences of partial LOT section are equally instructive. The cut fibres responded with proximal sprouting just as after complete LOT section. However, the fibres left untouched did not simply make their normal diffuse connections throughout the olfactory cortex. Rather, they formed a relatively dense innervation in the zone just behind the cut and failed to innervate the most distal part of the olfactory cortex at all (Fig. 3.1). This foreshortening occurred only when the LOT was partially cut before 17 days of age. In older hamsters the severed LOT fibres degenerated, but the surviving ones were not redisposed. Schneider's principle of axon arbor conservation neatly explains both proximal sprouting and distal foreshortening. In the first case the 'pruning' of distal branches would increase growth pressure proximally. In the second, more-than-normal terminal elaboration in the first empty zone encountered just distal to a partial LOT cut would require the sacrifice of growth further distally as a compensation. (Devor & Schneider, 1975).

After early (complete) section of the LOT, the far distal olfactory cortex remains without LOT input. Adjacent intact intracortical fibres respond by occupying the dendritic region left vacant by the LOT (Westrum, 1975; Leonard, 1975; Price *et al.*, 1976). Such synaptic replacement is minimal in the adult (Caviness *et al.*, 1977) and in consequence the denervated dendrites and sometimes the whole postsynaptic neuron atrophies and is resorbed (Jones & Thomas, 1962; White & Westrum, 1964; Heimer, 1968). Something about the presence of LOT or even of anomalous inputs has a sustaining effect on the target cell. An even more dramatic example of this type of interaction comes from the developing rodent somatosensory cortex (van der Loos & Woolsey, 1973; Weller & Johnson, 1975; Rice & van der Loos, 1977). In cortical lamina IV there is a field

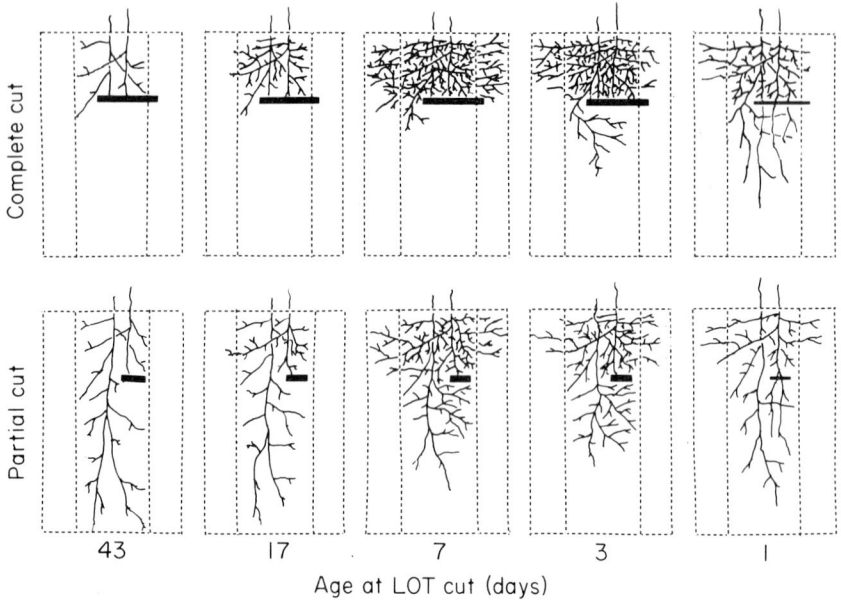

Fig. 3.1 Schematic representation of the rearrangement of lateral olfactory tract (LOT) axon collaterals following complete or partial transection of the tract in hamsters 1–43 days of age. LOT axon branches normally fill the whole olfactory projection cortex, represented by the middle panel in each of the drawings. In newborn animals the cut is bridged. In slightly older pups, fibres fail to cross the cut, but there is a substantial increase in the growth of proximal axon collaterals ('compensatory sprouting'). If the LOT is only partially severed the cut fibres undergo 'compensatory sprouting' and the uncut fibres are also affected. They make excessive branches in the zone just behind the cut at the expense of normal growth further distally ('compensatory stunting'). These forms of rearrangement are no longer seen if the LOT is injured in adulthood. (From Devor, 1976b, reprinted with permission, *Journal of Comparative Neurology*.)

of characteristic barrel-like cell aggregates, each barrel being associated with a single mystacial vibrissa (whisker). In mice, if a particular whisker and its follicle on the snout are destroyed before the time of barrel formation (five days of age) the corresponding barrel fails to develop. Later whisker removal does not cause barrels to degenerate. Note that this effect acts across three synapses.

EXAMPLE 3: THE VISUAL CORTEX

The peturbation that brings about a reordering of axonal and synaptic arrangement need not be a physical lesion. Altered neural activity may be sufficient. Studies in monkey (Hubel *et al.*, 1977; Rakic, 1977) have shown that in the normal course of development, geniculo-cortical fibres representing the two eyes terminate in the primary visual cortex in alternating stripes. Adjacent stripes overlap broadly. Beginning in the late prenatal period the afferent axons move away from one another until the stripes of alternating input are segregated— right eye, left eye, right eye. None the less, because of dendritic spread and intracortical connections, most cortical cells receive input equally, or nearly equally, from the two eyes. Segregation of inputs proceeds in the absence of visual stimulation. However, abnormal visual input, monocular occlusion for example, can disrupt segregation. In this situation, cortical afferents driven by the open eye come to dominate the cortex at the expense of the interdigitated stripe from the closed eye. Most cortical cells then respond to visual stimuli delivered through the opened eye, but sluggishly at best to stimuli delivered through the eye that had been occluded.

Behaviourally, too, the deprived eye is all but blind (von Noorden *et al.*, 1970). Such functional suppression (occlusion amblyopia) occurs only if the eye is occluded during a critical period—birth to about 12 weeks of age in kittens and monkeys (Dews & Wiesel, 1970; von Noorden, 1973). Even extended monocular occlusion in adulthood does not cause amblyopia, shift the occular dominance distribution of cortical cells, or affect the relative prominence of the alternating stripes of cortical afferents.

Monocular domination of the cortex and amblyopia can be partly or fully reversed if the occluded eye is given visual experience before the end of the critical period. After this time, however, the cortex loses its lability. Even if the animal is forced to use its previously occluded eye, the previously open one being shut, there is only minimal improvement (Dews & Wiesel, 1970; Blakemore *et al.*, 1978). Cortical lability during the critical period is thought to be related to catecholamine fibres in the cortex. Kasamatsu & Pettigrew (1976) have shown that catecholamine depletion by intraventricular 6-hydroxydopamine eliminates the development of monocular dominance following eye occlusion. Noradrenaline replacement by intraventricular application or local infusion restores this form of plasticity (Pettigrew & Kasamatsu, 1978). Application of the GABA blocker bicuculline, or enucleation of the dominant eye, has also been reported to enhance the effectiveness of the suppressed eye (Kratz *et al.*, 1976; Duffy *et al.*, 1976).

Monocular occlusion occurs in human children as a consequence of congenital cataract and has also been used over the years in the treatment of external eye disease, strabismic amblyopia etc. Unfortunately, if the occluded eye was un-covered too late, its acuity was often permanently impaired. In fact, even very brief periods of occlusion in very young children can cause amblyopia. In the light of these clinical and experimental findings it is now well known that congenital cataracts must be removed early and that continuous monocular occlusion in children must be avoided. Data available from such 'natural' experiments place the critical period for occular dominance lability in humans at birth to about four years of age (von Noorden, 1973). In addition to mono-cular occlusion, early visual deprivations of many other sorts (e.g. of vertically orientated lines, movement, binocular visual experience) can result in altered functional connectivity in the visual cortex and corresponding perceptual deficits.

PLASTICITY IN THE ADULT PERIPHERAL NERVOUS SYSTEM (PNS)

With maturity, the CNS loses a good deal of its former lability. This is much less so for the PNS. In fact, the processes of growth after peripheral nerve injury in the adult are reminiscent of initial axon outgrowth in the developing nervous system. The major difference, of course, is that the surrounding milieu is mature and not itself unfolding. The present discussion will concentrate on plastic reorganization in the somatosensory system. Relatively little reference will be made to the large literature on plasticity in motor and autonomic systems. For this material several review articles are recommended (Edds, 1953; Guth, 1956; Sunderland, 1978; Purves, 1976; Grinnell, 1977; Rosenthal, 1977).

Response to Injury

In all but the most minimal forms of nerve injury, nutritive contact between the proximal and distal parts of the axon is disrupted and the distal part degenerates along with its myelin sheath ('Wallerian' degeneration). This contrasts with many invertebrate preparations in which glial cells can maintain the severed axon for months (Bittner & Johnson, 1974). In the distal nerve segment Schwann cells, which survive, proliferate and become aligned in strands (bands of Bunger) that will serve as guides along which regenerating sprouts will grow.

Looking centrally from the point of injury, the axon dies back a variable distance, up to a few millimetres, with accompanying fragmentation and/or blistering of the myelin sheath (Cajal, 1928; Spencer & Thomas, 1970; Spencer & Lieberman, 1971; Morris *et al.*, 1972). The remainder of the proximal axon remains functional although it undergoes retrograde changes such as reduction of conduction velocity and diameter and widening of nodes. These changes are reversed upon successful regeneration, but tend to be progressive in its absence (Weiss *et al.*,1945; Cragg & Thomas, 1961; Anderson *et al.*, 1970; Devor & Govrin-Lippmann, 1979a). The most significant retrograde effects that have been described are the 'chromatolytic' changes in the cell body, dendritic retractions, and the stripping of some afferent synapses off of dendrites (for reviews see Cragg, 1970; Lieberman, 1971; 1974; Watson, 1974; Grafstein, 1975). Once considered a degenerative process, the retrograde cell reaction is now understood as a process of metabolic mobilization in preparation for axon repair. If regeneration is delayed or prevented, however, the cell may die. The incidence of retrograde cell death depends on a number of other factors including time after axotomy, the particular neural system involved, the distance of the injury along the axon, age, the existence of axon collateral branches, etc. (Lieberman, 1971; 1974).

Regenerative Sprout Outgrowth

Axonal elongation begins after a latent period of a day or two, the time required for modification of biosynthetic activity in the cell body. If a second more proximal axotomy is made at the end of the latent time, sprout outgrowth from the new cut is accelerated (Gutmann, 1942; McQuarrie *et al.*, 1977). The severed axon stump, or the zone just proximal to this, may emit anywhere from 1 to about 20 sprouts (Cajal, 1928; Shawe, 1955). The fate of these sprouts depends upon their success at entering the distal nerve stump and reaching an appropriate peripheral target. Regeneration is most satisfactory after crush injuries where the perineurial sheath remains intact and axons have easy access to the distal stump. It is least satisfactory when a large gap exists between proximal and distal stumps. Attempts at surgical repair of severed nerves generally concentrate on closing or bridging the gap while minimizing tissue obstructions and maintaining as good a fascicular alignment as possible (Campbell, 1970; Sunderland, 1978). In the process of crossing the zone of injury, fibres are strongly influenced by local mechanical factors. Many grow in a retrograde direction back along the proximal nerve, often forming spirals around parent axons or blood vessels. Others are arrested or escape from the nerve bundle (Cajal, 1928). Sprouts that do reach the distal stump, however, track along the Schwann cell guides with few such errors and at impressive rates. Successful sprouts of myelinated parent axons can advance at 2–4 mm/day; of unmyelinated fibres at about 1 mm/day (reviewed by Sunderland, 1978). Sprouts of small diameter myelinated fibres tend to lag behind sprouts of large diameter fibres, although much of the delay may be in crossing the zone of the injury (Thulin, 1960; Devor & Govrin-Lippmann, 1979a).

It is not trivial to determine the proportion of parent fibres that eventually cross the level of the lesion. It is impractical to trace single axons and their sprouts for substantial distances and the comparison of axon profile counts proximal and distal to the lesion can be misleading because individual fibres may have many crossing sprouts. Finally, because of changes in axon calibre, measurements of the compound action potential elicited by stimulation distal to the injury gives only a crude indication. The best method to date involves recording from large numbers of single axons in appropriate spinal roots and asking what percentage of axons that respond to electrical stimulation just proximal to the point of injury also respond to stimulation distally. For crush injury in rat sciatic nerve, this method has shown that 100% of myelinated fibres eventually regenerate (Devor & Govrin-Lippmann, 1979a). For sciatic nerve section with immediate end-to-end resuture anywhere from 25% to 75% of fibres regenerated in different rats (Seltzer & Devor, unpublished). Using similar methods, Burgess & Horch (1973) found at least 87% recovery in cut sural nerve in cats.

Although there is a massive overproduction of sprouts at first, relatively few fibres are thought to maintain more than one to maturity. The mechanism for culling the 'unsuccessful' sprouts during regeneration may be like that involved in the natural death of excess sensory, motor and autonomic neurons in developing organisms (Hamburger & Levi-Montalcini, 1949; Presige, 1967; Hughes, 1968; Landmesser & Pilar, 1974; Chu-Wang & Oppenheim, 1978), and the elimination of polyneuronal innervation in maturing muscle fibres (Brown *et al.*, 1976). It is tempting to speculate that the first outgrowing sprouts to become successfully connected to the periphery somehow signal this fact back to the cell body, perhaps by means of a trophic substance picked up in the periphery and transported by retrograde axoplasmic flow. Such a stream of trophic substance could shunt the flow of structural metabolites selectively towards the connected sprout to foster its maturation.

As in developing nerve, regenerating sprouts conduct impulses in the continuous (non-saltatory) mode of normal unmyelinated axons (Bostock *et al.*,1977). Shortly after reconnection a wave of diameter increase and myelinization sweeps over the axon from the point of injury distalward and conduction becomes saltatory and gradually accelerates (Quilliam, 1958; Devor & Govrin-Lippmann, 1979b). It is thought that internodal membrane in myelinated axons is inexcitable and that voltage-dependent sodium channels are concentrated almost exclusively on nodal membrane (Ritchie & Rogart, 1977). If this is true, the wave of maturation must be accompanied by major spatial shifts in sodium channel density.

Target Selectivity in Regenerating Nerve

The most clear-cut data on target selectivity are from invertebrates where individual neurons can be identified by their position in segmental ganglia. Following nerve crush injury in the leech (van Essen & Jansen, 1977), most cutaneous fibres returned to their original territory. Following nerve section, however, there were about 50% location errors, and after section with avulsion of the distal stump, 70% The most common type of error was for a fibre to innervate the first patch of skin encountered along its path of outgrowth. Stimulus sensitivity (touch, pressure, noxious) following regeneration was always normal, but this says little for specificity, because stimulus selectivity in the leech is determined by the fibre itself rather than by a transducer target within the skin.

In contrast, for many types of sensory fibres in mammals, stimulus sensitivity is at least partly determined by aggregates of non-neural cells in the skin in which the axon is embedded (Iggo, 1978). Examples are hair follicles, taste-buds and Merkel domes (Haarscheibe). The sensory structure generally atrophies upon denervation and recovers, usually in the original location, upon reinnervation (e.g. Burgess *et al.*, 1974). Fibres with a particular response sensitivity also share other distinguishing features: conduction velocity, terminal branch pattern within the dorsal horn grey matter, and the spinal segment to which they ascend in the dorsal columns (Petit & Burgess, 1968; Brown *et al.*, 1977). In experiments on cats recovered from sural nerve transection, Burgess and Horch (1973) failed to detect significant numbers of fibres with conduction velocity and central projections of one fibre class, but stimulus sensitivity of another. This suggests that sensory fibres returned to their original receptor type. It is not known whether the specificity resides in the axon, the target cells, or both.

As for locus specificity, cutaneous nerves tend to return to their own domain when reconnected to the appropriate distal nerve stump. They will not, however, seek out a patch of their skin transplanted elsewhere. Within a given area of skin fibres of a particular class return to the correct cutaneous cell stratum and type of receptor as discussed above and even re-form characteristic terminal branch patterns with characteristic interdigitations in the correct portion of the non-neural cell aggregate. It is not known, however, whether a particular fibre shows any special affinity towards the particular specialization it once occupied (Jacobson, 1971; Grinnell, 1977). In contrast to sensory fibres, regenerating motor fibres appear to exercise little specificity in terms of muscle block (Bernstein & Guth, 1961), or type (Miledi & Stefani, 1969, but see Brown & Butler, 1976), but they are precise in their choice of junctional membrane and the form of their terminal arbor (Letinsky *et al.*, 1976).

Despite their target preference, regenerating sensory fibres are capable of remarkable lability when their freedom of choice is restricted. Deflected cutaneous nerve, for example, will readily innervate foreign skin and even muscle, but without synapse formation (Zalewski, 1970). Similarly grafts of foreign skin receive innervation from local fibre plexes. Lability also extends to innervation to heterotypic receptor specializations. Schiff and Loewenstein (1972) found that cat hypogastric nerve can reinnervate mesenteric Pacinian corpuscles even though its normal target, the bladder, contains none. Other examples are innervation of Grandry corpuscles in duck bill skin transplanted to the leg (Dijkstra, 1933), the reinnervation of hair follicles transplanted to hairless skin on the soles of feet of mice and guinea pigs (Kadanoff, 1925) and the innervation of taste buds from the tongue by lumbar dorsal root ganglion cells in an anterior eye chamber co-culture system (Zalewski, 1973). It is still not clear whether axons necessarily take on the stimulus sensitivity of the heterotypical receptor, but this appears to be the case for Pacinian corpuscles (Schiff & Loewenstein, 1972) and taste buds (Oakley, 1967). Finally, there is evidence from cross-reinnervation experiments in muscle that in some cases axons modify functional properties of their target cells (Hnik *et al.*, 1967) and that in others the target can modify the axon (Lewis *et al.*, 1977).

Reactive (Collateral) Sprouting

It usually takes at least weeks or months before regenerating sprouts return to the denervated tissue. During this period there are important changes in intact fibres that normally share the distribution field of the injured ones, or that innervate adjacent zones. Specifically, extra sprouts may branch out from intact axon collaterals or from the juxtaterminal region and extend into the area of denervation. Once again, examples will be drawn mostly from the somatosensory system.

In a series of classic papers on skin and cornea in rabbits, Weddell and co-workers (e.g. Weddell *et al.*, 1941) reported seeing fine collateral sprouts extending from the intact fibres into the denervated zone. The return of touch sensitivity followed within about 1mm behind the advancing fibre front. Sensory return based on sprouting of neighbouring nerves also occurs in man (Livingston, 1947).

More recent experiments have focused on the regulation of the process. Diamond and co-workers (Diamond *et al.*, 1976) found that after cutting the middle of three nerves to the hindlimb in salamanders the remaining two expanded into the denervated skin, but only until they reached a new common boundary. Within the reinnervated zone the normal complement of receptor spots was formed, but no more. These results suggest a competitive interaction between the invading nerves. Sprouting also occurred after blocking axoplasmic flow in the middle nerve with colchicine. However, because colchicine does not destroy the nerve's own terminals, its territory became hyperinnervated (Cooper *et al.*, 1977). Not all fibre types within a nerve need react in the same way. In the rat, transection of the sciatic nerve makes the foot anaesthetic except for a narrow dorsomedial strip served by the saphenous nerve. Over the next few weeks, the saphenous nerve distribution expands and sensation returns to much, but not all, of the denervated zone (Devor *et al.*, 1979). Electrophysiological recordings showed that the only myelinated fibres that sprouted were high threshold mechano-receptors.

In the discussion of collateral sprouting in the developing CNS (above), we saw evidence that neurons tend to make a limited total arbor and that excess sprouting in one location may require reduction elsewhere (Devor & Schneider, 1975). Some PNS neurons appear to be similarly limited. In the superior cervical sympathetic ganglion, for example, preganglionic fibres normally make an average of 1100 ganglionic synapses each (Ostberg *et al.*, 1976). In rats in which the nerve was cut and resutured a variable fraction (mean 30%) of its fibres successfully regenerated. These failed to restore the normal synaptic complement of the ganglion.

On the other hand, qualitative descriptions suggest that at least some types of peripheral neurons can expand their total axonal distribution considerably. This may be achieved by increasing the metabolic output of the parent neuron pool. For example, when the tail is amputated in lizards several caudal dorsal root ganglia come off as well. Those that survive must reinnervate the new tail when it regenerates, in addition to their normal territory. This expansion in cutaneous territory innervated is accompanied by cell hypertrophy. In addition, there are ultrastructural changes that resemble those caused by axotomy (Pannese, 1963). In mammals, too, intact cells undergoing reactive sprouting in their terminal arbor show parikaryal changes similar to axotomized neurons preparing for regenerative growth (Lieberman, 1971; 1974).

Ectopic Impulses and Denervation Supersensitivity

Injured nerves, in addition to failing to conduct information faithfully, may actually introduce spurious impulses into the CNS (Wall & Devor, 1978). Immediately upon transection, axons produce an intense 'injury discharge' lasting seconds to minutes and then they fall silent. Over the next few days, however, an impulse volley originating in the region of the nerve end begins to appear (Wall & Gutnick, 1974; Govrin-Lippmann & Devor, 1978). In rats whose sciatic nerve was ligated or encapsulated so as to prevent regeneration, up to 29% of all fibres in the nerve fired spontaneously by the second week after the injury. The incidence fell back to about 4% by the end of the third week and then levelled off. Abnormal activity occurred mostly in sensory axons and took the form of repetitive bursts, or a steady discharge usually ranging from 1 to 50 impulses per second.

In addition to nerve end neuromas, ectopic impulse generation is known to occur in patches of demyelination in peripheral nerve and spinal roots and in regenerating sprouts (Calvin *et al.*, 1977; Rasminsky, 1978; Devor, unpublished data). These sites are also mechanosensitive. The essential pathophysiological change in these situations is likely to be the loss of membrane accommodation. In normal nerve, sustained depolarization as by mechanical distortion produces only a brief discharge. Here, sustained depolarization produces a sustained discharge. Such a repetitive firing capability is normally restricted to special sites such as sensory receptor endings and the axon hillock region of neurons. Nerve end neuromas are also abnormally sensitive to chemical stimulation, particularly by catecholamines (Wall & Gutnik, 1974). This raises the possibility that response to blood-borne adrenaline or direct sympathetic innervation contributes to ongoing discharge. Similarly, abnormal chemosensitivity may account for the pain relief afforded by sympathectomy and sympathetic blockade in causalgia and related conditions in man (Wall, 1979).

An additional abnormality, recently found in neuromas, regenerating nerve, and partially demyelinated nerve is the breakdown in the normal isolation between adjacent axons. Impulse activity on one fibre may, by electrical (ephaptic) interaction, cause activity in its neighbours (Rasminsky, 1978; Seltzer & Devor, 1979). Such crosstalk can take two forms, either one-for-one duplication of impulses, or 'afterdischarge' where a volley of impulses entering the altered zone stirs up asynchronous activity in adjacent fibres. The mechanism underlying the first form of crosstalk is probably close apposition of adjacent axonal membrane in sprouts or patches of myelin loss. The second is less well understood, but may result from changes in the extracellular ionic environment during the initial impulse volley. Renewed isolation between axons as by remyelinization in regenerating nerve stops crosstalk. For many years there has been speculation in the clinical literature that ephaptic interaction in damaged nerve is the underlying cause of pain in causalgia (Doupe *et al.*, 1944; Nathan, 1947).

A final important category of plastic change secondary to axonal damage is the increase in chemosensitivity of postsynaptic elements. The best studied example of denervation supersensitivity is in striated muscle fibres, but it clearly occurs in autonomic ganglia, viscera, blood vessels, etc., as well (reviewed by Purves, 1976). It is less well established whether denervation supersensitivity occurs in the CNS (see below). In normal skeletal muscle fibres, receptors for acetylcholine are concentrated in the narrow gutters of postjunctional membrane. Upon denervation, acetylcholine sensitivity spreads over the whole membrane surface probably by a combination of lateral spread from the junctional area and implantation of new receptor molecules from a continuously renewed intrafibre pool. The process is reversed with reinnervation. The mechanism underlying denervation supersensitivity is not completely understood, but seems to have something to do both with muscle contraction and trophic factors. Both blockage of transmitter release from the nerve terminal with botulinum toxin (Thesleff, 1960) and receptor blockade with α-bungarotoxin (Berg & Hall, 1975) are followed by the creation of extra-junctional receptors if more slowly and less completely than by denervation. Impulse conduction block in the afferent nerve is also effective and direct electrical stimulation of the muscle fibre partially prevents or reverses supersensitivity caused by conduction block and by denervation (Lomo & Rosenthal, 1972). Evidence for the involvement of a trophic substance includes the importance of the length of distal nerve stump to the time of onset of denervation changes (Luco & Eyzaguirre, 1955) and the effectiveness of axoplasmic transport blockers in normally conducting nerve (Hoffman & Thesleff, 1972; Albuquerque *et al.*, 1972; but see Cangiano & Fried, 1977).

PLASTICITY IN THE ADULT CNS—SPROUTING

In the brain of some lower vertebrates, even in their adult forms, severed fibre trunks such as optic and spinal tracts may regenerate much as in the PNS (Jacobson, 1978). For evolutionary reasons that are entirely unclear the mammalian CNS has lost much of this lability. A great deal of anatomical evidence from the last century, culminating in Cajal's (1928) monumental work, showed that central fibres may begin to sprout in mammals, but that growth is soon arrested and damaged tracts are not renewed. The only well-established exceptions are the hypothalamo-hypophyseal fibres (Adams *et al.*, 1969) and, in a limited sense, several fine fibre systems (see below, also see Marks, 1972). This fact placed a damper on research interest in neuromorphological plasticity in adult CNS. Interest has only recently been revived by new evidence that, despite the lack of long tract regeneration, substantial reorganization may none the less occur at short range within the neuropil.

Sprouting in the Spinal Cord and Somatosensory Pathways

Liu & Chambers (1958) reported rearrangement of spinal cord connections in cats using degeneration techniques. For example, about 9 months after cutting all dorsal roots, caudal to T_9 except for L_7, intact L_7 fibres appeared to increase their terminal density within their normal territory and in addition extended branches up to five segments (about 5 cm) rostrally beyond their then known limits. Correspondingly dramatic changes, also suggestive of short- and long-range collateral sprouting, followed hemisection of the cord. Several factors, however, demand that these observations, particularly of long-range sprouting, be interpreted with caution.

First, despite the authors' care, residual degeneration debris from the original lesion may still have confounded the estimate of distribution of the intact test root. Second, replication of these experiments using methods more sensitive than those available to Liu & Chambers (1958) has resulted in much more conservative claims of anomalous intersegmental spread. Local increase in terminal density, however, has been confirmed (Illis, 1973; Goldberger & Murray, 1974; Murray & Goldberger, 1974; Prendergast & Stelzner, 1976; Bernstein *et al.*, 1978). Even local sprouting is minimal or absent in the spinal trigeminal nucleus and the dorsal column nuclei (Westrum & Black, 1971; Kerr, 1872; Rustioni & Molenaar, 1975; Beckerman & Kerr, 1976). Finally, and most important, recent histological and electrophysiological studies have extended the known limits of dorsal root distribution in normal cats (see Wall & Werman, 1976). This raises the possibility that the partial deafferentation simply caused fringe fibres, always present, to become visible.

The problems involved in interpreting light microscopic evidence of sprouting are highlighted by recent electrophysiological studies of second-order sensory neurons in the dorsal horn following dorsal rhizotomy (Basbaum & Wall, 1976; Mendell *et al.*, 1978). In acute experiments, as expected, the deafferented cells failed to respond to cutaneous stimulation. Within 30 days, however, many cells became responsive once again, but now to skin served by distant intact dorsal roots. Response latencies of some cells suggest monosynaptic input. These changes might be caused by the sort of long-distance sprouting claimed by Liu and Chambers (1958). The authors, however, preferred an alternative explanation. It is known that many dorsal horn cells in normal cats can be driven by synchronous (electrical) stimulation of distant dorsal roots even though they cannot be driven by natural stimulation of the skin in the corresponding dermatome (Merrill & Wall, 1972; Devor *et al.*, 1977). A distant input channel therefore exists in intact cats, but it is normally ineffective and requires massive stimulation to influence postsynaptic cells. Is it possible that (partial) deafferentation simply unmasks or strengthens this pre-existing channel?

Corresponding studies of the somatosensory map at the level of the dorsal column nuclei (Millar *et al.*, 1976) and the ventrobasal complex of the thalamus (Wall & Egger, 1971) echo the ambiguity between sprouting and unmasking. In fact, morphological studies of these nuclei have tended to discount sprouting as the relevant mechanism (Rustioni & Molenaar, 1975; Tripp & Wells, 1978). For a small proportion of cells in the dorsal column nuclei (nucleus gracilis) sprouting can be ruled out conclusively. These are cells that normally respond to localized stimulation on the hindlimb, but that become responsive to the forelimb *immediately* as hindlimb input is (cold) blocked (Dostrovsky *et al.*, 1976; also see Fadiga *et al.*, 1978). The concept of unmasking will be discussed further below.

Because of its clinical importance, a good deal of research has been devoted to plastic changes related to spinal cord transection (reviewed by Windle, 1956; Pettegrew & Windle, 1976; Berry, 1978). In general, the results have been disappointing for those seeking a cure for paraplegia, but they have produced worthwhile data on fundamental aspects of sprouting. Like Cajal (1928), most authors have seen the beginnings of sprout outgrowth at the cut ends of spinal tracts. Growth is soon aborted, however, and at best only a handful of fibres eventually crosses the gap. Several explanations for this growth failure have been proposed. The most widely held hypothesis is that gliosis, fibrosis and cavitation create an impenetrable scar at the wound margin. None of the various drug treatments and surgical protocols designed to reduce scar formation, however, has yet proved useful at substantially increasing the number of axons that successfully cross the cut. Attempts to increase regeneration with anti-inflammatory drugs (e.g. corticosteroids), metabolic stimulants (e.g. thyroxin and growth hormone), application of mucolytic and proteolytic enzymes, immunosuppression, and nerve growth factor have also proved inconsistent so far.

Bernstein and Bernstein (1967; 1973) have offered an intriguing new explanation for the failure of long tract regeneration. Looking in the first few millimetres of neuropil rostral to transected spinal cord, they found rapid replacement of degenerating synapses. Most of the new synapses arose from local neuron populations, but a significant minority were from dorsal roots and long descending tracts (see also Pullen & Sears, 1978). This means that sprouts, although arrested at the spinal scar, proliferated within the proximal grey matter and formed numerous synaptic complexes. Bernstein and Bernstein (1967; 1973) proposed that this synaptogenesis discourages further growth on the presumption, discussed above, that axons are programmed to make only a fixed amount of total arbor (or number of synapses).

Sprouting in Cortex and Cortical Projections

Rose and his co-workers (Rose *et al.*, 1960) used a focused nuclear particle beam to make lesions restricted to discrete layers of (rabbit) neocortex. Silver-stained sections taken at intervals after the irradiation showed distinct axonal invasion of the damaged layer and, perhaps more surprisingly, the extension of dendritic processes from neighbouring intact cell layers. Dendritic sprouting has been seen by others (Bernstein & Bernstein, 1973) but has received little attention in comparison to axonal sprouting. Where it occurs, axonal and dendritic re-arrangement on the borders of cortical defects may be related to functional restitution after focal injury. Glees and Cole (1950) reported rapid recovery of limb movements after localized damage in the sensorimotor cortex in monkeys. Excision of cortex immediately surrounding the original lesion recalled the deficit suggesting a role for this tissue in the initial recovery.

The most labile cortical system described to date is the hippocampal formation (Cotman & Lynch, 1976). Like the olfactory cortex, the dentate gyrus receives a number of different classes of afferent input, each arranged along the length of the pyramidal cell dendrites, in a largely non-overlapping laminar arrangement. This stratification allows one to investigate changes in the various inputs when any particular one is eliminated. The most closely studied example is elimination of the ipsilateral entorhinal input (perforant pathway). In this case, terminals of most of the remaining afferent systems sprout and replace about 80% of the synaptic population of the deafferented dendate lamina. Some of the inputs (e.g. contralateral hippocampal fibres) sprout profusely in the neonate and poorly in the adult; others (e.g. contralateral entorhinal fibres) sprout equally well in neonate and adult.

An interesting system initially discovered with electrophysiological rather than histological tools is the dual input to neurons of the red nucleus (Tsukahara *et al.*, 1974). Sensorimotor cortex afferents end on dendrites; cerebellar (nucleus interpositus) afferents end on the cell body. The position of these inputs makes for characteristic patterns of intracellularly recorded synaptic potentials. Distal inputs produce a slowly rising waveform; proximal inputs a rapidly rising waveform. By 10 days after cerebellar excision, the distally terminating cerebral inputs begin to produce rapidly rising synaptic potentials suggesting a proximal shift in their location on the dendrite. Morphological evidence supports this interpretation (Nakamura *et al.*, 1974).

Another well-documented instance of synaptic rearrangement in the adult mammalian CNS is the case of the rat medial septal nucleus (Raisman, 1969; Moore *et al.*, 1971; Raisman & Field, 1973). Here, axon terminals of hypothal-amic, and other, fibres arriving along the medial forebrain bundle sprout to replace synaptic endings eliminated by transection of the fornix. Additional light and electron microscopic evidence for local sprouting within partially denervated neuropil has been obtained in the visual thalamus (Goodman & Horel, 1966; Goodman *et al.*, 1973; Ralston & Chow, 1973) and superior colliculus (Lund

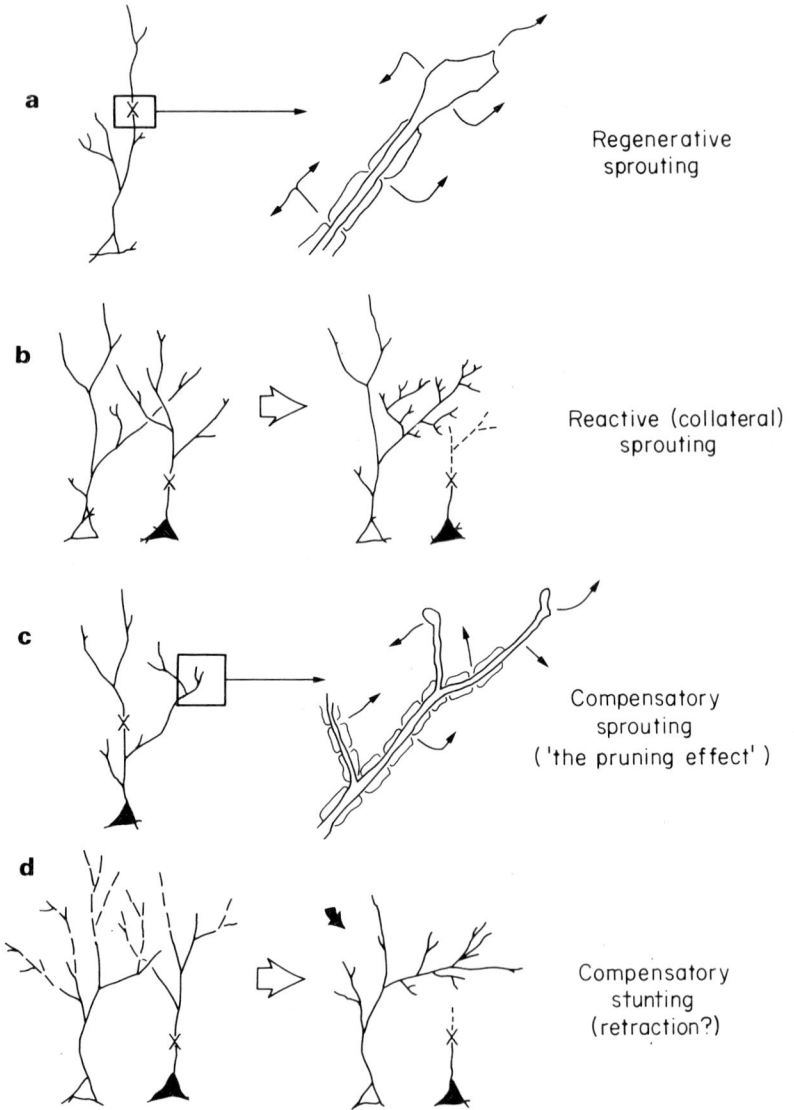

Fig. 3.2 Different circumstances under which there can be new growth in the developing or adult nervous system after injury. The branched figures represent the axonal arbors of CNS or PNS neurons.

a. 'Regenerative sprouting' refers to new growth from near the cut end (X) of a severed axon.

b. 'Reactive sprouting', often called 'collateral sprouting', refers to new growth from an intact neuron whose axonal tree overlaps or abuts on that of the injured neuron. Sprouting of this sort may also occur in a neuron when axoplasmic flow in its neighbours is blocked (Diamond *et al.*, 1976).

& Lund, 1971), the spinal trigeminal nucleus (Westrum & Black, 1971) and the ventral cochlear nucleus (Gentschev & Sotelo, 1973) among others.

Sprouting in the Fine Fibre Pathways

Because of the small diameter of unmyelinated axons, near the resolution limits of the optical microscope, the classical anatomists knew relatively little about unmyelinated fibre pathways in the brain. These have recently become accessible with the development of fluorescent and histochemical staining procedures capable of making pathways with distinctive biochemical content stand out from the background feltwork of fibre tracts and neuropil. Four such systems have been studied closely and the discovery of others can safely be anticipated. The four are: acetyl cholinesterase- (and therefore probably acetylcholine-) containing fibres on the banks of the third ventricle, noradrenalin-containing fibres originating in the locus coeruleus, serotonin-containing fibres of the brainstem raphe, and dopamine-containing fibres of the substantia nigra and scattered brain sites (Dahlstrom & Fuxe, 1964; Shute & Lewis, 1967; Ungerstedt, 1971).

The fine fibre pathways are remarkably labile in the face of injury. The widely branched adrenergic system is a prime example. When central adrenergic fibres are severed in the hypothalamus, spinal cord and elsewhere, there is a rapid swelling of the axon stump and an accumulation within the end-bulb of fluorescent material (e.g. Stenevi *et al.*, 1973). Over the next week or two the swollen structures fade and large numbers of fine, intensely fluorescent varicose processes, outgrowing sprouts, begin to appear proximal to the lesion. Many of these skirt the edges of the scar and some have been followed for substantial distances along the local blood vessels and myelinated fibre tracts. Because the sprouts appear to emerge from near the severed axon stump they are usually called regenerative sprouts (Fig. 3.2). Furthermore, in favourable circumstances, they can return to their original sites of termination (Björklund *et al.*, 1973).

The most dramatic examples of fine fibre sprouting come from experiments in

    c. 'Compensatory sprouting' may occur in one branch of an axonal tree when a distant branch is injured.

    d. 'Compensatory stunting' refers to the failure of a developing axon to make connections it would normally make (dashed line), as a result of excessive axonal growth in another location. Although it has not yet been described, reactive sprouting in one part of a mature axonal tree might be expected to result in compensatory retraction in other parts.

    Newly growing processes may emerge from several locations, for example, a motor or sensory axon terminal (ultraterminal sprouting), or an axon end-club in the case of regeneration. Alternatively, the sprout may emerge from a nearby node of Ranvier, or from a terminal or node of a distant axon collateral. Note that these four terms do not necessarily imply four different mechanisms. Regenerative sprouting, for example, might be a form of reactive sprouting in response to local degeneration, or it might be a form of compensatory sprouting initiated at a site very near to the point of injury.

which bits of peripheral tissue are implanted alongside central aminergic and/or cholinergic pathways. An elegant example is an experiment by Svendgaard *et al.* (1976) involving implantation of a fragment of dissected iris into the caudal diencephalon in adult rats. The iris normally receives peripheral adrenergic and cholinergic innervation. Within two to four weeks of implantation, central fibres of both types invaded the implant, in many cases tracking along pre-existing neural sheaths, and made terminal plexes characteristic of the normal sympathetic and parasympathetic iris innervation respectively. Destruction of the locus coeruleus on the side of the implant elimated the anomalous adrenergic input, but did not affect the cholinergic fibres. Activity in regenerated fibres can cause contractions in smooth muscle implants (Björklund *et al.*, 1975).

In addition to regenerative growth after damage, there is good evidence for reactive collateral sprouting in intact fine fibre pathways. Degeneration of aminergic or even non-aminergic terminals can result in proliferation of remaining adjacent aminergic terminals (Moore *et al.*, 1971; Stenevi *et al.*, 1973). Finally, denervation is not a precondition for collateral sprouting. Rather, as in the developing CNS (see above), it is sufficient for damage to part of the axonal arbor of aminergic neurons to occur for remaining branches to proliferate, even at a great distance. For example, Pickel *et al.* (1974) partially severed the superior cerebellar peduncle in adult rats, thus cutting the cerebellar branch of locus coeruleus neurons that innervate both cerebellar and cerebral cortex. One of the results was increased adrenergic input in the hippocampus as determined by histofluorescence and autoradiography. The phenomenon of compensatory sprouting (Fig. 3.2) is of particular importance for the fine fibre systems because of their wide-ranging branch pattern. By virtue of this effect, a lesion in one area could cause important and otherwise unpredictable rearrangement in far distant areas.

THE REGULATION OF SPROUTING

Each of the 10^{11} neurons in the adult nervous system is unique in form and connectivity. In development, however, there are probably only a small number of fundamental rules of cell interaction determined by the genome. Diversity is the outcome of the genetic programme of individual cells being played out in a complex and continuously varying milieu. The investigation of changes in neural connections caused by discrete insults at various stages of development has provided many clues as to the general properties of these fundamental rules, although we are still far from understanding them on a molecular level. Several of these developmental rules also seem to apply to neuroanatomical changes that occur after injury in the adult nervous system (Schneider, 1976; Barondes, 1976). In this section we shall make a brief inventory of some of the proposed principles of neural development and plasticity, and discuss some factors that constrain them.

Some Principles of Neural Development and Plasticity

The following list is elaborated from one published previously (Devor & Schneider, 1975). It should be kept in mind that each of these 'principles' is a vector; none is absolute law. Several may act simultaneously, or in temporal sequence, and when they constitute opposing 'forces', the final outcome depends upon the resolution of forces.

1.   Outgrowing axons are partially directed by pre-existing chemical 'fields' or gradients whose nature remains unknown. These gradients may comprise diffusible substances in the intercellular spaces to which growing axonal tips are sensitive, but it is more likely that differential affinities between cell and substrate elements are involved (Cajal, 1928; Weiss, 1969).

2.   Axons and cells may recognize their proper target by means of specific 'cytochemical position markers' made up of specific tissue-target recognition molecules (Sperry, 1963; Hunt & Jacobson, 1972; Moscona, 1976).

3.   Neurons and their processes tend to move in 'mechanical' adherence to pre-existing axonal or glial processes, but can be deflected by abnormal tissue configurations. Deflected axons can sometimes form connections at anomalous locations (Cajal, 1928; Sidman & Rakic, 1973; Schneider & Jhaveri, 1974; Letourneau, 1975).

4.   Individual axons in an outgrowing population may interact with one another, each constraining the growth of its neighour, by mutually attractive and/or repulsive 'forces'. This may result in the axons distributing in a fixed relation to one another within their terminal area (Dunn, 1971; Udin, 1977).

5.   The establishment of axonal terminations may in some cases be subject to temporal factors such as that the earliest arriving axons form connections to the exclusion of later arriving ones (Gottlieb & Cowan, 1972).

6.   Axonal systems compete for the exclusive occupation of available terminal space, that left vacant by the degeneration of neighbouring axons and that arising naturally from the expansion of the neuropil during growth. Chemical factors associated with degeneration may affect sprout outgrowth (for references, see end of chapter).

7.   Members of at least certain axonal populations tend to conserve the total amount of their axonal arborization (or synaptic complement). If growth in one part of the tree is limited or stopped, branches in another part will sprout extra collaterals. If exaggerated growth occurs in one part of the axonal tree, growth in another part may be stunted in compensation (Devor & Schneider, 1975).

8.   In some systems neurons and neuronal processes are produced in excess. Those that fail to form functional connections are eliminated (see this chapter).

9.   Neural elements may be mutually dependent such that, in the absence of one, the second may fail to differentiate, or if it already exists, may change or

atrophy. The dependence may involve physical contact, chemical signals, impulse activity etc. (Rosenthal, 1977).

10.   Neurons and their processes may be altered by the milieu through which they pass on their way to their final target (Douarin & Teillet, 1974; Patterson *et al.*, 1975).

Signals That Elicit Sprouting

It is not known what induces axons to sprout in the event of injury. One of the longest-standing hypotheses (Forssman, 1900; Cajal, 1928; Edds, 1953) is that debris or metabolites from degenerating axon and/or myelin stimulates growth either by direct action on the nerve ends or after retrograde transport back to the cell body. Variants of the hypothesis relate the stimulating substance to the denervated postsynaptic cells, Schwann cells, proliferating glia, etc. The proposal is attractive, of course, because of the tendency for sprouts to invade deserted terminal space. Furthermore, it has some experimental backing. For example, Hoffman (1950) injected extracts of degenerating nerve into intact muscle and saw ultraterminal sprouting. The putative trophic factor in the extract was given the name 'neurocletin'. Growth was not incisive, however, and sprouts failed to form neuromuscular junctions. In retrospect, the observed sprouting may well have been secondary to an immune neuritic reaction. More recently, Olson and Malmfors (1970) used an anterior eye chamber culture system to compare the sprouting of sympathetic axons into freshly denervated explants with growth into explants denervated some time earlier. There was less sprouting into the chronically denervated explants, suggesting that once degenerating debris had been removed, the signal for sprouting was gone. Unfortunately, many other trophic changes occur during the course of denervation, and any one of these might affect the competence of grafts to accept entering sprouts.

Whether or not products associated with denervation can promote growth, it is clear that such substances are neither necessary nor sufficient to account for sprouting in all situations. We have seen that in both developing and adult CNS, injury in one part of an axonal tree can induce sprouting in another part, even in the absence of degeneration in the region of the sprouts (compensatory sprouting). Similarly, axonal transport block in cutaneous nerves can induce neighbours to sprout, again, in the absence of degeneration (Diamond *et al.*, 1976). On the other hand, there can be massive degeneration and no detectable sprouting (e.g. Kerr, 1972; Guillery, 1972; Rustioni & Molenaar, 1975; Stelzner & Keating, 1977).

There is a second class of hypotheses that is, in essence, the converse of the degeneration hypothesis. By this, axon terminals in their resting state have a continuous tendency to sprout (under intrinsic or extrinsic stimulation), but growth is limited by an inhibitory trophic substance in the local tissue. The removal of this substance releases sprouting (Cajal, 1928; Weddell & Zander, 1951). The most likely source of inhibiting substance is adjacent axon terminals, inhibition among axonal systems being mutual (Diamond *et al.*, 1976). In different versions of the hypothesis, the growth-inhibiting substance is released in soluble form into the interstitial space, or is retained on the surface membrane. Similarly, the interaction between outgrowth and inhibition may be dynamic with axon terminals in a continuous state of remodelling (Sotelo & Palay, 1971), or it may be static with connections changing only in the event of injury.

The inhibition hypothesis, in its various forms, has a number of properties useful in explaining diverse neuroplastic phenomena. For example, it accounts for competition between adjacent axon populations and for the establishment of boundaries during development and regeneration. Mutual inhibition within an axon population can account for the even distribution of axonal endings within a terminal field. Adding appropriate specificities to the hypothesis, different axonal systems can share a single terminal field. The likelihood that the trophic substance is transported from the cell body to the axon terminal would explain why reactive collateral sprouting can be induced by blocking axoplasmic transport in cutaneous nerves (Diamond *et al.*, 1976).

Another difficult problem that can be handled with the help of the inhibition hypothesis is understanding the fate of collateral sprouts upon regeneration of the original nerve. Weddell & Zander (1951), for example, elicited collateral invasion in the cornea of rabbits by severing part of its natural innervation. When the cut fibres finally regenerated, the former invaders disappeared, presumably by a process of retraction. They did not leave degenerating debris. In the rat foot preparation discussed above (Devor *et al.*, 1979) regeneration of the crushed sciatic nerve caused the expanded field of the neighbouring saphenous nerve to shrink back to its original proportions. Similar reversal of sprouting has been described by some authors in muscle and autonomic ganglia while others claim that the alien sprouts persist but are functionally repressed (see below). Under the inhibition hypothesis, the priority of the original nerve would be a natural consequence of its having a greater local supply of inhibiting factor than neighbouring nerves, already over-extended in terms of territory held.

Why is the Brain More Labile in the Newborn than in the Adult?

Most hypotheses that attempt to account for critical periods of plasticity (see also Schneider, 1976; Cotman & Lynch, 1976; So & Schneider, 1978; Pettigrew, 1978) fall into one of two categories: those involving changes intrinsic to the neuron under consideration and those involving factors extrinsic to it. In the first category is the simple fact that in the developing brain the neuron is already growing. There is no need to remobilize the metabolic machinery of growth. A closely related factor is the intrinsic limitation on total axonal arbor (Devor & Schneider, 1975). In the developing neuron, extra growth in one area may be compensated for by a failure or stunting of growth in another (Devor, 1976b). In the mature neuron, already near or at its pre-programmed maximal size, anything more than a minor extension in one region might require retraction of an already well-established branch network elsewhere.

Along somewhat different lines, developmental changes in cell surface molecules may disrupt axonal guidance, cause a loss in the ability of an outgrowing fibre to recognize or induce postsynaptic specializations, or affect the ability of target cells to accept new synapses (Schachner & Hammerling, 1974; Merrell *et al.*, 1976). Likewise, the stabilization of maturing pre-terminal arbors and synaptic contacts may mitigate against renewed growth from these structures (Changeux & Danchin, 1976). Stabilizing factors may include a gradual change in membrane fluidity, an increase in structural adhesiveness to the target cell or to surrounding cells, myelinization and collateral neurite differentiation, etc.

Included in the second category, factors extrinsic to the neuron in question, is the stabilization and entrenchment of neighbouring and competing axonal systems. Similarly, the increasing density of the maturing neuropil (Bondareff & Narotzky, 1972) is likely to impede penetration by newly growing axonal processes. Local tissue reaction and scar formation, which is far more abundant in the adult, may form an additional impediment. The importance of this factor, however, is often over-rated. In neonates, there is little evidence that severed fibres, in contrast to newly ingrowing ones, can cross the cut despite minimal gliosis. Treatments that reduce scarring have not been found to greatly augment regeneration in the adult CNS, and sprouting can proceed vigorously in the PNS despite scarring (see above, also Berry, 1978).

Another difference in the response of neonatal and adult nervous tissue to injury is the rate at which degeneration products are removed. Debris cleared within hours or days in the newborn may persist for months in the adult. In fact, Leonard (1974; 1975) has claimed that the appearance of long-lasting axonal debris after injury in the rodent visual and olfactory systems coincides with the end of the critical period for axonal rearrangement. Finally, the demonstration that catecholamine pathways play a key role in the maintenance of plasticity in the visual cortex (Kasamatsu & Pettigrew, 1976; Pettigrew & Kasamatsu, 1978) raises the possibility that the where and when of CNS lability is itself under CNS control.

Why is the PNS More Labile than the CNS?

Over the years that this question has been considered, each significant morphological and physiological difference between PNS and CNS has given rise to an hypothesis (see also Raisman, 1977; Kiernan, 1978). Unfortunately, none can account for all instances of sprouting or the lack of it, nor can any be definitely ruled out as a contributing factor. A few examples will suffice. Cajal (1928) and others have proposed that the Schwann cell, found only in the periphery, is crucial to sprout growth. Indeed, regenerating nerve fibres follow Schwann cell guides closely and grow poorly in their absence. Similarly, dorsal and ventral root fibres induced to regenerate towards the spinal cord are mostly arrested at the Schwann cell-oligodendroglial transition (Kimmel & Moyer, 1947). On the other hand, peripheral nerve tissue, including Schwann cells, does not promote growth when implanted into brain (see Clark, 1942, however, this point ought to be reinvestigated with more modern techniques), and, as we have seen, some central fibres do sprout successfully in neonatal and adult CNS in the absence of Schwann cells.

Bernstein and Bernstein (1967; 1973) proposed that premature synapse formation prevents long-distance regeneration (see above). This, of course, does not account for the failure of peripheral fibres to enter the CNS, or the lack of regeneration in pure fibre tracts such as the optic nerve and corpus callosum.

Finally, differences between the blood–brain and blood–nerve barrier have been exploited in a new hypothesis by Kiernan (1978). He holds that sprouting is fostered by a trophic substance in the general circulation. Damaged CNS fibres have access to this for only two to three weeks until the blood–brain barrier is sealed (Persson *et al.*, 1976), whereas peripheral fibres are exposed for several months until the blood–nerve barrier is repaired (Motte & Allt, 1976). Unfortunately, among other things, this hypothesis does not account for collateral sprouting which often occurs in areas where the circulatory system is intact, or for the fact that in PNS, regenerating fibres can cover quite large distances in two to three weeks.

PLASTICITY IN THE ADULT CNS— CHANGES OTHER THAN SPROUTING

Increased Synaptic Effectiveness

The excitability of neural channels surviving CNS injury can be altered by several mechanisms other than expansion of existing synapses or sprouting of new ones. One promising, if still speculative, example is the uncovering of pre-existing ineffective or 'silent' synapses. The concept of silent synapses originated with studies by Mark and collaborators (e.g. Mark *et al.*, 1972) on the reinnervation of extraocular muscles in goldfish and salamanders. They claimed that regenerating abducens fibres suppressed sprouts of collateral invaders without actually removing them. The neuromuscular junctions of the sprouts remained morphologically sound, but were functionally 'silent', presumably because of reduced transmitter release (Harris & Ziskind, 1977). This story has been challenged recently by several groups who have data indicating that reinvasion is followed either by dual functional innervation or by the removal of alien inputs (e.g. Scott, 1977; Dennis & Yip, 1978).

The concept of silent synapses, however, has found application in the mammalian CNS. Based on evidence that many dorsal horn and dorsal column nucleus cells respond to electrical stimulation of dorsal roots and skin far outside the cells' cutaneous receptive field, Wall and collaborators (reviewed by Wall, 1977) have suggested that a substantial proportion of contacts in the adult CNS may be relatively ineffective. The strengthening or uncovering of these contacts following destruction of the cells' main input conveniently accounts for the emergence of a new receptive field in distant dermatomes (see above). It is unclear why the brain should be constructed with 'silent' synapses. Perhaps they play an important role not yet discovered, e.g. in special behavioural states? Or perhaps, as Merrill and Wall (1972) have suggested, they are 'ghosts' left over from an early stage of development. There are a number of mechanisms that could render synaptic efficacy low, but that could be reversed without recourse to sprouting. The input may be under tonic pre- or post-synaptic inhibition, or it may sit over an insensitive junctional membrane. It may be located far out on a dendrite, or be otherwise electrically distant from the spike initiation zone. Finally, it may simply release minimal transmitter per impulse.

A mechanism often enlisted to account for the strengthening of synapses surviving partial deafferentation is increased sensitivity of the postsynaptic membrane. In muscle and ganglion cells, chemosensitivity spreads over the cell surface as has been discussed above. It has been presumed that something similar takes place in the CNS on the grounds that deafferented neurons in many locations have elevated ongoing activity (Teasdale & Stravraky, 1953; Loeser & Ward, 1967; Kjerulf & Loeser, 1973; Black 1974), and that deafferented nuclei show elevated sensitivity to systemically or intraventricularly applied drugs (Sharpless, 1964; 1975). Unfortunately, the hypothesis of denervation supersensitivity has not, thus far, been supported by more direct tests. Specifically, partially deafferented neurons in neocortex, hippocampus, caudate nucleus and spinal trigeminal nucleus have failed, for the most part, to show elevated responsiveness to presumptive transmitters applied iontophoretically (reviewed by Macon, 1978).

More subtle mechanisms are suggested by recent experiments in which dorsal horn neurons in the lumbar enlargement in cats are deafferented by cutting the (sciatic and saphenous) nerves serving their natural receptive field (Devor & Wall, 1978). As after dorsal rhizotomy, the cells become responsive to distant cutaneous inputs (Fig. 3.3). The synapses of the originally effective input, however, do not, for the most part, degenerate and terminal space is not freed. This conclusion is based on evidence that, after axotomy of sciatic nerve afferents distal to the dorsal root ganglion, there is retrograde cell reaction, but very little ganglion cell death (Carlson *et al.*, 1978), virtually no degeneration is seen in the dorsal horn in light (Carmel & Stein, 1969; Devor & Wall, 1978 and unpublished data) or electron microscopic preparations (Knyihar & Csillik, 1976; but see Goode, 1977) and the first central synapse continues to conduct (Devor & Wall, 1978 and unpublished data). In this respect, hindlimb nerves are unlike forelimb nerves, intercostal nerves, trigeminal nerves and vestibular nerves in which a large proportion of the primary sensory neurons die following peripheral axotomy (reviewed by Arvidsson & Grant, 1978). The difference may depend on the

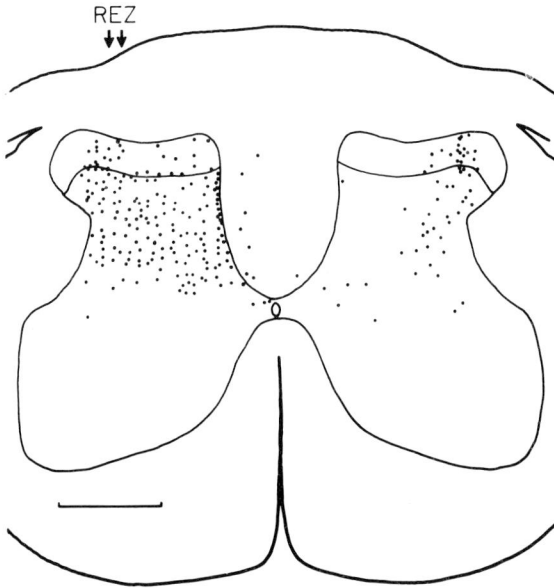

Fig. 3.3 Spinal cord secondary sensory neurons in adult mammals can acquire a 'new' receptive field (RF) after the nerve supplying the original RF is severed. Cells in the medial part of the L_{6-7} dorsal horn in cats normally receive their synaptic input from the toes and foot. Acutely after section of the major hindlimb nerves (sciatic and saphenous nerves) these cells have no RF (right). After one month, however, the cells once again respond to peripheral stimulation (left), but now in skin of the thigh or lower back.

Dots mark all satisfactorily isolated cells encountered in 164 penetrations in 12 acutely deafferented dorsal horns and 89 penetrations in 7 chronically deafferented dorsal horns (28–105 days survival). The arrows (upper left) mark the approximate location of the root entry zone (REZ) as seen from above. Its exact location varies somewhat between cats. Search penetrations began near the midline and continued to about the REZ but not much beyond it. The lack of cells in the far lateral edge of dorsal horn therefore does not indicate the absence of cells with proximal RFs there. (From Devor & Wall, 1978 reprinted with permission, *Nature, London.*)

larger distance from the point of injury in the hindlimb to the dorsal root ganglion (Lieberman, 1974).

If the synapses of the original input fibres are not removed, what signals plastic rearrangement, be it uncovering of distant silent afferents or sprouting of new ones? Four possibilities suggest themselves. First, there may be retrograde influence via axotomized sciatic nerve motoneurons, perhaps relayed by the stripping of afferent synapses off altered dendrites. Motoneurons themselves are not known to send axons or dendrites into the dorsal horn, nor do they have a substantial polysynaptic link in this direction (Gutnick *et al.*, 1975). Second, biochemical and subtle morphological changes in central synapses of axotomized sciatic nerve afferents may constitute a signal (Knyihar & Csillik, 1976).

Third, the signal may be the cessation of flow of some trophic substance originating in the skin (see also Rothshenker, 1978). Finally, the signal may be a reduction in afferent impulse traffic. In this case, however, it is not simply a cessation of synaptic usage, because it is known that the nerve end neuroma itself generates impulses that are conducted centrally (Wall & Gutnick, 1974; Govrin-Lippmann & Devor, 1978). The time integral of synaptic traffic or impulse patterning may be important.

There is substantial independent evidence that synaptic efficacy may be dependent upon use over a long period in addition to the well-known short- and long-lasting post-tetanic phenomena (Lloyd, 1949; Bliss & Lomo, 1973). The reduction of input traffic along muscle spindle afferents by transection of the muscle nerve decreases the monosynaptic reflex in corresponding motoneurons, and also in agonist motoneurons that have not themselves been axotomized (Eccles *et al.*, 1959). Unfortunately, in these experiments, the sensory neuron was axotomized and not simply silenced. This problem was avoided in a series of experiments in which proprioceptive afferents to the ventral horn and to Clark's column were silenced by tenotomy or bone fracture (reviewed by Spencer & April, 1970). Here, there was an *increase* in the efficacy of chronically underused synapses. This result has recently been confirmed for spinal motoneurons by blocking nerve conduction with tetrodotoxin (Gallego *et al.*, 1979). Returning to sensory neurons in the dorsal horn, one can only speculate on how an increase or a decrease in the strength of sciatic nerve input could increase the effectiveness of inputs from neighbouring nerves.

Closely related to the concept of uncovering 'silent' synapses is the possibility of post-lesion changes in the efficacy of normally functioning synaptic channels. An interesting example comes from experiments on the control of head–eye coordination during visual target acquisition. In primates, the counter-rotation of the eyes as the head turns towards the target is normally accomplished mostly by vestibular input, with only a small contribution from neck muscle afferents. Immediately following labyrinthectomy compensatory eye rotation is nearly lost. Within a few weeks, however, coordination is restored by means of an increase in the effectiveness of proprioceptive feedback (Dichgans *et al.*, 1973).

Although the foregoing example of gain compensation occurred in response to a lesion, it appears to have evolved as a normal physiological process. For example, in normal hand–eye coordination, when a visual target is presented 20° to the left, the arm will be extended at this same angle. If the subject is wearing prism goggles that displace the visual field by + 10°, the object will be seen at 30° and the corresponding arm extension of 30° will be + 10° off the real target. After a brief period of (active) experience wearing such goggles, however, the gain of the hand–eye system is adjusted. An object seen at 30° will now elicit arm extension of 20°, on target (Held, 1965). The effect of sensory signals may even be reversed in sign if reversing goggles are used (Melvill-Jones, 1977). It is at this level that mechanisms of neural plasticity following injury merge with mechanisms of normal learning.

Decreased Synaptic Efficacy

There are several instances in which nervous system lesions dramatically reduce excitability in related surviving structures. Excitability may recover spontaneously after a short interval, after a substantial interval, or not at all. The best-known case is 'spinal shock'. Sudden transection of the upper spinal cord in humans results in immediate areflexia below the level of the lesion which passes off over several weeks or months. In monkeys, spinal shock lifts in days, in the cat, hours. In rodents it is barely manifest at all (Fulton, 1949). Shock probably results from the removal of tonic descending excitation and the mechanism of its passing is obscure.

A related phenomenon was described by Sprague (1966) in cases of unilateral visual decortication in cats. Here there is permanent failure to attend to stimuli presented in the contralateral visual field ('cortical blindness'). If the superior colliculus on the side opposite to the cortical lesion is subsequently destroyed, or if the collicular commissure is split, however, visual attention instantly returns. There is good evidence that the effect results from an imbalance of excitation in the superior colliculi (see also Berman & Stirling, 1976). This colliculus ipsilateral to the lesion is normally inhibited by the contralateral colliculus and excited by the ipsilateral cortex. Removal of the ipsilateral cortex results in unbalanced inhibition and therefore visual neglect in the corresponding hemifield. Reduction of this crossed inhibition restores equilibrium, permitting collicular function to be expressed. The 'extinction' phenomenon in cortically injured humans (Denny-Brown *et al.*, 1953) may have a similar basis. In these patients there is a failure to 'see' one of two objects presented simultaneously in the two visual fields, even though when presented separately the objects are equally visible. A final example has recently been seen in nerve-injured rats (Devor *et al.*, 1979). Some rats have a completely anaesthetic foot 24 h after sciatic nerve transection even though the saphenous nerve innervating the medial edge of the foot is intact. By 48 h sensitivity returns to the medial foot.

OUTLOOK

The Functional Role of Anomalous Connections

There is evidence in many systems that synaptic junctions formed after injury in the PNS and CNS can release neurotransmitter and have postsynaptic effects. Likewise, both correct and anomalous connections can have behavioural consequences (Eidelberg & Stein, 1974; Schneider, 1976; Cotman, 1978). In many instances synaptic remodelling is correlated with full or partial restitution of function. In others, however, synaptic remodelling is detrimental.

In the PNS, satisfactory nerve regeneration is common, and in its absence, collateral growth can partially compensate for lost sensory, motor and automatic function (Sunderland, 1978). On the other hand, inappropriate regeneration such as the reconnection of salivatory parasympathetic fibres to lacrimal glands in Bell's palsy can cause disturbing symptoms such as 'crocodile tears'. In skin, collateral sprouts grow only from selective populations of afferent fibres (Devor *et al.*, 1979). Similarly, as discussed above, regrowing fibres sometimes innervate heterotypic receptor sites. Either of these phenomena could contribute to hyperaesthesia or hyperpathia. Ectopic impulse activity in injured nerves may likewise be a contributing factor in causalgia, phantom pain and anaesthesia dolorosa (see above, also Wall *et al.*, 1979).

In the CNS, too, anomalous connections can have favourable or unfavourable consequences. Goldberger and Murray (1974) found that after hindlimb deafferentation in cats, locomotor and postural use of the limbs was lost and, along with it, reflexes dependent upon descending pathways, such as the vestibular reflex and the (ear) scratch reflex. Both the local propriospinal and the supraspinal reflexes returned over the first post-operative month, some in exaggerated form. These functional changes correspond qualitatively and temporally to synaptic proliferation in local and descending pathways. Similarly, there was a correlation between the return of suppressed reflexes mediated by peripheral input following spinal cord hemisection and sprouting of ipsilateral dorsal roots (Murray & Goldberger, 1974). On the other hand, McCouch and co-workers (1958), also based on correlated anatomical, electrophysiological and functional changes, argued that abnormal sprouting and synapse formation in injured spinal cord results in spasticity. Along the same line, it has been proposed that catecholamine fibre sprouting around cortical insults can cause an epileptic focus (Bowen *et al.*, 1975) and that hyperactivity in deafferented CNS neurons can account for many central pains (e.g. Black, 1974).

Devor (1975) showed that after complete lateral olfactory tract transection in hamster pups up to three days of age, the critical period for reinnervation of prepyriform cortex distal to the cut (Fig. 3.1), there is partial restitution of olfactory function. Function is lost once again if the expanded part of the olfactory tract distribution is eliminated in adulthood. Tract lesions at later ages produce a severe and permanent deficit. In contrast, *partial* tract section has more serious effects when performed in neonates than in adults. This is probably because synaptic reorganization in the neonate ('compensatory stunting') results in a reduction in the total area of olfactory complex receiving input (Fig. 3.1).

The dramatic lability of the hippocampal formation has inspired a search for behavioural consequences of reorganization. Loesche and Steward (1977), for example, found that spontaneous alternation behaviour in rats with unilateral entorhinal cortex injury recovers in parallel with the sprouting of surviving (contralateral) entorhinal fibres in the dentate gyrus. Secondary destruction of the remaining entorhinal area, or transection of its efferent fibres, reinstates the deficit, this time permanently.

Perhaps the most elegant instance of correlated structure and functional plasticity is the after effect of unilateral superior colliculus injury in hamster pups (Schneider & Jhaveri, 1974; Schneider, 1976). Anomalous visual input directly to the deep layers of the damaged colliculus provides a substrate for the sparing of visual target acquisition. In the same animals, however, fibres that cross to the contralateral colliculus cause maladaptive wrong-direction turning to targets presented in the part of the visual field corresponding to abnormal (re)crossing fibres. Wrong-direction turning can be eliminated in this case by 'corrective surgery', cutting the anomalous commissure (Schneider, 1976).

It has been known for a long time that slowly progressive CNS lesions, such as caused by tumour growth, often produce less functional disturbance than equivalent injury inflicted suddenly. This phenomenon has been studied experimentally by comparing single-stage and serial lesions. There is still no comprehensive explanation of the effect. Most authors, however, have suggested that incremental injury somehow facilitates reorganization of surviving tissues (see Eidelberg & Stein, 1974; Scheff *et al.*, 1977).

Prospects for the Future

Genetic information in myriad individual neurons orchestrates the complex process of nervous system development. This process evolved under pressure of natural selection with the end goal of producing a functionally adaptive organism. Changes upon nervous system injury are likewise an expression of the genetic code. There is little reason to suspect, however, that neuroplasticity is the outcome of an evolutionary process with rehabilitation as its end product. Indeed, as evolution has progressed, the functional lability of the intact brain has increased greatly, but its regenerative capacity in the face of injury has, if anything, declined. The brain was 'designed' to avoid injury, not to recover from it. Why, then, is there any recovery at all? In all likelihood, neuroplasticity is simply an epiphenomenon, a hangover from mechanisms of embryonic development on the one hand and normal learning processes on the other. Under fortunate circumstances plastic changes may result in functional restitution, and in fact the tendency for fibres to invade vacated terminal space may bias the process in this direction. On the other hand, as we have seen, plastic rearrangement may just as well make things worse.

Despite the fact that at the organism level recovery of function may be fortuitious rather than planned, neuroplastic mechanisms are not capricious. Inasmuch as we understand them, post-lesion changes at the cellular level appear to be lawful, and in many cases they are predictable (see above). Attempts to use our knowledge of the principles of plasticity in order to engineer patterns of rearrangement favourable to functional sparing have only just begun. We can safely anticipate further developments in the direction of such 'corrective' treatments including surgery, the use of drugs or, some day, trophic factors, and the use of special environmental conditions.

Finally, we must recall that the normal, uninjured brain is intrinsically labile. Some neural functions, respiration for example, are prewired and require minimal learning or experience. For most, however, e.g. skilled movement and language, the genome has provided a substrate exquisitely receptive to programming, but one that must be programmed in order to function. Neural mechanisms that have undergone plastic morphological or physiological changes after injury are similar. For some, function may return spontaneously with minimal outside intervention. For others, special training routines may be necessary. Unlike the training of children and would-be typists, however, optimal teaching methods do not come to us through long periods of cultural evolution or practical experience. They must be sought with diligence and an eye towards the unexpected.

SUMMARY

The neuroanatomical and neurophysiological picture after nervous system injury is not static. Although killed neurons are not replaced, new growth can occur among neuronal processes (axons and dendrites) of partially damaged neurons and also of associated intact neurons. Such growth is very prominent in the peripheral nervous system (PNS) and in the developing central nervous system (CNS), but it also occurs in some locations in the CNS in adults. Surviving neurons may also have altered levels of excitability and, for example, introduce spurious impulses into the CNS. Plastic changes in morphology and physiology are lawful and determined by mechanisms at the cellular level. They are probably not designed to foster behavioural recovery of function. In fact, they may often be detrimental. As we gain a deeper understanding of fundamental neuroplastic processes, our ability to predict and to control the progress of rehabilitation after brain injury is likely to improve.

ACKNOWLEDGEMENT

This chapter was written with the support of the Fritz Thyssen Stiftung and the Israel Centre for Psychobiology. The helpful comments of M. Kaitz, P. D. Wall and R. Werman are gratefully acknowledged.

REFERENCES

ADAMS J.H., DANIEL P.M. & PRITCHARD M.M.L. (1969) Degeneration and regeneration in the neurohypophysis after pituitary stalk section in ferret. *Journal of Comparative Neurology*, **135**, 121–44.

ALBURQUERQUE E.X., WARNICK J.E., TASSE J.R. & SANSONE F.M. (1972) Effects of vinblastine and colchicine on neural regulation of the fast and slow skeletal muscles of the rat. *Experimental Neurology*, **37**, 607–34.

ANDERSSON M.H., FULLERTON P.M., GILLIATT R.W. & HERN J.E.C. (1970) Changes in the forearm associated with median nerve compression at the wrist in the guinea pig. *Journal of Neurology, Neurosurgery and Psychiatry*, **33**, 70–9.

ARVIDSSON J. & GRANT G. (1979) Further observations on transganglionic degeneration in trigeminal primary sensory neurons. *Brain Research* **162**, 1–12.

BARONDES S.H. (ed.) (1976) *Neuronal Recognition.* Plenum Press, New York.

BASBAUM A.I. & WALL P.D. (1976) Chronic changes in the response of cells in adult cat dorsal horn following partial deafferentiation: the appearance of responding cells in a previously nonresponsive region. *Brain Research,* **116**, 181–204.

BECKERMAN S.B. & KERR F.W.L. (1976) Electrophysiologic evidence that neither sprouting nor neuronal hyperactivity occur following long term trigeminal or cervical primary deafferentation. *Experimental Neurology,* **50**, 427–38.

BERG D.K. & HALL Z.W. (1975) Increased extrajunctional acetylcholine sensitivity produced by chronic post-synaptic blockade. *Journal of Physiology, London,* **244**, 659–76.

BERMAN N. & STERLING P. (1976) Cortical suppression of the retino-collicular pathway in the monocularly deprived cat. *Journal of Physiology, London,* **255**, 263–73.

BERNSTEIN J.J. & BERNSTEIN M.E. (1967) Effect of glial-ependymal scar and Teflon arrest on the regenerative capacity of goldfish spinal cord. *Experimental Neurology,* **19**, 25–32.

BERNSTEIN J.J. & GOODMAN D.C. (eds.) (1973) *Neuromorphological Plasticity.* Karger, Basel. (*Brain, Behaviour and Evolution,* **8**, 1973.)

BERNSTEIN J.J. & GUTH L. (1961) Nonselectivity in establishment of neuromuscular connections following nerve regeneration in the rat. *Experimental Neurology,* **4**, 262–75.

BERNSTEIN J.J., WELLS M.R. & BERNSTEIN M.E. (1978) Spinal cord regeneration: synaptic renewal and neurochemistry. In *Neuronal Plasticity* (Ed. Cotman C.W.). Raven Press, New York.

BERNSTEIN M.E. & BERNSTEIN J.J. (1973) Regeneration of axons and synaptic complex formation rostral to the site of hemisection in the spinal cord of the monkey. *International Journal of Neuroscience,* **5**, 15–26.

BERRY M. (1978) Regeneration in the central nervous system. In *Recent Advances in Neuropathology.* Churchill Livingstone, Edinburgh.

BITTNER G.D. & JOHNSON A.L. (1974) Degeneration and regeneration in crustacean peripheral nerves. *Journal of Comparative Neurology,* **89**, 1–21.

BJÖRKLUND A., JOHANSSON B., STENEVI U. & SVENDGAARD N-A. (1975) Re-establishment of functional connections by regenerating central adrenergic and cholinergic axons. *Nature, London,* **253**, 446–8.

BJÖRKLUND A., NOBIN A. & STENEVI U. (1973) Regeneration of central serotonin neurons after axonal degeneration induced by 5,6-dihydroxytryptamine. *Brain Research,* **50**, 214–20.

BLACK R.G. (1974) A laboratory model for trigeminal neuralgia. *Advances in Neurology,* **4**, 561–659.

BLAKEMORE C., FAREY L.J. & VITAL-DURAND F. (1978) The physiological effects of monocular deprivation and their reversal in the monkey's visual cortex. *Journal of Physiology, London,* **238**, 223–62.

BLISS T.V.P. & LOMO T. (1973) Long-lasting potentiation of synaptic transmission in the dentate area of the anaesthetized rabbit following stimulation of the perforant path. *Journal of Physiology, London,* **232**, 331–56.

BONDAREFF W. & NAROTZKY R. (1972) Age changes in the neuronal microenvironment. *Science,* **176**, 1135–6.

BOSTOCK H., FEASBY T.E. & SEARS T.A. (1977) Continuous conduction in regenerating myelinated nerve fibres. *Journal of Physiology, London,* **269**, 88P–89P.

BOWEN F.P., KARPIAK S.E., DEMIRJIAN C. & KATZMAN R. (1975) Sprouting of noradrenergic nerve terminals subsequent to freeze lesions of rabbit cerebral cortex. *Brain Research,* **83**, 1–14.

BROWN A.G., ROSE P.K. & SNOW P.J. (1977) The morphology of hair follicle afferent fibre collaterals in the spinal cord of the cat. *Journal of Physiology, London,* **272**, 779–97.

BROWN M.C. & BUTLER R.G. (1976) Regeneration of afferent and efferent fibres to muscle spindles after nerve injury in adult cats. *Journal of Physiology, London,* **260**, 253–66.

BROWN M.C., JANSEN J.K.S. & VAN ESSEN D. (1976) Polyneuronal innervation of skeletal muscle in new-born rats and its elimination during maturation. *Journal of Physiology, London,* **261**, 387–422.

BURGESS P.R., ENGLISH K.B. & HORCH K.W. (1974) Patterning in the regeneration of type I cutaneous receptors. *Journal of Physiology, London*, **236**, 57–82.

BURGESS P.R. & HORCH K.W. (1973) Specific regeneration of cutaneous fibres in the cat. *Journal of Neurophysiology*, **36**, 101–14.

RAMON y CAJAL S. (1928) *Degeneration and Regeneration of the Nervous System* May R.M. (Trans. 1968.) Hafner, New York, reprint of 1928 edition.

CALVIN W.H., HOWE J.F. & LOESER J.D. (1977) Ectopic repetitive firing in focally demyelinated axons and some implications for trigeminal neuralgia. In *Pain in the Trigeminal Region* (Eds. Anderson & Matthews.) Elsevier/North Holland Publishing Company, Amsterdam.

CAMPBELL J.B. (1970) Peripheral nerve repair. *Clinical Neurosurgery*, **17**, 77–98.

CANGIANO A. & FRIED J.A. (1977) The production of denervation-like changes in rat muscle by colchicine, without interference with axonal transport of muscle activity. *Journal of Physiology, London*, **265**, 63–84.

CARLSON J., LAIS A.C. & DYCK P.J. (1978) How are numbers and sizes of motor and spinal ganglion neurons altered when their distal axons are transected in adult cats. *Journal of Neuropathology and Experimental Neurology*, **37**, 597.

CARMEL P.W. & STEIN B.M. (1969) Cell changes in sensory ganglia following proximal and distal nerve section in the monkey. *Journal of Comparative Neurology*, **135**, 145–66.

CAVINESS V.S. JR, KORDE M.D. & WILLIAMS R.S. (1977) Cellular events induced in the molecular layer of the piriform cortex by ablation of the olfactory bulb in the mouse. *Brain Research*, **134**, 13–34.

CHANGEUX J-P. & DANCHIN A. (1976) Selective stabilization of developing synapses as a mechanism for the specification of neuronal networks. *Nature, London*, **264**, 705–12.

CHU-WANG I-W. & OPPENHEIM P.W. (1978) Cell death of motoneurons in the chick embryo spinal cord. *Journal of Comparative Neurology*, **177**, 33–86.

CLARK W.E. LE G. (1942) The problem of neuronal regeneration in the central nervous system. 1. The influences of spinal ganglion and nerve fragments grafted into the brain. *Journal of Anatomy*, **77**, 20–48.

COOPER E., DIAMOND J. & TURNER C. (1977) The effect of nerve section and of colchicine treatment on the density of mechanosensory nerve endings in salamander skin. *Journal of Physiology, London*, **264**, 725–49.

COTMAN C.W. (ed.) (1978) *Neuronal Plasticity*, pp. 335. Raven Press, New York.

COTMAN C.W. & LYNCH G.S. (1976) Reactive synaptogenesis in the adult nervous system: the effects of partial deafferentation on new synapse formation. In *Neuronal Recognition* (Ed. Barondes S.), pp. 69–108. Plenum Press, New York.

CRAGG B.G. (1970) What is the signal for chromatolysis? *Brain Research*, **33**, 1–21.

CRAGG B.G. & THOMAS P.K. (1961) Changes in conduction velocity and fibre size proximal to peripheral nerve lesions. *Journal of Physiology, London*, **157**, 315–27.

DAHLSTROM A. & FUXE K. (1964) Evidence for the existence of monoamine containing neurons in the central nervous system. I. Demonstration of monoamines in the cell bodies of brain stem neurons. *Acta Physiologica Scandinavica*, **62**, Suppl. 232, 1–55.

DENNIS M.J. & YIP J.W. (1978) Formation and elimination of foreign synapses on adult salamander muscle. *Journal of Physiology, London*, **274**, 299–310.

DENNY-BROWN D., MEYER J.S. & HORENSTEIN S. (1953) The significance of perceptual rivalry resulting from parietal lesion. *Brain*, **75**, 433–71.

DEVOR M. (1975) Neuroplasticity in the sparing or deterioration of function after early olfactory tract lesions. *Science*, **190**, 998–1000.

DEVOR M. (1976a) Fibre trajectories of olfactory bulb efferents in the hamster. *Journal of Comparative Neurology*, **166**, 31–48.

DEVOR M. (1976b) Neuroplasticity in the rearrangement of olfactory tract fibres after neonatal transection in hamsters. *Journal of Comparative Neurology*, **166**, 31–48.

DEVOR M. & GOVRIN-LIPPMANN R. (1979a) Selective regeneration of sensory fibres following nerve crush injury. *Experimental Neurology* **65**, 243–54.

Devor M. & Govrin-Lippmann R. (1979b) Maturation of axonal sprouts after nerve crush. *Experimental Neurology*, **64**, 260–70.

Devor M., Merrill E.G. & Wall P.D. (1977) Dorsal horn cells that respond to stimulation of distant dorsal roots. *Journal of Physiology, London*, **270**, 519–31.

Devor M. & Schneider G.E. (1975) Neuroanatomical plasticity: the principle of conservation of total axonal arborization. In *Aspects of Neural Plasticity* (Eds. Vital-Durand F. & Jeannerod M.), pp. 191–200. [see Vital-Durand & Jeannerod p. 84].

Devor M., Schonfeld D., Seltzer Z. & Wall P.D. (1979) Two modes of cutaneous reinnervation following peripheral nerve injury. *Journal of Comparative Neurology*, **185**, 211–20.

Devor M. & Wall P.D. (1978) Reorganisation of spinal cord sensory map after peripheral nerve injury. *Nature, London*, **275**, 75–6.

Dews P.B. & Wiesel T.N. (1970) Consequences of monocular deprivation on visual behaviour in kittens. *Journal of Physiology, London*, **206**, 437–55.

Diamond J., Cooper E., Turner C. & Macintyre L. (1976) Trophic regulation of nerve sprouting. *Science*, **193**, 371–7.

Dichgans J., Bizzi E., Morasco P. & Tagliasco V. (1973) Mechanisms underlying recovery of eye-head coordination following bilateral labyrinthectomy in monkeys. *Experimental Brain Research*, **18**, 548–62.

Dijkstra C. (1933) Die De- und Regeneration der sensiblen Endkorperchen des Enterschnabels (Grandry und Herbst-Korperchen) nach Durchschneidung des Nerven, nach Fortnahme der ganzen Haut und nach Transplantation des Hautstuckchens. *Zeitschrift für mikroskopisch-anatomische Forschung (Leipzig)*, **34**, 75–158.

Dostrovsky J.O., Millar J. & Wall P.D. (1976) The immediate shift of afferent drive of dorsal column nucleus cells following deafferentation: a comparison of acute and chronic deafferentation in gracile nucleus and spinal cord. *Experimental Neurology*, **52**, 480–95.

Douarin N.M. le & Teillet M.M. (1974) Experimental analysis of the migration and differentiation of neuroblasts of the autonomic nervous system and of neuroectodermal mesenchymal derivatives using a biological cell marking technique. *Developmental Biology*, **41**, 162–84.

Doupe J., Cullen C.H. & Chance G.Q. (1944) Post traumatic pain and the causalgic syndrome. *Journal of Neurology, Neurosurgery and Psychiatry*, **7**, 33–48.

Duffy F.H., Snodgrass S.R., Burchfiel J.L. & Conway J.L. (1976) Bicuculline reversal of deprivation amblyopia in the cat. *Nature, London*, **260**, 256–7.

Dunn G.A. (1971) Mutual contact inhibition of extension of chick sensory nerve fibres in vitro. *Journal of Comparative Neurology*, **143**, 491–508.

Eccles J.C., Krnjevic K. & Miledi R. (1959) Delayed effects of peripheral severance of afferent nerve fibres on the efficacy of their central synapses. *Journal of Physiology, London*, **145**, 204–20.

Edds M.V. (1953) Collateral nerve regeneration. *Quarterly Review of Biology*, **28**, 260–76.

Eidelberg E. & Stein D.G. (Eds.) (1974) Functional recovery after lesions of the nervous system. *Neurosciences Research Program Bulletin*, **12**, (2).

Essen D.C. van & Jansen G.K.S. (1977) The specificity of reinnervation by identified sensory and motor neurons in the leech. *Journal of Comparative Neurology*, **171**, 433–54.

Fadiga E., Haimann C., Margnelli M. & Sotgiu M.L. (1978) Variability of peripheral representation in ventrobasal thalamic nuclei of the cat: effects of acute reversible blockade of the dorsal column nuclei. *Experimental Neurology*, **60**, 484–98.

Forssman H. (1900) Zur Kenntnis des Neurotropismus. *Ziegler's Beiträge zur pathologischen Anatomie, Bd.*, **27**, Cited by Cajal (1928).

Fullerton P.M. & Gilliatt R.W. (1965) Axon reflex in human motor nerve fibres. *Journal of Neurology, Neurosurgery and Psychiatry*, **28**, 1–11.

Fulton J.F. (1949) *Physiology of the Nervous System*, 3e. Oxford University Press, New York.

Gallego R., Kuno M., Nunez R. & Snider W.D. (1979) Disuse enhances synaptic efficacy in spinal motoneurons. *Journal of Physiology, London*, **291**, 191–205.

Gentschev T. & Sotelo C. (1973) Degenerative patterns in the ventral cochlear nucleus of the rat after primary deafferentation. An ultrastructural study. *Brain Research*, **62**, 37–60.

GLEES P. & COLE J. (1950) Recovery of skilled motor functions after small repeated lesions of motor cortex in macaque. *Journal of Neurophysiology*, **13**, 137–148.

GOLDBERGER M. & MURRAY M. (1974) Restitution of function and collateral sprouting in cat spinal cord: the deafferented animal. *Journal of Comparative Neurology*, **158**, 37–54.

GOODE G.E. (1977) The ultrastructural identification of primary and suprasegmental afferents in the margin and gelatinous layers of lumbar spinal cord following central and peripheral lesions. *Neuroscience Abstracts*, **2**, 975.

GOODMAN D.C., BOGDASARIAN R.S. & HOREL J.A. (1973) Axonal sprouting of ipsilateral optic tract following opposite eye removed. *Brain, Behaviour and Evolution*, **8**, 27–50.

GOODMAN D.C. & HOREL J.A. (1966) Sprouting of optic projections in the brain stem of the rat. *Journal of Comparative Neurology*, **127**, 71–88.

GOTTLIEB D.I. & COWAN W.M. (1972) Evidence for a temporal factor in the occupation of available synaptic sites during development of the dentate gyrus. *Brain Research*, **41**, 452–6.

GOVRIN-LIPPMANN R. & DEVOR M. (1978) Ongoing activity in severed nerves: sources and variation with time. *Brain Research*, **159**, 406–10.

GRAFSTEIN B. (1975) The nerve cell body response to axotomy. *Experimental Neurology*, **48**, 32–51.

GRAZIADEI P.P.C. & GRAZIADEI G.A.M. (1977) Continuous nerve cell renewal in the olfactory system. In *Handbook of Sensory Physiology*, Vol. IX (Ed. Jacobson M.). Springer-Verlag, Berlin.

GRINNELL A.D. (1977) Specificity of neurons and their interconnections. In *Handbook of Physiology*, Section 1. *The Nervous System*. Vol. 1. *Cellular Biology of Neurons*, Section 2 (Ed. Kandel E.R.). American Physiological Society, Bethesda.

GUILLERY R.W. (1972) Experiments to determine whether retinogeniculate axons can form translaminar collateral sprouts in the dorsal lateral geniculate nucleus of the cat. *Journal of Comparative Neurology*, **146**, 407–20.

GUTH L. (1956) Regeneration in the mammalian peripheral nervous system. *Physiological Reviews*, **36**, 441–78.

GUTH L. (Ed.) (1969) Trophic effects of vertebrate neurons. *Neurosciences Research Program Bulletin*, **7**, 1–71.

GUTMANN E. (1942) Factors affecting recovery of motor function after nerve lesions. *Journal of Neurology, Neurosurgery and Psychiatry*, **5**, 81–95.

GUTNICK M., RUDOMIN P. & WALL P.D. (1975) Is there interaction between motoneurons and afferent fibres in the spinal cord? *Brain Research*, **23**, 507–10.

HAMBURGER V. & LEVI-MONTALCINI R. (1949) Proliferation, differentiation and degeneration in the spinal ganglia of the chick embryo under normal and experimental conditions. *Journal of Experimental Zoology*, **111**, 457–501.

HARRIS A.J. & ZISKIND L. (1977) Spontaneous release of transmitter from 'repressed' nerve terminals in axolotl muscle. *Nature, London*, **268**, 265–7.

HEIMER L. (1968) Synaptic distribution of centripetal and centrifugal nerve fibres in the olfactory system of the rat. An experimental anatomical study. *Journal of Anatomy*, **103**, 413–32.

HELD R. (1965) Plasticity in sensory-motor systems. *Scientific American*, **213**, 84–94.

HICKEY T.L. (1975) Translaminar growth of axons in the kitten dorsal lateral geniculate nucleus following removal of one eye. *Journal of Comparative Neurology*, **161**, 359–82.

HNIK P., JIRMANOVA I., VYKLICKY L. & ZELENA J. (1967) Fast and slow muscles of the chick after nerve cross-union. *Journal of Physiology, London*, **193**, 309–25.

HOFFMAN H. (1950) Local re-innervation in partially denervated muscle: a histo-pathological study. *Australian Journal of Experimental Biology and Medical Science*, **28**, 383–97.

HOFFMANN W.W. & THESLEFF S. (1972) Studies on the trophic influence of nerve on skeletal muscle. *European Journal of Pharmacology*, **20**, 256–60.

HUBEL D.H., WIESEL T.N. & LEVAY S. (1977) Plasticity of ocular dominance columns in monkey striate cortex. *Philosophical Transactions of the Royal Society of London*, Series B, **278**, 377–410.

HUGHES A.F.W. (1968) *Aspects of Neural Ontogeny*. Logos, London.

HUNT R.K. & JACOBSON M. (1972) Development and stability of positional information in Xenopus retinal ganglion cells. *Proceedings of the National Academy of Sciences of the United States of America (Washington)*, **69**, 780–3.

IGGO A. (1978) Is the physiology of cutaneous receptors determined by morphology? In *Progress in Brain Research*, Vol. 43. *Somatosensory and Visceral Receptor Mechanisms* (Eds. Iggo A. & Ilyinsky O.B.), pp. 15–34. Elsevier, Amsterdam.

ILLIS L.S. (1973) Experimental model of regeneration in the central nervous system. *Brain*, **96**, 47–60.

JACOBSON M. (1971) Formation of neuronal connections in sensory systems. In *Handbook of Sensory Physiology*, Vol. 1. *Principles of Receptor Physiology* (Ed. Loewenstein W.R.). Springer-Verlag, Berlin.

JACOBSON M. (1978) *Developmental Neurobiology*, 2e, pp. 574. Plenum, New York.

JONES W.H. & THOMAS D.B. (1962) Changes in the dendritic organisation of neurons in the cerebral cortex following deafferentation. *Journal of Anatomy*, **96**, 375–81.

KADANOFF D. (1925) Untersuchungen über die Regeneration des sensiblen Nervenendigungen nach Vertauschung verschieden innervierten Haustucke. *Archiv für Entwicklungsmechanik der Organismen*, **106**, 249–78.

KALIL R.E. (1973) Formation of new retino-geniculate connections in kittens: effects of age and visual experience. *Anatomical Record*, **175**, 353.

KASAMATSU T. & PETTIGREW J.D. (1976) Depletion of brain catecholamines: failure of ocular dominance shift after monocular occlusion in kittens. *Science*, **194**, 206–8.

KENNARD M.A. (1940) Relation of age to motor impairment in man and in subhuman primates. *Archives of Neurology and Psychiatry*, **44**, 377–97.

KERR F.W.L. (1972) The potential of cervical primary afferents to sprout in the spinal nucleus of V following long term trigeminal denervation. *Brain Research*, **43**, 547–60.

KIERNAN J.A. (1978) An explanation of axonal regeneration in peripheral nerves and its failure in the central nervous system. *Medical Hypotheses*, **4**, 15–26.

KIMMEL D.L. & MOYER E.K. (1947) Dorsal roots following anastomosis of the central stump. *Journal of Comparative Neurology*, **87**, 289–320.

KJERULF T.D. & LOESER J.D. (1973) Neuronal hyperactivity following deafferentation of the lateral cuneate nucleus. *Experimental Neurology*, **39**, 70–85.

KNYIHAR E. & CSILLIK B. (1976) Effects of peripheral axotomy on the fine structure and histochemistry of the Rolando substance: degeneration atrophy of central processes of pseudounipolar cells. *Experimental Brain Research*, **26**, 73–78.

KRATZ K.E., SPEAR P.D. & SMITH D.C. (1976) Postcritical period reversal of effects of monocular deprivation on striate cortex cells in the cat. *Journal of Neurophysiology*, **39**, 501–11.

LANDMESSER L. & PILAR G. (1974) Synaptic transmission and cell death during normal ganglionic development. *Journal of Physiology, London*, **241**, 737–49.

LEONARD C.M. (1974) Degeneration argyrophilia as an index of neural maturation: studies on the optic tract of the golden hamster. *Journal of Comparative Neurology*, **156**, 435–58.

LEONARD C.M. (1975) Developmental changes in olfactory bulb projections revealed by degeneration argyrophilia. *Journal of Comparative Neurology*, **162**, 467–86.

LETINSKY M.S., FISHBECK K.H. & MCMAHAN U.J. (1976) Precision of reinnervation of original postsynaptic sites in frog muscle after a nerve crush. *Journal of Neurocytology*, **5**, 691–718.

LETOURNEAU P.C. (1975) Cell-to-substratum adhesion and guidance of axonal elongation. *Developmental Biology*, **44**, 92–101.

LEWIS D.M., BAGUST J., WEBB S.N., WESTERMAN R.A. & FINOL H.J. (1977) Axon conduction velocity modified by reinnervation of mammalian muscle. *Nature, London*, **270**, 745–6.

LIBERMAN A.R. (1971) The axon reaction. A review of the principle features of perikaryal responses to axon injury. *International Review of Neurobiology*, **14**, 49–124.

LIEBERMAN A.R. (1974) Some factors affecting retrograde neuronal responses to axonal lesions. In *Essays on the Nervous System* (Eds. Bellairs R. & GRAY E.G.), pp. 71–105. Clarendon Press, Oxford.

LIU C-N. & CHAMBERS W.W. (1958) Intraspinal sprouting of dorsal root axons. *Archives of Neurology and Psychiatry*, **79**, 46–61.

LIVINGSTON S.K. (1947) Evidence of active invasion of denervated areas by sensory fibres from neighbouring nerves in man. *Journal of Neurosurgery*, **4**, 140–5.

LLOYD D.P.C. (1949) Post-tetanic potentiation of response in mono-synaptic reflex pathways of the spinal cord. *Journal of General Physiology*, **33**, 147–70.

LOESCHE J. & STEWARD O. (1977) Behavioural correlates of denervation and reinnervation of the hippocampal formation of the rat: recovery of alternation performance following unilateral entorhinal cortex lesions. *Brain Research Bulletin*, **2**, 31–9.

LOESER J.D. & WARD A.A. (1967) Some effects of deafferentation on neurons of the cat spinal cord. *Archives of Neurology*, **17**, 629–36.

LOMO T. & ROSENTHAL J. (1972) Control of Ach sensitivity by muscle activity in the rat. *Journal of Physiology, London*, **221**, 493–513.

LOOS H. VAN DER & WOOLSEY T.A. (1973) Somatosensory cortex: structural alterations following early injury to sense organs. *Science*, **179**, 395–8.

LUCO J.V. & EYZAGUIRRE C. (1955) Fibrillation and hypersensitivity to Ach in denervated muscle: effect of length of degenerating nerve fibres. *Journal of Neurophysiology*, **18**, 65–73.

LUND R.D. & LUND J.S. (1971) Synaptic adjustment after deafferentation of the superior colliculus of the rat. *Science*, **171**, 804–7.

MACON J.B. (1978) Neuronal responses to amino acid iontophoresis in the deafferented spinal trigeminal nucleus. *Experimental Neurology*, **60**, 522–40.

MARK R.F., MAROTTE L.R. & MART P.E. (1972) The mechanism of selective reinnervation of fish eye muscles. IV. Identification of repressed synapses. *Brain Research*, **46**, 149–57.

MARKS A.F. (1972) Regenerative reconstruction of a tract in a rat's brain. *Experimental Neurology*, **34**, 455–64.

McCOUCH G.P., AUSTIN G.M., LIU C.N. & LIU C.Y. (1958) Sprouting as a cause of spasticity. *Journal of Neurophysiology*, **21**, 205–16.

McQUARRIE I.G., GRAFSTEIN B. & GERSHON M.D. (1977) Axonal regeneration in the rat sciatic nerve: effect of a conditioning lesion and of dbcAMP. *Brain Research*, **132**, 443–53.

MELVILL-JONES G. (1977) Plasticity in the adult vestibulo-ocular reflex arc. *Philosophical Transactions of the Royal Society of London*, Series B, **278**, 241–436.

MENDELL L.M., SASSOON E.M. & WALL P.D. (1978) Properties of synaptic linkage from 'distant' afferents onto dorsal horn neurons in normal and chronically deafferented cats. *Journal of Physiology, London*, **285**, 299–310.

MERRELL R., GOTTLIEB D.I. & GLASER L. (1976) Membranes as a tool for the study of cell surface recognition. In *Neuronal Recognition* (Ed. Barondes S.H.), pp. 249–74. Plenum Press, New York.

MERRILL E.G. & WALL P.D. (1972) Factors forming the edge of a receptive field. The presence of relatively ineffective afferents. *Journal of Physiology, London*, **226**, 825–46.

MILEDI R. & STEPHANI E. (1969) Non-selective re-innervation of slow and fast muscle fibres in the rat. *Nature, London*, **222**, 569–71.

MILLAR J., BASBAUM A.I. & WALL P.D. (1976) Restructuring of the somatotopic map and appearance of abnormal neuronal activity in the gracile nucleus after partial deafferentation. *Experimental Neurology*, **50**, 658–72.

MILNER B. (1974) Hemispheric specialisation: scope and limits. In *The Neurosciences: Third Study Program* (Eds. Schmitt F.O. & Worden F.G.), pp. 75–89. MIT Press, Cambridge, Mass.

MONAKOW C. VON (1914) Die Grosshirn und der Abban Funktion durch Kortikale. Herde, Wiesbaden, Bergmann.

MOORE R.Y., BJORKLUND A. & STENEVI U. (1971) Plastic changes in the adrenergic innervation of the rat septal area in response to denervation. *Brain Research*, **33**, 13–35.

MORRIS J.H., HUDSON A.R. & WEDDELL G. (1972) A study of degeneration and regeneration in the divided rat sciatic nerve based on electron microscopy. *Zeitschrift Zellforsch*, **124**, 76–203.

MOSCONA A.A. (1976) Cell recognition in embryonic morphogenesis and the problem of neuronal specificities. In *Neuronal Recognition* (Ed. Barondes S.H.), pp. 205–23. Plenum Press, New York.

MOTTE D.J. DE LA & ALLT G. (1976) Crush injury to peripheral nerve. An electron miscroscopic study employing horseradish peroxidase. *Acta Neuropathologica*, **36**, 9–16.

MURRAY M. & GOLDBERGER M. (1974) Restitution of function and collateral sprouting in cat spinal cord. The partial hemisected animal. *Journal of Comparative Neurology*, **158**, 19–36.

NAKAMURA Y., MIZUNO N., KONISHI A. & SATO M. (1974) Synaptic reorganisation of the red nucleus after chronic deafferentation from cerebellorubral fibres: an electron microscopic study in the cat. *Brain Reasearch*, **82**, 298–301.

NATHAN P.W. (1947) On the pathogenesis of causalgia in peripheral nerve injuries. *Brain*, **70**, 145–70.

NOORDEN G.K. VON (1973) Experimental amblyopia in monkeys. Further behavioural observations and clinical correlations. *Investigative Ophthalmology*, **12**, 721–6.

NOORDEN G.K. VON, DOWLING J.E. & FERGUSON D.C. (1970) Experimental amblyopia in monkeys. I. Behavioural studies of stimulus deprivation amblyopia. *Archives of Opthalmology*, **84**, 206–14.

OAKLEY B. (1967) Altered temperature and taste responses from cross-regenerated sensory nerves in the rat's tongue. *Journal of Physiology, London*, **188**, 353–71.

OLSON L. & MALMFORS T. (1970) Growth characteristics of adrenergic nerves in the adult rat. *Acta Physiologica Scandinavica*, Suppl. 348.

OSTBERG A.J.C., RAISMAN G., FIELD P.M., IVERSEN L.L. & ZIGMOND R.E. (1976) A quantitative comparison of the formation of synapses in the rat superior cervical sympathetic ganglion by its own and by foreign nerve fibres. *Brain Research*, **107**, 445–70.

PANNESE E. (1963) Investigations of the ultrastructural changes of the spinal ganglion neurons in the course of axon hypertrophy. *Zeitschrift für Zellforchung*, **61**, 561–86.

PATTERSON P., REICHARDT L. & CHUN L. (1975) Biochemical studies on the development of primary sympathetic neurons in cell culture. *Cold Spring Harbor Symposia on Quantitative Biology*, **40**, 389–98.

PERSSON L., HANSSON H.A. & SOURANDER P. (1976) Extravasation, spread and cellular uptake of Evans blue-labelled albumin around a reproducible small stab wound in the rat brain. *Acta Neuropathologica*, **34**, 125–36.

PETIT D. & BURGESS P.R. (1968) Dorsal column projection of receptors in cat hairy skin supplied by myelinated fibres. *Journal of Neurophysiology*, **31**, 849–55.

PETTEGREW R.K. & WINDLE W.F. (1976) Factors in recovery from spinal cord injury. *Experimental Neurology*, **53**, 815–29.

PETTIGREW J.D. (1978) The paradox of the critical period for striate cortex. In *Neuronal Plasticity*, (Ed. Cotman C.W.), pp. 311–30. Raven Press, New York.

PETTIGREW J.D. & KASAMATSU T. (1978) Local perfusion of noradrenaline maintains visual cortical plasticity. *Nature, London*, **271**, 761–63.

PICKEL V.M., SEGAL M. & BLOOM F.E. (1974) Axonal proliferation following lesions of cerebellar peduncles: a combined fluorescence microscopic and autoradiographic study. *Journal of Comparative Neurology*, **155**, 43–60.

PRENDERGAST J. & STELZNER D.J. (1976) Increases in collateral axonal growth rostral to a thoracic hemisection in neonatal and weanling rat. *Journal of Comparative Neurology*, **166**, 145–62.

PRESTIGE M.C. (1967) Differentiation, degeneration and the role of the periphery: quantitative considerations. In *The Neurosciences Second Study Program* (Ed. Schmitt F.O.), pp. 73–82. Rockefeller University Press, New York.

PRICE J.L., MOXLEY G.F. & SCHWOB J.E. (1976) Development and plasticity of complementary afferent systems to the olfactory cortex. *Experimental Brain Research Supplement*, **1**, 148–54.

PULLEN A.H. & SEARS T.A. (1978) Modification of 'c' synapses following partial central deafferentation of thoracic motoneurons. *Brain Research*, **145**, 141–6.

PURVES D. (1976) Long-term regulation in the vertebrate peripheral nervous system. In *Neurophysiology II*, Vol. 10 (Ed. Porter R.). University Park Press, Baltimore.

QUILLIAM T.A. (1958) Growth changes in sensory fibre aggregates undergoing remyelination. *Journal of Anatomy*, **92**, 383–98.

RAISMAN G. (1969) Neuronal plasticity in the septal nuclei of the adult rat. *Brain Research*, **14**, 25–48.

RAISMAN G. (1977) Formation of synapses in the adult rat after injury: similarities and differences between a peripheral and a central nervous site. *Philosophical Transactions of the Royal Society of London*, Series B, **278**, 349–59.

RAISMAN G. & FIELD P.M. (1973) A quantitative investigation of the development of collateral reinnervation after partial deafferentation of the septal nuclei. *Brain Research*, **50**, 241–64.

RAKIC P. (1977) Prenatal development of the visual system in rhesus monkey. *Philosophical Transactions of the Royal Society of London*, Series B, **278**, 245–60.

RALSTON H.J. & CHOW K.L. (1973) Synaptic reorganisation in the degenerating lateral geniculate nucleus of the rabbit. *Journal of Comparative Neurology*, **147**, 321–50.

RASMINSKY M. (1978) Ectopic generation of impulses and cross-talk in spinal nerve roots of 'dystrophic' mice. *Neurology*, **3**, 351–7.

RICE F.L. & VANDER LOOS H. (1977) Development of the barrels and barrel field in the somatosensory cortex of the mouse. *Journal of Comparative Neurology*, **171**, 545–60.

RITCHIE J.M. & ROGART R.B. (1977) Density of sodium channels in mammalian myelinated nerve fibres and nature of the axonal membrane under the myelin sheath. *Proceedings of the National Academy of Sciences of the United States of America (Washington)*, **74**, 211–15.

ROSE J.E., MALIS L., KRUGER I. & BAKER C.P. (1960) Effects of heavy ionizing monoenergetic particles on the cerebral cortex. II. Histological appearance of laminar lesions and growth of nerve fibres after laminar destruction. *Journal of Comparative Neurology*, **115**, 243–95.

ROSENTHAL J. (1977) Trophic interactions of neurons. In *Handbook of Physiology*. Section 1. The nervous System. Vol. 1. Cellular Biology of Neurons. Part 2 (Ed. Kandel E.R.), pp. 775–802. William and Wilkins, Baltimore.

ROTSHENKER S. (1978) Sprouting of intact motor neurons induced by neuronal lesions in the absence of degenerated muscle fibres and degenerating axons. *Brain Research* **55**, 354–6.

RUSTIONI A. & MOLENAAR I. (1975) Dorsal column nuclei afferents in the lateral funiculus of the cat: distribution pattern and absence of sprouting after chronic deafferentation. *Experimental Brain Research*, **23**, 1–12.

SCHACHNER M. & HAMMERLING U. (1974) The postnatal development of antigens on mouse brain cell surfaces. *Brain Research*, **73**, 362–71.

SCHEFF S., BERNADO L. & COTMAN C. (1977) Progressive brain damage accelerates axon sprouting in adult rats. *Science*, **197**, 795–7.

SCHIFF J. & LOEWENSTEIN W.R. (1972) Development of a receptor on a foreign nerve fibre in a Pacinian corpuscle. *Science*, **177**, 712–15.

SCHNEIDER G.E. (1970) Mechanisms of functional recovery following lesions of visual cortex or superior colliculus in neonate and adult hamsters. *Brain, Behaviour and Evolution*, **3**, 295–323.

SCHNEIDER G.E. (1973) Early lesions of superior colliculus: factors affecting the formation of abnormal retinal projections. *Brain, Behaviour and Evolution*, **8**, 73–109.

SCHNEIDER G.E. (1976) Growth of abnormal neural connections following focal brain lesions: constraining factors and functional effects. In *Neurosurgical Treatment in Psychiatry, Pain and Epilepsy* (Ed. Sweet W.H.). University Park Press, Baltimore.

SCHNEIDER G.E. & JHAVERI S.R. (1974) Neuroanatomical correlates of spared or altered function after brain lesions in the newborn hamster. In *Plasticity and Recovery of Function in the Central Nervous System* (Eds. Stein D.G., Rosen J.J. & Butters N.), pp. 65–109. Academic Press, New York.

SCOTT S.A. (1977) Maintained function of foreign and appropriate junctions on reinnervated goldfish extraocular muscles. *Journal of Physiology, London*, **268**, 87–109.

SELTZER Z. & DEVOR M. (1979) Ephaptic transmission in chronically damaged peripheral nerves. *Neurology* **29**, 1061–4.

SHARPLESS S.K. (1964) Reorganisation of function in the nervous system—use and disuse. *Annual Review of Physiology*, **26**, 357–88.

SHARPLESS S.K. (1975) Supersensitivity—like phenomena in the central nervous system. *Federation Proceedings*, **34**, 1990–7.

SHAWE G.D.H. (1955) On the number of branches formed by regenerating nerve fibres. *British Journal of Surgery*, **42**, 474–88.

SHUTE C.C.D. & LEWIS P.R. (1967) The ascending cholinergic reticular system: neocortical, olfactory and subcortical projections. *Brain*, **90**, 497–540.

SIDMAN R.L. & RAKIC P. (1973) Neuronal migration with special reference to developing human brain: a review. *Brain Research*, **62**, 1–35.

SO K.F. & SCHNEIDER G.E. (1978) Abnormal recrossing retinotectal projections after early lesions in Syrian hamsters: age related effects. *Brain Research*, **147**, 277–95.

SOTELO C. & PALAY S.C. (1971) Altered axons and axon terminals in the lateral vestibular nucleus of the rat. Possible examples of axonal remodeling. *Laboratory Investigation*, **25**, 653–71.

SPENCER P.S. & LIEBERMAN A.R. (1971) Scanning electron microscopy of isolated peripheral nerve fibres: normal surface structure and alterations proximal to neuromas. *Zeitschrift für Zellforchung*, **119**, 534–51.

SPENCER P.S. & THOMAS P.K. (1970) The examination of isolated nerve fibres by light and electron microscopy, with observations on demyelination proximal to neuromas. *Acta Neuropathologica*, **16**, 177–86.

SPENCER W.A. & APRIL R.S. (1979) Plastic properties of monosynaptic pathways in mammals. In *Short-term Changes in Neural Activity and Behaviour* (Eds. Horn G. & Hinde R.A.). Cambridge University Press, Cambridge.

SPERRY R.W. (1963) Chemoaffinity in the orderly growth of nerve fibre patterns and connections. *Proceedings of the National Academy of Sciences in the United States of America (Washington)*, **50**, 703–10.

SPRAGUE J.M. (1966) Interaction of cortex and superior colliculus in mediation of visually guided behaviour in the cat. *Science*, **153**, 1544–7.

STEIN D.G., ROSEN J.J. & BUTTERS N. (Eds.) (1974) *Plasticity and Recovery of Function in the Central Nervous System*. Academic Press, New York.

STELZNER D.J. & KEATING E.G. (1977) Lack of intralaminar sprouting of retinal axons in monkey LGN. *Brain Research*, **126**, 201–10.

STENEVI U., BJORKLUND A. & MOORE R.Y. (1973) Morphological plasticity of central adrenergic neurons. *Brain, Behaviour and Evolution*, **8**, 110–34.

SUNDERLAND S. (1978) *Nerves and Nerve Injuries*. 2e. Churchill Livingstone, London.

SVENDGAARD N-A., BJÖRKLUND A. & STENEVI U. (1976) Regeneration of central cholinergic neurons in the adult brain. *Brain Research*, **102**, 1–22.

TEASDALL R.D. & STRAVRAKY G.W. (1953) Responses of deafferented spinal neurones to corticospinal impulses. *Journal of Neurophysiology*, **16**, 367–76.

TEUBER H-C. (1974) Recovery of lesions of the central nervous system: history and prospects. *Neurosciences Research Program Bulletin*, **12**, 197–211.

TEUBER H-L. & RUDEL R.G. (1962) Behaviour after cerebral lesions in children and adults. *Developmental Medicine and Child Neurology*, **4**, 3–20.

THESLEFF S. (1960) Supersensitivity of skeletal muscle produced by botulinum toxin. *Journal of Physiology, London*, **151**, 598–607.

THULIN C-A. (1960) Electrophysiological studies of peripheral nerve regeneration with special reference to the small diameter (gamma) fibres. *Experimental Neurology*, **2**, 598–612.

TRIPP L.N. & WELLS J. (1978) Formation of new synaptic terminals in the somatosensory thalamus of the rat after lesions of the dorsal column nuclei. *Brain Research*, **155**, 362–7.

TSUKAHARA N., HULTBORN H. & MURAKAMI F. (1974) Sprouting of corticorubral synapses in red nucleus neurons after destruction of the nucleus interpositus of the cerebellum. *Experientia*, **30**, 57–8.

UDIN S.B. (1977) Rearrangements of the reginotectal projection in Rana Pipens after unilateral candal half-tectum ablation. *Journal of Comparative Neurology*, **173**, 561–82.

UNGERSTEDT U. (1971) Stereotaxic mapping of the monoamine pathways in the rat brain. *Acta Physiologica Scandinavica*, Suppl. 367.

VITAL-DURAND F. & JEANNEROD M. (Eds.) (1975) *Aspects of Neural Plasticity*. INSERM 43.

WALL P.D. (1977) The presence of ineffective synapses and the circumstances which unmask them. *Philosophical Transactions of the Royal Society of London*, Series B, **278**, 361–72.

WALL P.D. (1979) Changes in damaged nerve and their sensory consequences. In *Advances in Pain Research and Therapy*, Vol. 3 (Eds. Bonica J.J., Liebeskind J.C. & Albe-Fessard D.G.). Raven Press, New York.

WALL P.D. & DEVOR M. (1978) Physiology of sensation after peripheral nerve injury, regeneration and neuroma formations. In *Physiology and Pathobiology of Axons* Ed. Waxman S.G.). Raven Press, New York.

WALL P.D., DEVOR M., INBAL R., SCADDING J.W., SCHONFELD D., SELTZER Z. & TOMKIEWICZ M.M. (1979) Autotomy following peripheral nerve lesions: experimental anaesthesia dolorosa. *Pain*, **7**, 103–13.

WALL P.D. & EGGER M.D. (1971) Formation of new connections in adult rat brains after partial deafferentation. *Nature, London*, **232**, 542–5.

WALL P.D. & GUTNICK M. (1974) Ongoing activity in peripheral nerves: the physiology and pharmacology of impulses originating from a neuroma. *Experimental Neurology*, **43**, 580–93.

WALL P.D. & WERMAN R. (1976) The physiology and anatomy of long ranging afferent fibres within the spinal cord. *Journal of Physiology, London*, **255**, 321–34.

WATSON W.E. (1974) Cellular responses to axotomy and to related procedures. *British Medical Bulletin*, **30**, 112–15.

WEDDELL G., GUTTMANN L. & GUTMANN E. (1941) The local extension of nerve fibres into denervated areas of skin. *Journal of Neurology, Neurosurgery and Psychiatry*, **4**, 206–25.

WEDDELL G. & ZANDER E. (1951) The fragility of nonmyelinated nerve terminals. *Journal of Anatomy*, **85**, 242–50.

WEISS P. (1969) *Principles of Development*. Hafner, New York.

WEISS P., EDDS M.V. & CAVANAUGH M. (1945) The effect of terminal connections on the caliber of nerve fibres. *Anatomical Record*, **92**, 215–33.

WELLER W.L. & JOHNSON J.I. (1975) Barrels in cerebral cortex altered by receptor disruption in newborn, but not in five-day-old mice. (Cricetidae and Muridae). *Brain Research*, **8**, 504–8.

WESTRUM L.E. (1975) Axonal patterns in olfactory cortex after olfactory bulb removal in newborn rats. *Experimental Neurology*, **47**, 442–7.

WESTRUM L.E. & BLACK R.G. (1971) Fine structural aspects of the synaptic organisation of the spinal trigeminal nucleus (pars interpolaris) of the cat. *Brain Research*, **25**, 265–87.

WHITE L.E.J. & WESTRUM L.E. (1964) Dendritic spine changes in prepyriform cortex following olfactory bulb lesions—rat, Golgi method. *Anatomical Record*, **148**, 410–11.

WINDLE W.F. (1956) Regeneration of axons in the vertebrate central nervous system. *Physiological Reviews*, **36**, 427–40.

WOODS B.T. & TEUBER H-L. (1973) Early onset of complementary specialization of cerebral hemispheres in man. *Transactions of the American Neurological Association*, **98**, 113–17.

ZALEWSKI A.A. (1970) Reinnervation of denervated skeletal muscle by axons of motor, sensory and sympathetic neurons. *The Physiologist*, **13**, 354.

ZALEWSKI A.A. (1973) Regeneration of taste buds in tongue grafts after reinnervation by neurons in transplanted lumbar sensory ganglia. *Experimental Neurology*, **40**, 161–9.

Chapter 4
Clinical Neurophysiology in Rehabilitation

There are those who see no need for neurophysiology in rehabilitation and no need for research, or at least for technical methods of research. By implication these people must either be satisfied with the existing state of neurological rehabilitation or regard the situation as hopeless. The aim of this chapter is to disenchant the former and encourage the latter.

It is difficult to begin without admitting that clinical neurophysiology has contributed rather little to the rehabilitation of the CNS damaged patient in the past. Perhaps this has been because the only widely applied technique has been electroencephalography (EEG) which relates only distantly to the rehabilitation process. Electromyography (EMG) on the other hand and nerve conduction studies have been successfully used by rehabilitation specialists themselves to observe denervation, re-innervation and other changes. There are many excellent texts available which the interested reader may consult.

In this chapter some ideas and lines of research which are being pursued in clinical departments or in laboratories devoted to animal work and which seem pertinent to rehabilitation are summarized and discussed. In many cases direct application of the ideas or techniques into rehabilitation practice may seem remote, but remote ideas have been developed into important practices by gifted persons, often in a rather short space of time. Should none of this happen, neurophysiology still offers objective methods for studying the function of a damaged nervous system and how it changes as the CNS adapts to damage. Just as the function of the heart is to pump blood, so the function of the nervous system is to adapt to changing circumstances. Even though the dead nerve cells are not replaced, the CNS still adapts to injury; imperfectly to be sure, but it changes none the less, and one role of the neurophysiologist is to observe and understand these changes. Another role is to measure carefully any beneficial or harmful change which might have been wrought by treatment and to suggest possible procedures which may alleviate particular problems.

WHY NEUROPHYSIOLOGY?

It might be asked why neurophysiology should be thought at all relevant to rehabilitation, as it is a study of events within the nervous system whereas rehabilitation is concerned with the restoration of capabilities which lie outside the nervous system. We all possess a nervous system which is more or less the same as that of our fellows in terms of anatomy and physiology. This applies whether our lives have developed the skills of force (labouring, physical sports), the skills of dexterity and aestheticism (artist, musician) or merely the skills of daily living. Whatever the skills, the same neurophysiological processes are common to all. Impairment can therefore be expressed in physiological terms while functional limitation, handicap and disability are all compounded concepts developed from the interaction between impairment and life style, social status, ideas of normality and premorbid skills.

Diagnosis

Clinical neurophysiology is, at present, a diagnostic service whereas rehabilitation begins after a diagnosis has been made. Perhaps this is the reason why the two fields have not interacted very much in the past. The neurophysiologist who would become interested in rehabilitation must approach clinical problems differently; he needs to try and define the precise extent of impairment and the extent of physiological adaptation or maladaptation to the original disease or injury. The problems become those of assessment and progress.

Assessment

The first meeting point of neurophysiology and rehabilitation could be in the neurological assessment of a patient entering a course of rehabilitation. The diagnosis has been firmly established, all appropriate acute treatments have been applied and the prognosis is known to an acceptable level of probability. One begins with an evaluation and assesses degrees of paralysis, spasticity, lack of coordination etc. It is here that neurophysiological techniques allow a more detailed evaluation than clinical methods. Readers of this book are no doubt aware of the need for better, more thorough and more relevant methods of assessment. It must be appreciated that the clinical neurological signs probably will not change, but the immutability of signs such as extensor plantar responses and brisk tendon reflexes do not preclude significant functional changes which can favourably alter life style.

   Assessment of patients at the beginning of a programme of rehabilitation is a fundamental activity of the rehabilitation team and must extend across all aspects of human function and behaviour, from an assessment of a person's financial status, his family and home circumstances through to personal activities such as sexual, physical and vegetative functions, sometimes going into extreme details such as whether a particular muscle can produce any tension and how much. The team frequently have to take decisions which have moral implications that often colour one's approach to a particular patient. There is a need to assess an apparent lack of function as due to fear of pain, to hysterical overlay, to malingering, to overemphasis on matters of legal compensation, and to separate such factors from more organic problems. In this area objective tests of function can be very valuable in helping to resolve doubts.

One neurophysiological test which has been used for many years in assessing head-injury patients is the EEG. It must be admitted that its usefulness is limited, and it is well known that a successfully rehabilitated patient may possess a very abnormal EEG and the converse is not infrequently seen. There is a very important role for EEG in the management of post-traumatic epilepsy.

Signal processing techniques have been applied to the EEG and this work is of potential interest to rehabilitation for it demonstrates features in the brain waves which cannot be assessed by eye such as the coherence of rhythms in two areas. Psychiatric interest has been stimulated by work which shows an apparent lack of coordination between the two hemispheres in certain schizophrenic states (Shaw *et al.*, 1977; Wexler, 1980). In the past such technology has been expensive, but the coming of microprocessors brings sophisticated signal analysis within financial reach.

Evoked potentials are a method of assessing the response of the nervous system to stimuli. These techniques may well be more relevant to the study of the rehabilitation process than the EEG which records only the activity of an awake but otherwise inactive brain. The short latency components of evoked potentials are an indication of activity in the subcortical pathways. Next are potentials reflecting early cortical and cortico–thalamo–cortical pathways and finally a group of potentials, the late potentials, are seen which vary according to the 'set' or expectation of the subject. It is possible therefore to trace the sensory volley and integrative processes of the brain to the point where meaning is assigned to the signal, where decisions are made on the basis of the signal and even beyond. A number of pre-motor potentials have also been identified which can be traced back from a motor act to the motor command from the motor cortex and back to the time where the command signal is being prepared. It is too early to identify clinical uses of these techniques, but it is very encouraging to have them at one's disposal. Early studies on evoked potentials in head injuries have been concerned with assessing coma; there are indications, however, that the later components of evoked potentials may be very sensitive indicators of cerebral dysfunction after even mild head injuries.

Evoked potentials are fashionable at present and their shapes and sizes are being recorded in every conceivable condition. It is unfortunate that few workers have attempted to discover the precise generator mechanisms of the waves, for until an explanation rather than a description of the potentials is given this valuable new technique will only be of empirical use. Empirical techniques are useful in medicine, especially in diagnosis, but neurological rehabilitation demands greater insight into the CNS than can be offered by empiricism. Some workers have suggested possible explanations and it is now clear that the visual evoked potential can be used to estimate conduction time in the optic nerve (McDonald, 1977) and that different combinations of spinal and cortical potentials can also be used to estimate conduction times in the long ascending tracts. The spinal cord potentials (El-Negamy & Sedgwick, 1978) give an indication of the excitability of the first synapse in the somatosensory system while the early click-evoked brain-stem potentials provide similar information on the auditory system (Desmedt, 1977). A start has been made on following the changes in evoked potentials in chronic neurological disease and the findings suggest that evoked potentials will play an important role in evaluating progress and treatment (Matthews & Small, 1979; Robinson & Rudge, 1978; Sedgwick *et al.*, 1980).

One surprising outcome of neurophysiological assessment has been the discovery of surviving axons in patients who were thought to have complete traumatic spinal cord lesions. Using a technique called polyelectromyography (pEMG) to be described below, Dimitrijevic and his colleagues (1977; 1980) have shown that muscles below the lesion can be influenced to contract subclinically by Jendrassik's and similar manoeuvres even when the cord lesion is clinically complete.

The findings suggest that some fibres cross the traumatized area of cord and facilitate motoneurons in the surviving caudal segment. They are presumed to be small reticulospinal and propriospinal pathways. These surviving fibres are of no functional use and indeed they may be contributing to the spasticity which appears to be more severe in these patients than in those with clinically and neurophysiologically complete lesions.

Progress

Having made a thorough assessment of a patient one must selectively reassess certain functions from time to time to measure progress and the effects of treatment. One of the major problems in rehabilitation is to know just what effect, if any, treatment has and what changes are due to the natural history of the repairing process. To an outsider the unquestioned acceptance of very expensive and prolonged treatment regimes administered by physiotherapists is a continuing surprise. If the techniques of physiotherapy were subjected to rigorous assessment, like new drugs, then the services of well-trained physiotherapists could be used to greater effect and with more confidence. Neurophysiological techniques should be able to aid in showing the effectiveness, or otherwise, of different physical, pharmacological and surgical treatments.

Research

There has been so little use of neurophysiological techniques in rehabilitation that almost any series of investigations has a research element to it in the sense that similar work will not have been reported previously. That a project 'has not been done before' is not, however, sufficient reason for doing it. One has to construct an hypothesis which is testable by applying the techniques available in such a way that the results will unequivocally support or refute the starting hypothesis. All of this must be accomplished within the framework of ethical considerations for the patients. The role of neurophysiological techniques in research into the rehabilitation of the neurological patient is self evident, especially as nearly all the techniques are non-invasive and risk free.

WHAT NEUROPHYSIOLOGY?

The accompanying table lists neurophysiological techniques all of which involve the measurement of factors which are relevant to neurological rehabilitation. A lesion of the nervous system can alter the parameters of one or several of the functions listed. In this section a few of the more generally applicable techniques are described. The techniques are mostly non-invasive and risk free and the majority require little cooperation by the patient.

Table 4.1 List of neurophysiological investigations available.

	Test	CNS level
1.	Conduction velocity of muscle fibre	Muscle
2.	Neuromuscular transmission	Motor end plate
3.	Motor unit: firing pattern	Motor unit
	force generation	
	territory	
	recruitment	
	number	
4.	Nerve conduction velocity	Nerve
5.	Single fibre conduction velocity	
	Sensory nerve function	
	Autonomic fibre activity	
6.	Muscle spindle activity	Motoneuron
7.	F-response	Motoneuron and ventral root
	Monosynaptic reflex excitability	Spinal
	Flexor reflex	Spinal
	Cutaneous and other reflexes	Spinal
8.	Autonomic bladder reflexes	Spinal
9.	Presynaptic inhibition	Spinal
	1a. interneurone inhibition	Spinal
	1b. interneurone inhibition	Spinal
	Renshaw cell inhibition	Spinal
10.	Conduction times in central tracts	Long tracts
11.	Brain stem—auditory pathway	Brain stem
	Brain stem reflexes: Blink	
	Pinna	
	Stapedius	
12.	Respiratory centre—CO_2 response	Brain stem
13.	Long loop reflexes	Rostro-caudal tracts
14.	Sensory evoked responses	Sensory pathways
15.	EEG	Cortex
16.	Motor potentials	Cortex

The list (Table 4.1) gives a good indication of the range of neurophysiological techniques and measurements at present available. It is beyond the scope of this chapter to explain how each is performed or in which cases they should be used. Rather one would wish to encourage those proposing a course of treatment, whether physical or pharmacological, to identify and describe patients' problems in physiological terms as well as in medical and social terms. Then some objective test of the physiological process to be influenced is applied before, during and after treatment. An analogy might be the treatment of anaemia, which one would not begin without a haemoglobin measurement; in rehabilitation, however, extensive treatments are given for spasticity without any objective measure of spasticity and without any objective measure of the outcome. Only by detailed studies will rehabilitation be able to establish rational bases for treatment and show that they work.

Polyelectromyography

Polyelectromyography (pEMG) consists of recording many channels of EMG through surface electrodes on the arms or legs of a subject. An ink jet EEG recording machine is almost ideal for the purpose, but pen recorders can also be used. The electromyogram is a high frequency signal and much of the artefact produced by movement is of low frequency and can be reduced by adjustment of the amplifier bandwidth characteristics. Bipolar recordings from disc electrodes stuck 20–40 mm apart over the muscles are used, and low noise cable, together with arrangements to prevent lead sway and friction, helps to cut down movement artefact. We follow a similar convention to that used in EEG; the first channels at the top of the paper record from the most proximal muscles on the right side and the last channels will therefore record the most distal muscles on the left.

A standard recording protocol is used, but the physician and an experienced technician will add to it according to their findings and the idiosyncrasies of the subject. It is essential to record from normal subjects in order to learn the normal responses and to recognize artefacts and 'crosstalk' from deep muscles to the one immediately beneath the electrodes. An outline of a protocol is given in Fig. 4.1. Each procedure is repeated three times to get an estimate of habituation. In the course of one hour a very detailed and semi-quantitative estimate of spasticity and the response of motoneuron pools to various centripetal and centrifugal influences can be determined and recorded for comparison with later pEMGs. The initial recording can assist in planning therapy and subsequent ones help to determine if treatment has been effective. Of course techniques can be refined with quantitative forms of stimulation, i.e. constant force tendon hammers, goniometers and devices for moving joints at constant rates, and the resultant EMG can be quantified by signal analysis such as integration. pEMG can be used as an adjunct to drug trials in spasticity, trials of physiotherapeutic regimes,

OUTLINE SCHEME of THE pEMG EXAMINATION

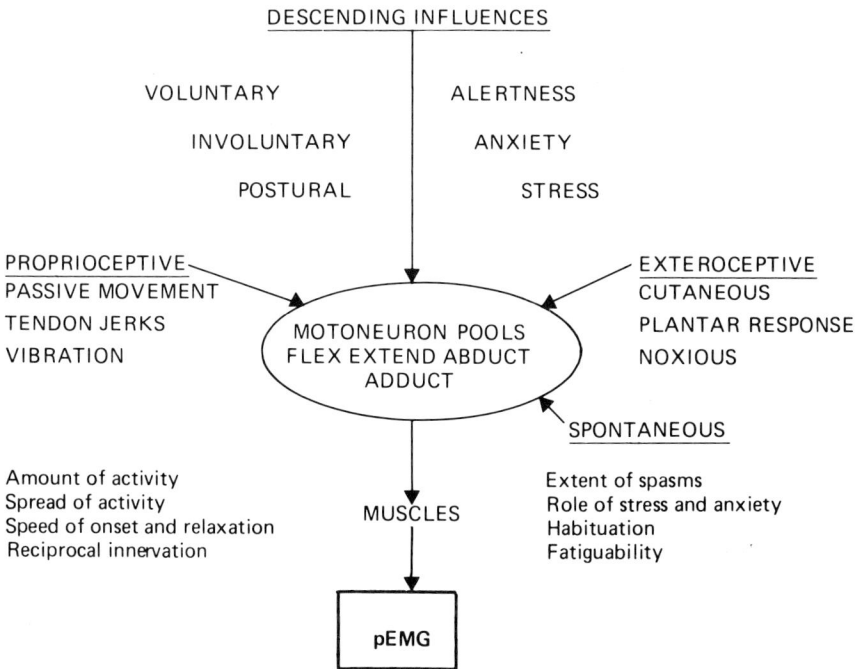

DESCENDING INFLUENCES

VOLUNTARY　　　　ALERTNESS

INVOLUNTARY　　　ANXIETY

POSTURAL　　　　　STRESS

PROPRIOCEPTIVE　　　　　　　　　　　　　EXTEROCEPTIVE
PASSIVE MOVEMENT　　　　　　　　　　　CUTANEOUS
TENDON JERKS　　MOTONEURON POOLS　PLANTAR RESPONSE
VIBRATION　　　　FLEX EXTEND ABDUCT　NOXIOUS
　　　　　　　　　　　　ADDUCT

SPONTANEOUS

Amount of activity　　　　　　　　　Extent of spasms
Spread of activity　　　MUSCLES　　Role of stress and anxiety
Speed of onset and relaxation　　　Habituation
Reciprocal innervation　　　　　　　Fatiguability

pEMG

Fig. 4.1 The diagram indicates the different central and peripheral influences on the motoneuron pools of flexor, extensors etc. which can be tested during a pEMG examination for their part in the production of spasticity. The record is examined also for the features noted in smaller type.

but more fundamentally just to observe the natural history of conditions as Twitchell (1951) did for hemiplegia.

It has been mainly through use of pEMG in patients with spinal cord trauma that has led to the demonstration by Dimitrijevic *et al.* (1977) that many patients with clinically complete spinal cord lesions do, in fact, have some preserved descending pathways which can influence motor unit and reflex activity caudal to the lesion. It is rare for a spinal cord to be severed completely; there is usually some tissue bridge across the region and this may contain surviving nerve tracts, possibly propriospinal or small reticulospinal fibres. The demonstration of surviving pathways is of extreme theoretical importance as it maintains the possibility of using impulses in these pathways to trigger some of the automatic functions in the distal cord. It has also been proposed that the isolated spinal cord can respond only phasically to peripheral stimuli and that regular stimuli soon lose their effect or habituate. Patients with complete lesions tend not to experience sustained spasticity but have flaccid limbs.

We have used pEMG to assess changes in motor function of patients with multiple sclerosis who were undergoing a trial of spinal cord stimulation. The technique is extremely valuable for assessing fatiguability of repetitive movements and the speed and regularity with which they can be carried out. Fig. 4.2 is an example of a portion of pEMG record of the muscles of one leg of a patient with an apparently clinically complete traumatic spinal cord lesion. All the muscles become active during a short period of breath holding and continue active after exhalation. The second trial gives a smaller response, indicating some degree of habituation.

pEMG is only semi-quantitative and it only records 45–60 minutes of a patient's day. Other techniques are necessary to follow fluctuations in spasticity throughout the day and according to medication. Small tape recorders are available which will monitor 24 hours of ECG or EEG over 1–4 channels and

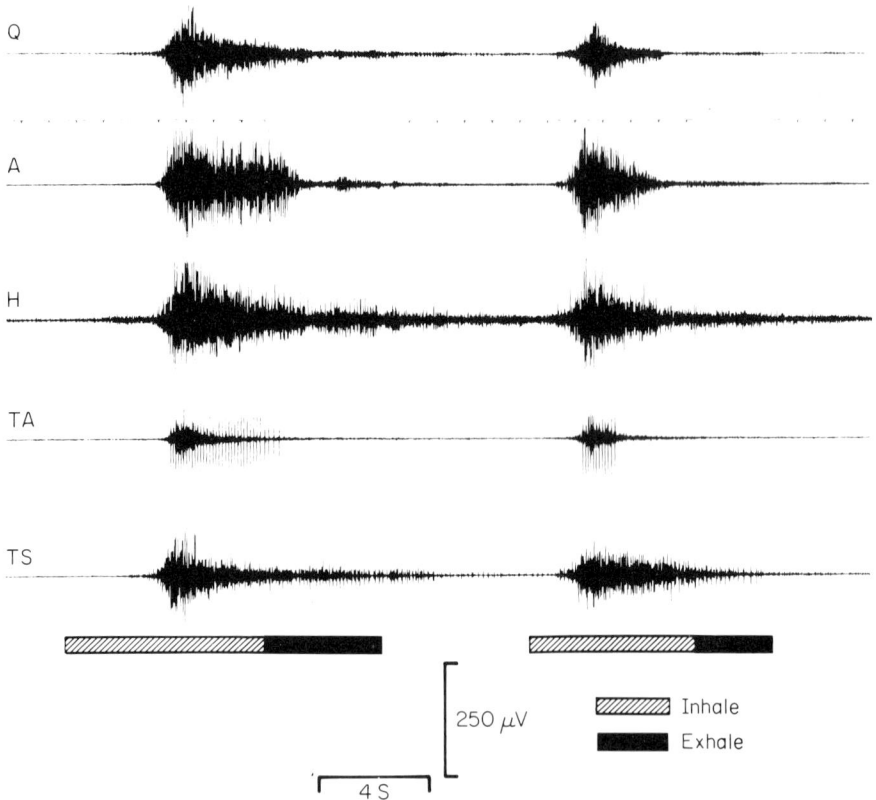

Fig. 4.2 Part of a pEMG recording of the activity in muscles of one leg of a patient with traumatic paraplegia: Q, quadriceps; A. adductors; H, hamstrings; TA, tibialis anterior; TS, triceps surae. Muscle spasm was triggered by a deep inhalation after a 3 second delay and continues after exhalation. (Kindly supplied by Professor M. R. Dimitrijevic.)

could, with minimal modification, be used to record EMG. One principle for artefact-free recording is to have the amplifier as close to the pickup electrode as possible and pickup electrodes which are an integral part of a small first-stage amplifier are now commercially available (Oxford Medical Systems Ltd, Oxford, England).

Interpretation is facilitated by considering a pEMG as measuring the responsiveness of motoneuron pools to different inputs and Fig. 4.1 gives an outline of how to organize a pEMG recording and how to interpret the findings. A series of pEMG observations very pertinent to spasticity have been made by Dimitrijevic and Nathan (1967a; b; 1968; 1970; 1971).

Inhibition in the Spinal Cord

Workers in animal physiology have shown very clearly the existence of three important groups of inhibitory interneurons in the spinal cord. They are: the Renshaw cell which is excited by collaterals from motoneurons and inhibits motoneurons of the same pool; the 1a inhibitory neuron which is excited by incoming volleys from muscle spindles and inhibits motoneurons of the antagonist muscle; the Golgi inhibitory neuron which is excited by impulses from Golgi tendon organs (tension receptors) and inhibits motoneurons of the same muscle. These neurons are shown diagrammatically in Fig. 4.3. Their existence in a similar form in human spinal cord is assumed and recently indirect methods of studying their functions have been devised.

Use of the size of the H reflex as a test of monosynaptic reflex excitability has permitted a study of no less than four different spinal segmental inhibitory mechanisms. The H reflex, so called after Hoffmann (1918) who first described it, is a reflex muscle twitch of soleus produced by electrical stimulation of the low threshold muscle afferent fibres of the tibial nerve; these are large diameter, fast conducting class 1a fibres from muscle spindles. Electrical stimulation of the muscle nerve therefore gives a precisely controlled afferent volley which monosynaptically excites the motoneurons in the same way as a tap on the Achilles tendon. At rest the H reflex occurs only in soleus, but it can also be obtained in arm and hand and other muscles which are actively contracting.

Under favourable conditions a single volley in the tibial nerve will excite 30–80% of the soleus motoneuron pool; the amplitude of soleus EMG is used as a measure of the number of motoneurons activated. Two closely spaced volleys, say up to 10 ms apart, will temporally summate to produce a larger response. With more widely spaced volleys the second shock fails to elicit a response until the shocks are 50 ms or so apart when a complex 'recovery' cycle begins and goes on for up to 3–5 s. This recovery cycle has been extensively studied and is of different form in hemiplegic spasticity, extrapyramidal disorders and cerebellar disease (Matthews, 1970). Interesting though these findings are they have led to no significant insight into the pathophysiology of these neurological

Spinal segmental inhibitory mechanisms

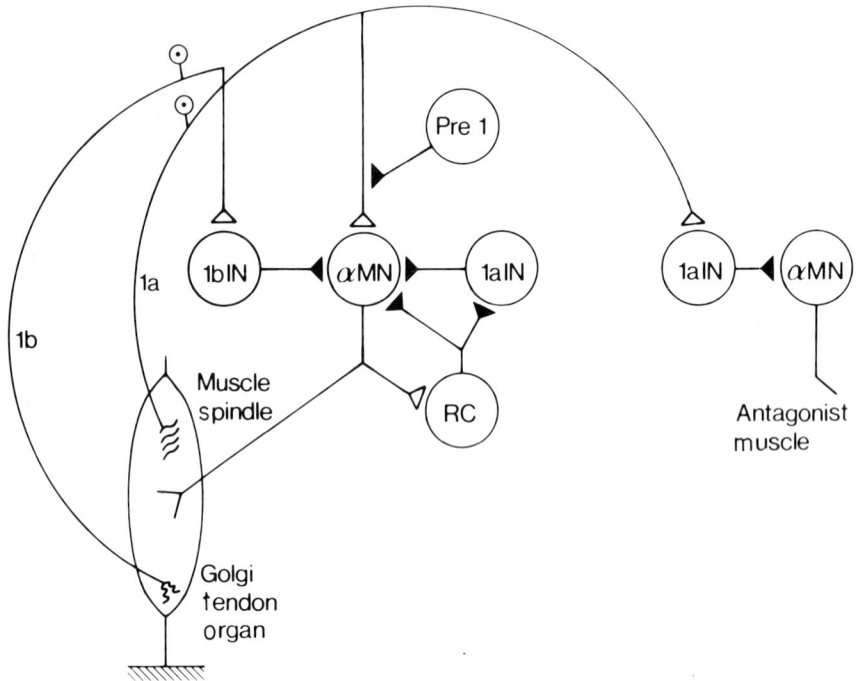

Fig. 4.3. Spinal segmental inhibitory mechanisms. The alpha motoneuron (α MN) is excited by 1a afferent fibres from muscle spindles of its own muscle which also inhibit the α MN of the antagonist muscle by activating the 1a inhibitory inter-neuron (1a IN). The Golgi tendon organs inhibit their own MN by way of the 1b interneurone (1b IN) and there is recurrent inhibition by the Renshaw cell (RC). The presynaptic inhibitory interneurons (Pre I) have not been anatomically or physiologically identified.

syndromes. The real interest in the H reflex now lies in its use in studying spinal segmental mechanisms. The segmental mechanisms to be mentioned here are shown diagrammatically in Fig. 4.3.

An interesting series of experiments by Tanaka and colleagues (Mizuno *et al.*, 1971; Simoyama & Tanaka, 1974; Tanaka, 1972; 1974; Yaragisawa *et al.*, 1976) used the size of the H reflex of soleus after stimulation of the tibial nerve as an indication of monosynaptic excitability of soleus motoneurons. A preceding stimulus to the peroneal nerve which supplies tibialis anterior, an antagonist of soleus, should, they argue, excite the 1a inhibitory neuron which projects on to soleus motoneurons and the soleus H reflex should therefore be reduced in size. By careful timing of the conditioning stimulus to the peroneal nerve and by adjustment of the stimulus strength so that it gave a maximal 1a volley and minimally excited other fibres, they were able to explore the nature of inhibition mediated by the 1a interneuron (IN). It is thought that the process of reciprocal innervation (relaxation of the antagonist muscle while the agonist contracts) is mediated by the 1a IN and, as reciprocal innervation fails in spasticity, a study of its mechanism is of great interest in clinical neurophysiology.

The studies show that, at rest, a single peroneal nerve volley fails to activate the 1a IN as the soleus H reflex remains unchanged. If, however, a small voluntary contraction of tibialis anterior is made, the 1a IN receives excitatory synaptic bombardment from two sources. First there is an excitatory input from the corticospinal tract and possibly from other descending motor pathways (Jankowska & Tanaka, 1974); the second excitatory input is from the muscle spindle afferents which are excited by contraction of the muscle (tibialis anterior in this case). Under these conditions an additional electrically induced volley in the peroneal nerve produces an inhibition of the soleus H reflex of about 30%.

Studies on neurological patients are incomplete and await confirmation, but the following pattern of 1a IN activity has emerged. In athetosis the 1a IN is active even at rest, while in spastic hemiplegia there is some evidence that the activity of the 1a IN is unbalanced. It seems that the 1a IN can be activated by the extensor muscle to inhibit the dorsiflexor but not by the flexor to inhibit the extensor; the normal reciprocal innervation is therefore disrupted. This could be one factor underlying the weakness of ankle dorsiflexors seen in hemiplegia.

Further alteration of the timing and strength of the conditioning stimulus to the peroneal nerve reveals another period of inhibition of the H reflex lasting from 7 to 30 ms after arrival of the peroneal nerve volley. Tanaka (1972; 1974) suggests that this is presynaptic inhibition because it has characteristics similar to presynaptic inhibition seen in animals. The concept of presynaptic inhibition is not fully established in the mammalian spinal cord and its physiological role is not clear. For the present, one should retain the term 'presynaptic' inhibition even though the name remote inhibition proposed by Frank (1959), who first described the phenomenon, seems more appropriate. Recently Carlen *et al.* (1980) have used modern techniques to show that 'presynaptic' inhibition is accompanied by post synaptic changes in the motoneuron which could explain some, if not all, the inhibitory phenomena and show that the inhibition occurs remote from the perikaryon and out on the dendrites. Whatever the precise mechanism may turn out to be, Tanaka has demonstrated motoneuron inhibition in man similar in time course to presynaptic inhibition by using an experimental protocol equivalent to that used in animals. It is not yet known if this type of inhibition is altered in disease states. Ashby *et al.* (1974) have suggested the absence of presynaptic inhibition in man suffering from chronic spinal lesions, but their methods were indirect and assumptions had to be made to relate their data to the presynaptic inhibitory mechanism.

A third inhibitory system, that from the Golgi tendon organs on to the homologous and synergist muscles, has been studied in normal subjects by Pierrot-Deseilligny *et al.* (1979), again using the H reflex as a test of motoneuron excitability. It is not yet known whether this type of inhibition is altered by upper motoneuron lesions.

Finally there is the recurrent inhibition provided by the Renshaw neurons; so called after the man who, on the basis of physiological experiment, postulated their existence. These neurons are excited by discharges of motoneurons and feedback inhibition into the homologous motoneuron pool. Their precise role, and even the extent of distribution of their axons, is unknown. Control engineers have been quick to point out, however, that they appear to form part of a negative feedback loop which would regulate and stabilize the firing of the motoneurons, perhaps matching the rate of firing to the physical properties of the muscle and smoothing recruitment of motoneurons to make for evenly regulated muscle tension. Bussel and Pierrot-Deseilligny (1977) and Hultborn and Pierrot-Deseilligny (1979) have demonstrated presumed Renshaw neuron inhibition in normal man, but no studies of disease states are yet available.

There are, then, four spinal segmental inhibitory mechanisms which can be studied non-invasively in man: the 1a IN, presynaptic inhibition, Golgi tendon organ inhibition and Renshaw inhibition. We teach students that spasticity is caused by a release of motoneurons from inhibitions; now there is an opportunity to demonstrate whether these four types of inhibition are the ones from which the motoneuron is released. If they are involved, as seems likely, in movement disorders and if their neurotransmitter mechanisms can be elucidated by animal experiments then a sensible pharmacological strategy for the treatment of spasticity could be evolved, tried and monitored objectively.

WHICH NEUROPHYSIOLOGY?

Scientific neurophysiology is a notoriously difficult field for the non-specialist. The literature is a bewildering collection of technical terms borrowed from control engineering, chemistry and physics with added abbreviations conspiring to make papers read like a foreign language. In this section some of the recent advances in neurophysiology are briefly reviewed. These topics have been selected for their potential importance to rehabilitation of the neurological patient. Nearly all the experimental work was done on animals so that interspecies assumptions have to be made; nevertheless a small but highly significant proportion of the work derives from human studies.

Trophic Factors

The close relationship between nerve and muscle is dramatically illustrated by the effects of denervation. The immediate result is paralysis as impulses no longer reach the muscle. The sarcolemma of muscle fibres begins to change immediately after denervation, and alterations in ionic permeability and sodium pump activity soon result in a lowered resting membrane potential. From the region of the end plate, acetylcholine receptors spread along the fibre. The end plate itself becomes unstable and spontaneously generated action potentials, fibrillation potentials, appear. The fibres loose contractile protein and a large number of histological atrophic changes begin culminating in replacement of muscle bulk by fibrous tissue, but small atrophic muscle fibres survive for many years. Subsequent contraction of the fibrous tissue results in contractures. If the denervation is partial, the remaining nerves will sprout collaterals which will innervate neighbouring denervated fibres.

To what extent are the atrophic changes attributable to disuse of the muscle and which, if any, can be attributed to the absence of a trophic substance? If there is a trophic substance, is it acetylcholine (ACh) or some other chemical? Disuse of a muscle results in wasting, which is mainly loss of contractile protein, and this well-known clinical phenomenon is reversible. Other changes such as fibrillation potentials and sprouting of innervating nerves do not occur in disuse atrophy, but these changes are not prevented by direct electrical stimulation of denervated muscle. These long established facts lead to the idea that nerve has a trophic or sustaining effect on muscle. Could this effect be simply the liberation of acetylcholine at the end plate? Liberation continues even during disuse as there is always some leakage of acetylcholine from the end plate even in the absence of impulses, there are leaked packages which evoke miniature end plate potentials at the muscle fibre as well as molecular leakage. If not acetylcholine, could there be a specific trophic substance, or group of substances, liberated at the same time as acetylcholine or perhaps leaking out continually? It is well established that axonal transport carries a considerable quantity of material down the axon. Much of this is protein and enzymes as these can only be manufactured in the perikaryon. Amino acids, prostaglandins and protein are known to leak out of the nerve at the motor end plate.

The cross re-innervation experiments beginning with those of Buller *et al.* (1960) boosted interest in trophic substances. They showed that a nerve taken from a fast-twitch muscle (e.g. flexor digitorum longus of the cat) would innervate a previously denervated slow-twitch muscle (soleus) and convert it into a fast-twitch muscle. The speed of muscle contraction depends on two factors, the speed of liberation and uptake of Ca^{2+} by sarcoplasmic reticulum and the rate of a reaction controlled by a calcium-dependent enzyme, myosin adenosine triphosphatase, which is involved in the formation of cross bridges between actin and myosin. The cross re-innervated muscles showed appropriate biochemical changes in their myosin adenosine triphosphatase and in the speed of movement of Ca^{2+} as well as other changes.

Slow muscles serve postural functions and tend to be excited by long steady trains of impulses at 10 Hz or so while fast muscles are only activated occasionally by fast short bursts of impulses (20–60 Hz). It has been shown that the speed of twitch of muscle can be altered by imposing upon it a particular firing pattern; this can be done experimentally by implanted stimulators. The trophic influence in this case seems to be a pattern of excitation and not a trophic substance (Buller & Pope, 1977).

Another aspect of trophic function which has come under close scrutiny in recent years is the production and distribution of ACh receptors on muscle fibres. Normally these are present in a high concentration only at the motor end plate. Shortly after denervation an increase in synthesis of these protein receptors has been observed in the muscle fibre. The receptors are transported to, and incorporated in, clusters or hot spots along the whole of the length of the muscle fibre membrane. Here they survive for 6–36 hours before being destroyed by usual lysosomal mechanisms but are replaced by continuing synthesis. Denervation therefore stimulates genetically controlled protein synthesis.

Direct electrical excitation of muscle early after denervation will prevent the increase in ACh receptors. The complete blocking of action potentials in the nerve by local anaesthetics or by botulinum toxin which prevents most ACh release results in some increase in ACh receptors. Muscle activity therefore seems to be the major regulator for production of ACh receptors and this is possibly mediated by the adenylcyclase system or by the concentration of intracellular Ca^{2+}.

Acetylcholinesterase (AChE), normally associated with ACh receptors at the motor end plate, does not appear at the newly formed ACh receptor hot spots unless the hot spot becomes innervated by a regenerating nerve. Re-innervation is independent of nerve or muscle activity but cannot occur in the absence of ACh receptor hot spots. When the muscle fibre is reactivated ACh receptor synthesis is turned off and receptors concentrate and stabilize at the new end plate. The fibre begins synthesis of AChE which also concentrates at the end plate.

Despite 20 years of vigorous investigation no trophic substance has been discovered, but the importance of muscle activity has been emphasized. The role of ACh release as a trophic agent is still not clear, but Drachman (1974) points out that, in the absence of ACh, any other trophic substance that may be released from a nerve is incapable of preventing degenerative change. Detailed molecular mechanisms such as these may seem remote from rehabilitation, but an understanding of the processes of disuse and denervation degeneration are fundamental to rehabilitation.

Trans-synaptic Degeneration

The occurrence or not of trans-synaptic degeneration has long been debated. There has been growing evidence of trans-synaptic degeneration of motoneurons in man for some years and a detailed review of it is given by McComas (1977). Standard electromyographic examination of muscles of patients with hemiplegia or spinal injury reveals fibrillation potentials in the muscles of the affected side for a few months after onset, beginning after 1–3 months. Care was taken to exclude any patients with pressure palsies, to which the partially paralysed are especially susceptible. McComas made estimates of the number of motor units in patients with hemiplegia and found a reduction of up to 50%. The findings are explained by a loss of motoneurons and this is borne out by motoneuron counts in autopsy studies of patients dying with hemiplegia. In explanation it is suggested that the upper motor neuron lesion deprives the motoneuron of some trophic influence and some of the motoneurons die as a result.

This phenomenon could be fruitfully studied in a rehabilitation department and much could be learned about the dynamics of trans-synaptic degeneration in man simply by applying routine electromyographic techniques to appropriate subjects at suitable times during their recovery.

Spinal injury would remove a considerable amount of descending influence, but the only tract from the cortex or internal capsule to the spinal cord is the corticospinal tract and most of its terminals are on interneurons rather than directly on to motoneurons. How, therefore, can its loss produce such considerable degeneration of motoneurons?

The Motor Unit

The concept of the motor unit as a functional and anatomical entity has been well established for many years. The recruitment of more and more motor units into activity to give greater muscle tension is well established and the size principle of Henneman is now widely accepted. This principle, arising first from animal experiments (Henneman *et al.*, 1965), is that, during graded muscular activity, units producing small tensions are recruited first and those producing large tensions are recruited later. The organization within the CNS to produce such an orderly pattern seems quite simple. The small motor unit consists of anatomically few muscle fibres which are innervated by a relatively small diameter axon which in turn arises from a small motoneuron. The membrane of motoneurons behaves electrically as a resistor and capacitor in parallel and therefore the larger the area of membrane the lower is its electrical resistance. A standard excitation will therefore produce a higher voltage excitatory post-synaptic potential in small motoneurons than in large ones. In the large ones the excitation current flows through the low resistance membrane and a high voltage cannot build up. The small neurons therefore will be the first to be depolarized to their excitation threshold. It has also been established that all the muscle fibres innervated by one motoneuron are of the same biochemical type and therefore have common mechanical properties such as twitch speed and fatigue resistance. With such a wealth of detailed physiological and biochemical knowledge about motor units the time is ripe to study them in man in health and disease. Fortunately recent technical developments enable exploration of new areas in man with usually no more inconvenience than the insertion of a needle.

Single fibre EMG (sfEMG) is a technique which has been pioneered by

Stalberg and Ekstedt (1973). To record a sfEMG a needle electrode with a very small recording surface (25 μm diameter) of dimensions similar to that of the diameter of a muscle fibre is inserted into the muscle; the recording surface is on the side of the needle to avoid recording from damaged fibres at the tip. With care, the needle can be adjusted to record two potentials from two fibres innervated by the same motoneuron.

The discharges of the two fibres will be separated in time due to the different conduction times in their innervating nerve terminals and different distances from the motor end plates to the recording site. The time between discharges on successive occasions is not constant but varies within a range of 50 μs. This variation is called jitter and it is a measure of the time taken for a nerve impulse to excite the muscle fibre. In myasthena gravis, nerve–muscle excitation is uncertain and a prolonged jitter is seen; sometimes only one fibre is excited, indicating a block of neuromuscular transmission to its companion. Increased jitter and blockage of impulses can be observed even in asymptomatic muscles in myasthenia gravis.

Another useful measure in sfEMG is fibre density. The small needle electrode can record potentials from fibres within a radius of about 270 μm. Normally there are one or two fibres within the area supplied by the same motor unit so that recording from multiple sites will yield an average of 1.5 fibres recorded per site; a fibre density of 1.5. After partial denervation and re-innervation the fibre density increases to 2–10 or even higher. The newly innervated fibres also show an increased jitter.

The technique is a very sensitive indicator of disturbances of nerve–muscle transmission and increased jitter has been noted in polymyositis, spinal muscular atrophy, neuropathies and a number of other conditions. So far it has not been applied in problems of rehabilitation, but its use as described or modified to test some aspect or motor unit function in rehabilitation can only be a matter of time.

To ask how many motoneurons supply a particular muscle in man has been an impossible question to answer, but McComas (1977) has described a very simple technique for motor unit counting. Carefully placed electrodes on the skin over a muscle record the very smallest potential following weak stimulation of the nerve. If the potential is a true 'all or none' phenomenon it must represent one motor unit. A slightly stronger stimulus will give an added all or none increment to the potential and by slowly adjusting the stimulus strength one tries to identify 5–10 or more increments and measure their voltage. One can then work out the average size of potential produced by one motor unit. Then a supramaximal stimulus is given and a maximal motor response recorded. It is then possible to work out how many individual motor units must have discharged to produce the maximal motor potential. There are, of course, assumptions and technicalities which lead to inaccuracies, but McComas believes this method counts correctly to within 20%.

These researches have shown that the number of motor units remains constant until the age of 60 years whereafter a steady decline is noted. The finding of reduced numbers of motor units in Duchenne dystrophy reopened the debate on the neural hypothesis of the disease and findings supporting either nerve or muscle hypotheses have been set out by McComas (1977). Although the neural hypothesis is losing ground the debate has stimulated research and led to an increased understanding of the motor unit.

By an ingenious application of signal processing techniques Milner-Brown *et al.* (1973a; b) have been able to define the contractile properties of single human motor units during isometric contraction. They were able to demonstrate quite clearly that the small motor units, producing low tensions, were always recruited into activity first and the larger ones were recruited when greater tensions were exerted. In subsequent papers (Milner-Brown *et al.*, 1974a; b) it was shown that this orderly recruitment was preserved after recovery from entrapment neuropathies but not after recovery from neurotmesis (nerve section). In motoneuron disease where high amplitude electrical potentials from surviving motor units are characteristic, one would expect these remaining motor units to produce large and fast twitches. However, this is not the case; the high amplitude units seem to be mechanically inefficient. Further application of this technique gives more insight into the nerve–muscle relationship in health and disease.

Axons

Axons in the CNS have been regarded by neurologists as passive transmission lines which work normally unless physically disrupted or demyelinated. The importance of the myelin sheath for rapid transmission of impulses has long been appreciated and the way impulses jump from node to node has been well established. Recent work, however, on experimentally demyelinated fibres in animals has revealed details of the relationship of axons and their myelin which allow explanations of certain clinical phenomena seen in demyelinating disease and indicate possible avenues for the search for therapeutic strategies. The work is reviewed by Rasminsky (1978), but it must be noted that the experimental methods use diphtheritic neuritis, certain genetic conditions in mice, compression blocks and experimental allergic encephalitis, which differ considerably in their clinical manifestations from multiple sclerosis, the most important demyelinating condition of the CNS in man. Computer models of nerve have also been used, and although these models cannot be better than the information used to build them, judicious testing of the model has revealed information which was not apparent from a consideration of the basic biological data.

Conduction of the action potential is a sequence of depolarization and repolarization of the axon membrane. Depolarization occurs when sodium channels in the axonal membrane open and permit sodium ions to flow into the fibre. The sodium channels are lipoprotein structures which, it is believed, can be visualized by the electron microscope after preparation of the specimen by a freeze-fracture technique. Their numbers can be estimated because they bind securely with certain toxins which can be isotope labelled. Using these methods it can be shown that there are about 500 times more sodium channels at nodes of Ranvier than on the internodal axon. It is thought that the paucity of sodium channels in a demyelinated segment would produce a small depolarization insufficient to trigger an action potential in the next part of the fibre. If demyelination is partial or the demyelinated segment very short the action potential may be conducted across the lesion at a slowed rate. The computer model shows such fibres exist on a knife edge between conduction and block. Conduction can be blocked by a slight rise in temperature, and it is thought that this is the basis of Uhthoff's phenomenon seen in multiple sclerosis where a patient's functional abilities decrease markedly if body temperature is raised by exercise, fever or climatic change. Reduction in Ca^{2+} can improve conduction and the clinical state of patients with multiple sclerosis.

It has been suggested (Schauf & Davis, 1974) that drugs which increase the time for which a sodium channel remains open, or decrease or delay the time of opening of potassium channels, would facilitate conduction of action potentials through areas of demyelination. So, too, would an increase in the number of sodium channels, but as yet we have no knowledge of how these are produced, although it is very probable that the oligodendrocytes which produce CNS myelin play a role in arranging the distribution of the sodium channels to concentrate at the nodes.

The altered function of demyelinated fibres underlies the use of evoked potentials in clinical diagnosis of multiple sclerosis. The visual evoked potential can be delayed in this condition thereby revealing a previously unsuspected lesion of the optic nerve; the demonstration of *multiple* lesions is fundamental to the diagnosis of *multiple* sclerosis. Few workers have yet studied the evolution of evoked potentials during the course of multiple sclerosis (Matthews & Small, 1979; Robinson & Rudge, 1978; Sedgwick *et al.*, 1980), but this is a simple procedure which could give valuable information about the state of the axons operating on a knife-edge. Such studies would be mandatory if an attempt were made to rehabilitate patients by modifying the sodium channels in their axons.

Muscle Spindles

Since the discovery of the role of these end organs in the stretch reflex they have been central to any consideration of spasticity, movement disorder or tremor. It is here that human studies have added so much to our understanding of muscle tone.

At rest the muscle spindle is not stretched and sends no impulses to the spinal cord. During contraction, however, the spindle shortens at the same rate as the muscle due to discharges in its own motor fibres (γ fibres) and sends a moderate barrage of impulses into the spinal cord where they contribute to the excitation of the motoneuron (α motoneuron). At the beginning of contraction both the α and γ motoneurons are excited simultaneously, called α/γ coactivation.

In any arresting disturbance of a planned movement the muscle spindle continues to attempt to shorten by stretching its elastic central region where the afferent fibre terminates; an increased barrage of afferent impulses is therefore induced and, on reaching the cord, will increase the activity of the α motoneurons thereby increasing the force of contraction and tending to overcome the arresting force. This mode of action is called the load compensation reflex because it provides the first immediate (30 ms or less) response to a disturbance (Phillips & Porter 1977).

Because, in spasticity, the muscles are so sensitive to slight manipulation it has been proposed that the γ motoneurons are overactive thereby enhancing the afferent discharge of the muscle spindles. This idea of an overactive γ system has received indirect experimental support (Rushworth, 1960) and has become firmly entrenched teaching. Unfortunately the idea has never been confirmed by modern experimental methods and is almost certainly incorrect. The Swedish neurophysiologists have devised microneuronography, a technique for recording individual nerve fibre activity in humans, and this has been applied to the study of muscle spindle activity in normal movement and in motor disorders. The limited experimental data so far available show that the γ motor system of spastic subjects at rest is not overactive (Vallbo *et al.*, 1979).

Physiological Tremor

Physiological tremor is a fine vibration of the limb at 8–12 Hz, the frequency being constant in any individual but the amplitude is extremely variable. The tremor is present when muscles are active and is produced by them; other factors such as the natural frequency of the oscillating limb and ballisto-cardiac effects are unable to account for it although they have a modulating effect. Physiological tremor increases with fatigue of the muscles, with the force of contraction, with anxiety, fright and with adrenaline, but not noradrenaline, infusion.

The role of the stretch reflex in physiological tremor has long been debated and now seems to be established as an important, but not necessarily the only, mechanism for its generation. Animal and human experiments have shown that the muscle spindle has a very much higher dynamic sensitivity to small perturbations of muscle length than to larger ones and the afferent discharges produced by spindles during tremor induce some degree of clustering of motoneuron discharge and hence small fluctuations in tension (Hagbarth & Young, 1979).

Muscle spindles and extrafusal muscle fibres have β adrenergic receptors which, when activated, cause increased sensitivity of spindles to stretch and faster extrafusal contraction. This has the effect of enhancing tremor. Tremors seen in thyrotoxicosis, benign essential tremor and alcohol withdrawal seem to

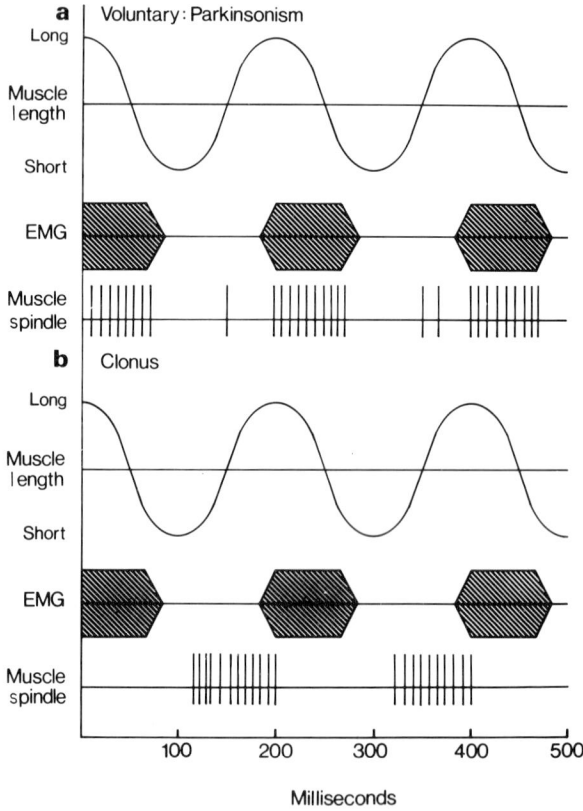

Fig. 4.4 The timing of afferent discharges from muscle spindles during voluntary and parkinsonian tremor is shown in A and they occur mainly during muscle contraction. During clonus, B, the discharges occur during the stretching phase.

have the same characteristics as exaggerated physiological tremor and can be attenuated by β adrenergic blocking drugs such as propanolol.

Pathological Tremor

Electromyographic recordings of pathological tremor show very clearly bursts of muscle activity indicating synchronization of motoneuron discharge. Whatever the pathological origin of tremor its rate is always slower than physiological tremor and usually falls in the 4–6 Hz range.

Clinicians know well the types of tremor associated with Parkinson's disease and cerebellar pathology, and physiologists and engineers have given a detailed and quantified picture of them. Drug therapies and destructive operations will modify tremor, but we are still ignorant of the local mechanisms which produce regular synchronous firing of motor units. The stretch reflex plays an important part in all theories, but the only direct physiological observations of the behaviour of the stretch receptors (muscle spindles) have been made by Hagbarth *et al.* (1975a; b).

During a voluntarily produced tremor, i.e. rapidly alternating movements, in a normal subject, the muscle is excited according to the principle of α/γ coactivation which produces impulses in the afferent fibres during muscle shortening. Sometimes the spindles will produce a second discharge during the lengthening phase when they are acting as stretch receptors (Fig. 4.4).

In parkinsonian tremor the α/γ link appears to behave in the same way as in the normal subjects during voluntary tremor. It seems that parkinsonian tremor cannot be explained in terms of a malfunctioning α/γ link but that a central generator must activate both α and γ motoneurons rhythmically.

Clonus

Clonus appears to be quite different from parkinsonian tremor. Recordings show that the α/γ link is broken because the muscle spindles only fire during the relaxation phase, i.e. they are acting as passive stretch receptors. It is quite reasonable to propose that the muscle spindle afferent bursts occurring during muscle stretch play an important part in exciting the α motoneurons to produce the next contraction. Clonus, however, cannot be explained just as an oscillating stretch reflex. Dimitrijevic *et al.* (1980) have shown that, although clonus is initiated by a burst of Ia afferent impulses produced by muscle stretch, the motoneurons are unresponsive to further Ia volleys for at least 120 ms. The mechanism of the refractory period is not known but seems to be too long to be attributed to Renshaw neuron inhibition. It is clear that the α/γ link is disturbed in clonus and that spindle afferent discharge and an oscillating excitability of the motoneurons both play a role in generating rhythmic activity.

Walking

Recent neurophysiological work on the coordinated act of walking or stepping has induced a move away from the old idea of successive reflexes coming into action, the 'chain reflex' hypothesis, and forced a re-examination of a much older idea called the 'reciprocal half centre hypothesis' which was first proposed by Brown in 1914. This latter hypothesis has been refined and modelled by Miller and Scott (1977) and their half centre or stepping generator is a simpler and more testable proposal than the 'ring' hypothesis set forth by Shik and Orlovsky (1976). The importance of recent work on stepping lies in the clear demonstration that the neurons of the spinal cord can act as generators of stepping movements within a limb and also, by propriospinal pathways, stepping generators of each limb can be coordinated to produce gait. Even spinal animals can produce coordinated stepping activity in certain circumstances (Shik & Orlovsky, 1976). All the experimental work has been on cats and it remains to be shown that a similar organization is present in primates and, indeed, in man.

The simplest effective model of a stepping generator is that proposed by Miller and Scott (1977) which involves just three types of neuron for each muscle group. The α motoneuron, the 1a inhibitory neuron (1a IN) and the Renshaw Cell (RC) make up a 'half centre' and are known to be anatomically connected in the manner shown in Fig. 4.5. The 1a IN and RC both send projections to the antagonist half centre and both half centres receive simultaneous tonic excitation on to the α MN and the 1a IN. The cycle can begin by tonic excitation which raises the extensor 1a IN to firing point. This will inhibit the flexor α motoneuron and the flexor 1a IN which results in disinhibition of the extensor MN. The extensor MN fires producing limb extension and the impulses are fed back on to the RC which is excited. The connections of the RC, which are inhibitory, are to the 1a IN of the extensor centre and to the RC of the flexor group. The RC

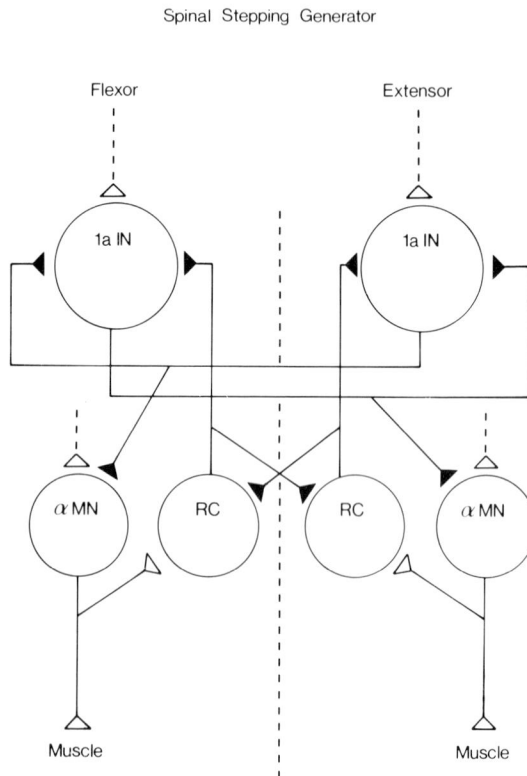

Fig. 4.5 The smallest assembly of neurons necessary to generate stepping movements according to Miller and Scott. For a functional description see text.

activity reduces or turns off the extensor 1a IN and thereby disinhibits the flexor 1a IN which is now able to become active and permit the flexor half of the cycle to begin. This very simple model can explain alternating flexion and extension of a limb. The necessary anatomical connections are known to exist and the neurons involved are known to be inhibitory, except for the α MN. Two, four or more generators can be modelled by computer and coupled together when they show coordinated activity between the generators within a limb or between limbs. Previously afferent input was regarded as essential for stepping, but this is not so, hence there was no need to include the gamma system or skin and joint sensors in the model. This must not be taken to imply that afferents play no part; rather they provide for maintenance of posture by modulating muscle force so that the body is carried smoothly even over rough ground.

Supraspinal control of the stepping generators appears to involve fine reticulospinal fibres, some of which release noradrenaline, some 5-hydroxytryptamine and other unspecified transmitters. The reticulospinal neurons are activated by a midbrain locomotor area which seems coterminous with the nucleus cuneiformis in the cat. Electrical stimulation of this region of a cat after removal of its forebrain (a mesencephalic animal) will produce coordinated stepping activity. A subthalamic locomotor region has also been described (Fig. 4.6).

This work on mesencephalic cats has emphasized the importance of the spinal stepping generator and the slow conducting reticulospinal systems. The role of the traditional motor pathways, corticospinal, vestibulospinal, cerebellum etc., has been relegated to subsidiary modulation. These fast conducting pathways are active during walking, but the effect of their impulses is dependent on the state or setting of the spinal locomotor generator. The afferent pathways have also been relegated as has the gamma motor system. Future work will examine the relationships between the different systems during walking and no doubt will investigate to what extent the walking mechanisms of primates, including man, are similar to those of quadrupeds and also to what extent the organization of a stepping centre can survive upper motoneuron lesions.

There have been many studies of gait in man; forces, speeds, accelerations and numerous other mechanical parameters have been measured accurately by sophisticated computerized systems. The data have been regurgitated in various forms and some is of great value in orthopaedic specialities. However, very little neurophysiological understanding has resulted although a recent attempt by Knutson and Richards (1979) to classify gait disorders in hemiplegia deserves mention. They found three types of abnormality:

1. premature activation of calf muscles in the stance phase
2. cases where two or more muscles were relatively more paralysed than others
3. those in which inappropriate co-contraction of several or all muscle groups in the leg occurred.

It was necessary to have a fourth group to accommodate unclassifiable varieties of gait disorder.

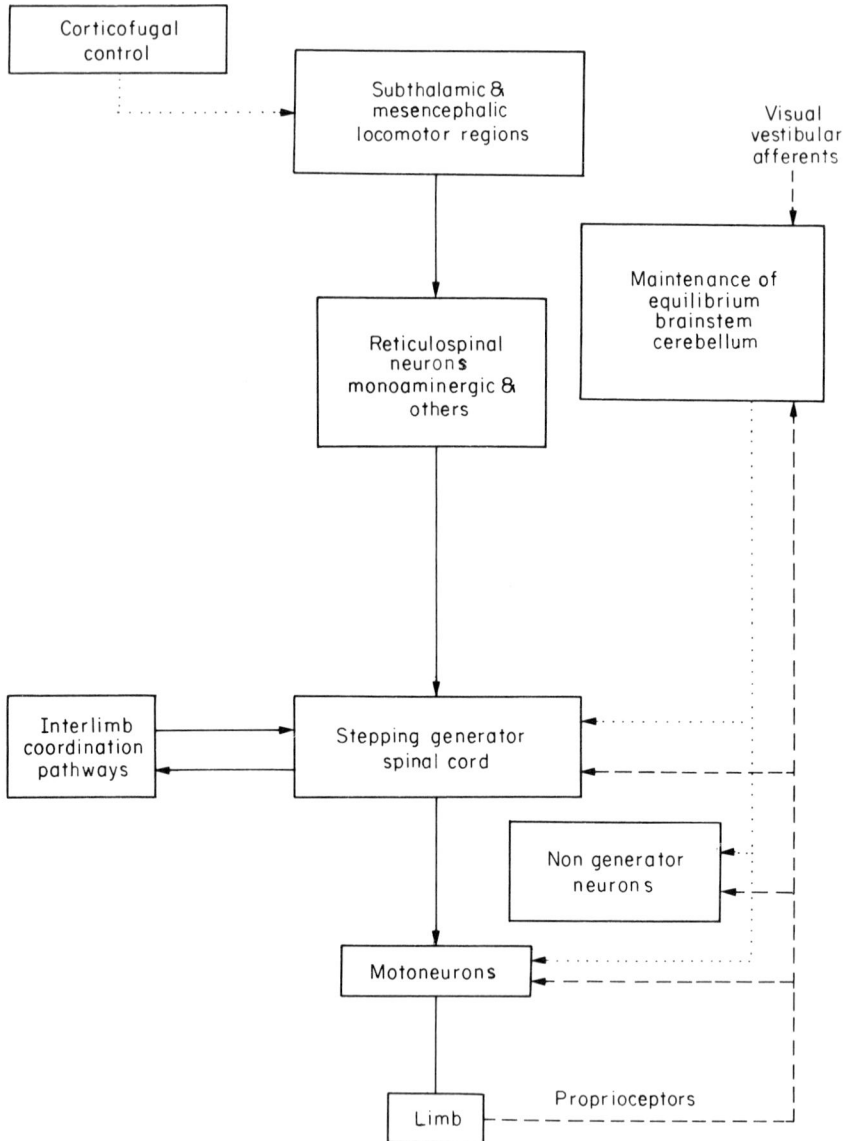

Fig. 4.6 Diagram of the organization of the locomotor system as revealed by experiments on stepping in cats.

Group 1 is interesting; it includes the common problem of foot drop due to upper motoneuron lesions. These patients could be fruitfully studied in the light of the work of Yanagisawa *et al.* (1976) who indicated that the 1a inhibitory neuron from the flexor (tibialis anterior) to the extensor (gastrocnemicus—soleus) is inactive in hemiplegia. If one set of neurons can be identified as responsible for a particular type of deficit then the challenge to rehabilitation is to find a means of facilitating the action of those neurons by drugs, by training, by electrical stimulation or by any other means.

MOVEMENT

In recent years it has been possible to study movement with more accuracy than previously and the findings have been interpreted using ideas and concepts borrowed from control engineering. Germinal to most modern work were the papers by Hammond *et al.* (1956) who proposed that muscle spindles operated as a feedback device for a follow-up length servo system. Earlier pioneers analysed movement in some detail, photographed and described locomotion accurately; Holmes (1922) carefully analysed the defects of movement following cerebellar lesions; the work of Bernstein (1966) deserves to be better known in the west.

Cortico-spinal Tract

Generations of students have been confused by the use of the word 'pyramidal' as an adjective for a type of neuron, a tract and a set of clinical manifestations of a cerebral lesion. The clinical terms, pyramidal lesion, pyramidal hemiplegia, pyramidal syndrome, upper motoneuron lesion of pyramidal type, pyramidal pattern of weakness, are so well entrenched that it will be years before alternative terms are introduced. There seems to be no reason to continue to refer to the corticospinal (CS) tract as pyramidal as it leads to the assumption that a lesion of it will produce a pyramidal syndrome.

Corticospinal tract lesions have been investigated rarely in humans but intensively in other primates. The clear and unequivocal finding is that a pyramidal syndrome, e.g. weakness or paralysis of voluntary movements, hyperactive tendon jerks and spasticity with reorganized cutaneous reflexes, does not occur. Monkeys with corticospinal tract lesions show very good visually directed voluntary movements but show poorly executed fine finger movements which are under proprioceptive control. The position of the corticospinal tract and indeed of the motor cortex in the hierarchy of the motor organization has been questioned. One suggestion has been that the corticospinal tract neurons are 'downstream' of the cerebellum.

The work of Evarts (1974) and others has shown what the cortex signals to the spinal cord along the CS tract. By recording from neurons whose axons run in the tract he has shown that the discharge of impulses precedes muscle activity and is proportional to the force and rate of change of force generated by an appropriate muscle. Phillips and Porter (1977) have shown that muscle spindle afferents feed back to the cortex but not directly to the motor cortex. They also have demonstrated the strong monosynaptic connections between the CS tract and the motoneurons of hand muscles. The old idea of the motor cortex as a director of willed activity is crumbling under the weight of modern physiological investigation, which is showing it to be a 'summing point' where peripheral events jostle with cerebellar input and higher nervous system activity to control a direct executive pathway to the spinal cord.

Anatomy of Movement

Voluntary movements can be divided into two main types which are quite different in their organization. These are the ramp movement and the ballistic movement. Ramp movements are slow and sustained and are under visual and proprioceptive feedback control which regulates the force developed to minimize external disturbances and to maximize accuracy. Ballistic movements are rapidly executed and there is no time for feedback control; the movement is planned as a whole in the CNS where local conditions, e.g. posture and ongoing movement, are taken into account with experience and the whole motor command is given with precise timing. If the outcome is inappropriate nothing can be done to correct it. An incorrect ballistic movement is experienced when one quickly picks up a suitcase which was thought to be heavy and is not.

Ramp Movements

Ramp movements have been profitably studied by a very ingenious method by Marsden *et al.* (1972; 1973). The subject's thumb was attached to a frame which allowed measurement of angle of the interphalangeal joint and force of flexion. A motor, attached to the frame, provided a resistance to movement and could produce a sudden increase or release of resistance. The subject was required to track a target on an oscilloscope by flexing his thumb slowly while the EMG activity of flexor policis longus was recorded.

The findings of this type of experiment are summarized in Fig. 4.7. When the ramp movement is disturbed by a sudden stretch four phases of muscle response can be identified. The first, SP, has a short latency of 23 ms and is the spinal segmental stretch reflex equivalent to a tendon jerk. Next are two peaks of EMG activity at 40 and 55 ms respectively labelled A and B. These are reflex events because they cannot be voluntarily suppressed and their size depends upon the magnitude and velocity of the displacement. There is then a short period of relative silence of EMG followed by a final EMG burst labelled V. This burst is under voluntary control and its size depends upon prior instruction to the subject, i.e. the 'set' of the motor system. When told to resist stretch as vigorously as possible V was large, when told to let go as soon as stretch occurred V was absent. At its earliest the latency of V was about 80 ms.

The second response to stretch at 40 ms, A, could be a transcortical stretch

Response of a contracting muscle to sudden stretch

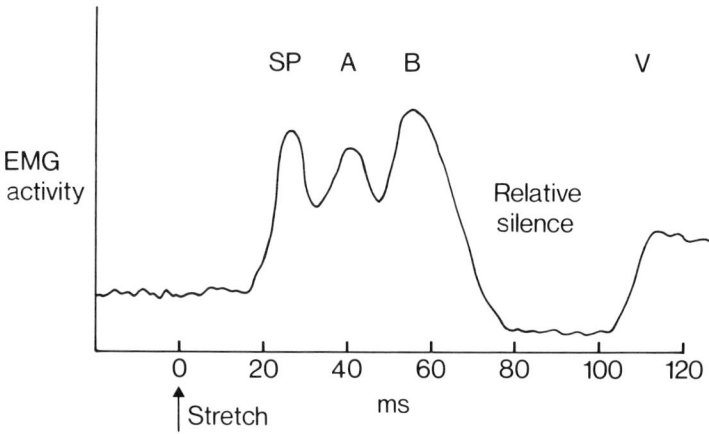

Fig. 4.7 Diagram compiled from the work of Marsden showing increased EMG activity after sudden unexpected muscle stretch during a tracking task. SP, spinal stretch reflex; A, probable transcortical reflex; B, a 'long-loop' reflex of uncertain origin; V, a voluntary contraction to overcome the stretch.

reflex. This hypothesis was proposed by Marsden *et al.* (1973) and is supported by a large body of circumstantial evidence. The latency time is appropriate; it is known that muscle spindles project to the cortex and can almost certainly excite pyramidal tract neurons in primates; lesions in the dorsal columns, sensory or motor cortex or internal capsule all abolish this response.

These precisely measured responses to muscle stretch are beginning to be made in patients with CNS disease. As mentioned above the 'A' response is abolished by lesions of the dorsal column, cortex and CS tract, but Lee and Tatton (1978) describe a case where the response recovered after a surgical lesion of the cortex. In extrapyramidal disease the findings are equivocal and publication of further work is awaited. In cerebellar disorders, where there is no pyramidal disturbance, the 'A' response occurs, but its latency is prolonged whereas the initial SP response is normal. These interesting experimental findings are still at an early stage, but it is clear that such precise measurements of the behaviour of the motor system will be relevant to rehabilitation where an accurate assessment of a disability is required and an equally accurate assessment of whether time and therapy can restore normal responses.

Ballistic Movement

When a ballistic movement is executed the first event is a relaxation of the antagonist muscle if that is active. The agonist muscle gives a short burst of activity followed by a silent period and then a second burst. During the silent interval of the agonist there is a short burst of activity in the antagonist (Fig. 4.8). The initial agonist burst of activity is of short and invariable duration; accuracy of movement is provided by variation in the amplitude rather than duration of muscle activity. The antagonist burst is important for arresting the movement but is not of variable amplitude. The final part of the movement is a second burst of acitivity in the agonist of variable size; this burst is probably feedback controlled and corrects any misalignment remaining after the initial burst. The timing of the bursts seems to be pre-programmed and the amplitude of them depends on experience and the expected force required.

Peripheral conditions must be taken into account in programming a ballistic burst, but some experiments suggest that the transcortical stretch response does not operate for a time after the initial burst of activity in the agonist muscle but a stretch occurring just before the movement results in a higher amplitude initial

EMG during a ballistic movement

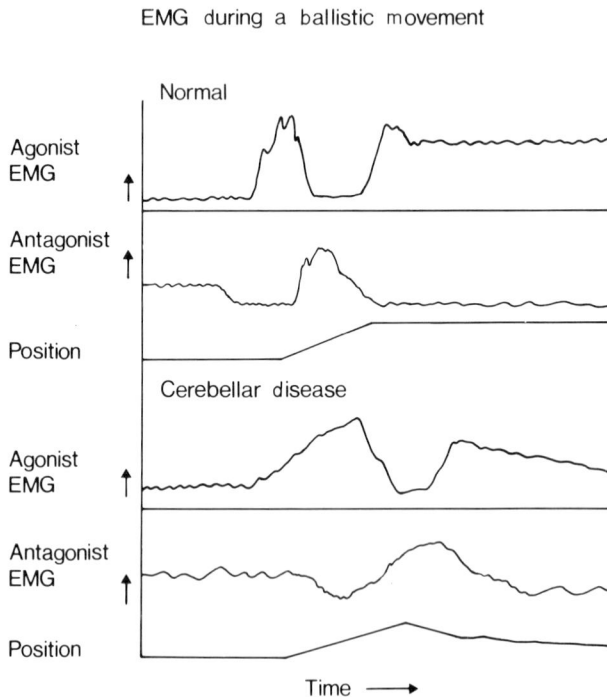

Fig. 4.8 The diagram shows the main features of an EMG recorded during a ballistic movement. In normal subjects, the antagonist muscle relaxes prior to agonist contraction. Movement follows a short burst of agonist activity and is arrested by a burst of the antagonist. Both muscles then become active to hold the new position. In cerebellar disease the events are much slower and the antagonist relaxation may not occur until the agonist is contracting. The level of contraction is not always appropriate for the task and the final position is not held.

EMG burst. The brain updates its ballistic movement programme with respect to peripheral conditions, but just before movement the updating ceases and the programme is put into effect. The onset and timing of the bursts of activity during ballistic movement are severely disturbed by cerebellar disease. The initial contraction of the agonist is delayed and sometimes occurs before appropriate inhibition of the antagonist. The durations of the agonist and antagonist bursts are prolonged. With these disturbances one can see how many of the clinical manifestations of abnormal movement of cerebellar disease can be explained.

These novel ways of examining willed movement have supported a model of motor control first proposed by Kornhuber (1971; 1974). The model proposes that there are generators in the brain for ramp and ballistic movements. The motor area simply executes the movement planned by the generators. Kornhuber identifies the posterior association cortex of the parietal lobe as the assessor of the movement required, i.e. 'the hand should not be too close to the table top or it will knock over the glass'. Lesions here produce loss of skill or apraxias. Ramp generation is thought to be a role of the basal ganglia and this is supported by the clinical picture of parkinsonism; akinesia is the absence of ramps and athetosis is continuous uncontrolled ramps. Ballistic movements are organized by the cerebellum and cerebellar failure results in dysmetria which can be interpreted as a disturbance of ballistic movement.

The novel feature of this model is that the basal ganglia and cerebellum are involved in the planning of a movement and are 'upstream' of the motor cortex. This role does not obviate their traditional role in responding to changing circumstances during a movement. These structures therefore become the repository of learned and skilled movement. The model may seem to be a remote conceptual affair of little relevance to the rehabilitation clinic. It is too recent a development to have had any impact on physical therapy techniques, but it is an important model for anyone intending to study the control of movement whether in the disabled or in the dancer or sportsman who wishes to achieve ultimate perfection in muscle control.

An ingenious method for studying the electrical events in the brain preceding a motor act has revealed a set of potentials which are generated by the motor system. The technique is similar to averaging evoked potentials, but the trigger for averaging is the onset of a prescribed movement and the electrical events preceding the movement are averaged—a process called opisthochronic averaging.

The potentials associated with movement have been identified as: the bereitschaftspotential (BP) or readiness potential, the pre-motion positivity (PMP) and the motor potential (MP). The first, BP, is a slowly developing surface negativity beginning 800 ms before a rapid finger movement or as long as 1300 ms before a ramp movement. It reaches $7\,\mu V$ in amplitude over the anterior parietal area and is bilateral even when only one finger is to be moved, but it eventually becomes higher in amplitude over the hemisphere contralateral to the moving side. The BP also precedes saccadic eye movements and speech as well as brisk finger movement. The PMP is not easily detected as it is less than $2\,\mu V$ in amplitude and cannot be seen in all subjects. It appears bilaterally, is spread widely over the scalp and begins 90 ms before the movement. The MP is also a small potential of less than $2\,\mu V$ beginning 60 ms before movement and located rather precisely over the contralateral motor cortex. It is believed to correspond to discharges of neurons in the motor cortex.

It is of some interest that BP and MP occur over those areas of cortex and in the order predicted by the Kornhuber model. It has also been reported that the BP is reduced over the affected hemisphere in unilateral parkinsonism with a lesser reduction over the unaffected hemisphere when the normal hand is moved. Both the MP and PMP were reduced when moving the affected side.

PAIN

Very great advances in our understanding of pain have been made in recent years and Melzack and Wall's (1965) gate control theory of pain stands as a germinal theory from which much physiological and therapeutic experimental work developed. Wall (1978) has recently taken a second look at the theory in the light of clinical and experimental discoveries since that time. More recent still have been the advances made beginning with the discovery of the enkephalins, the brain's endogenous analgesics (Hughes *et al.*, 1975). At the same time studies of human sensory nerves and of the responses of nerve fibres to injury have been pursued to great effect (Vallbo *et al.*, 1979; Devor & Govrin-Lippermann, 1979a; b). Chapters by Wynn Parry and Long discuss the management of pain.

In man A delta and C fibres carry impulses from nociceptors. Their activity has been recorded in man and the receptors showed increased responsiveness after heat injury which was accompanied by hyperalgesia. Impulses could occur at up to 15/s for a short period of time but pain was not perceived at discharge rates of less than 0.3/s. The fibres innervate an area of 1 mm^2 to 1 cm^2 within which there are several spots more sensitive to stimuli. The receptors are sensitive to many types of stimuli—thermal, cold, mechanical and chemical irritants such as histamine—but the stimuli had to be strong enough to fall in the painful intensity range. Without stimuli there is no impulse activity. There is evidence that group C nociceptor fibres release substance P in the spinal cord.

Nerve fibres in damaged nerves which have formed neuromas show spontaneous activity. Studies have been mainly on small myelinated fibres which are pressure sensitive as well as being spontaneously active. The spontaneous activity can be increased by hypoxia and by noradrenaline which can be released from sympathetic fibres in the neuroma. The activity can be blocked by antidromic stimulation and by sympathetic blockers such as guanethidine (Wall & Gutnik, 1974; 1978). Local chemical sympathectomy has proved a very simple and effective treatment for causalgic pain (Hannington-Kiff, 1974). Recent animal studies have shown ephaptic transmission in chronically damaged nerves; that is, impulses in one fibre electrically excite impulses in a neighbour in the damaged region. It would be difficult to argue that these spurious impulses play no part in paraesthesiae and dysaesthesiae which are associated with nerve damage.

Moving into the spinal cord brings one to a consideration of the gate control theory of pain. This theory was developed from well-known clinical facts about the interaction of pain and touch stimuli. Shafts of criticisms have been aimed at the theory, but it is more the interpretations and extrapolations from the theory which have been the target. Wall (1978) has restated the theory in the light of recent physiological work and it is quite clear that in lamina I and lamina V of the dorsal horn there are neurons which transmit impulses from primary noci-ceptor fibres. At this point transmission can be enhanced or reduced by activity in other segmental or descending neurons.

The descending nociceptor modulation system has been the subject of much recent research activity, for it is this system, originating from the nucleus raphe magnus, nucleus reticularis magnocellularis and possibly also from the region of locus caeruleus, which is activated by systemic opiates acting on neurons in the periaqueductal grey region (Basbaum & Fields, 1978). The system is normally activated by the release of enkephalins, a group of pentapeptide compounds naturally occurring in the brain of which β-endorphin is the most potent anal-gesic. There is probably another group of endorphin releasing neurons at the segmental level of the cord.

It is not known just how the pain-inhibiting system is normally activated, but there is evidence to suggest that it is active in painful states and this activity can perhaps be increased by acupuncture. No doubt a number of effective methods for activating the system will be proposed and some of them should be thera-peutically effective. It has already been shown that β-endorphin has profound analgesic properties when injected intrathecally (Oyama *et al.*, 1980).

Finally the dorsal horn of the spinal cord may become the site of origin of spurious impulses leading to pain. With certain insults dorsal horn neurons may fire spontaneous bursts of impulses rather like groups of cortical neurons in an epileptic focus (Somjen *et al.*, 1978). Such discharges, whether arising from ephaptic or other mechanisms, could explain the paroxysmal shooting pains seen in a number of conditions of which tabes dorsalis is the classic, but the root pains of the paraplegic and brachial plexus pain are more common examples.

It is in the area of intractable pain that neurological rehabilitation should be most successful in the near future. There seems to be no fundamental reason why the physiological advances and the advances in management as described by Long (Chapter 10) should not eradicate many forms of intractable pain during this decade.

HIGHER NERVOUS FUNCTION

It is in the area of higher mental function that advances in rehabilitation are most hoped for yet least likely to be achieved. Experimental physiologists have elaborated an operational policy or belief which may appear sterile and unduly mechanistic to many rehabilitationists. It is based on the idea of psychoneuronal identity, which is that the total neural events within the brain are, of themselves, the items we call sensation, perception, consciousness and behaviour. Mind, consciousness and their contents are physicochemical neural events occurring in reactive structures (brain) and cannot be separated from the material of the nervous system. The neural events obey physical laws and are not subject to interference from gods, ghosts or free-will.

Behaviour is based on the perceived environment and not on the real environment. Mountcastle (1975; 1978) forcibly explains how our image of the world depends upon a set of imperfect sensory maps drawn with the ink of action potentials on the sensory cortices. Abstractions and inferences from these maps give a perception of the environment on which behaviour is based. Work on the visual cortex has shown how groups of neurons respond to particular abstractions of a stimulus: edge, orientation, corner, direction of movement, colour etc. Mountcastle has begun to identify the abstractions represented by activity in neurons of the parietal cortex and has been able to indicate the positive features of neural activity which correspond reasonably well with the negative symptoms of the parietal lobe syndrome of spatial inattention seen not uncommonly after strokes.

If a behaviour pattern is identified as depending upon certain features in the environment and if the neurons which normally abstract that feature of the environment from the sensory map are damaged then that particular behaviour pattern will never follow regardless of the state of drive or need of the individual. The organism may develop alternative strategies and thereby achieve the same ends on some occasions, but the total behaviour pattern will be degraded to a greater or lesser extent.

One of the first questions to which a rehabilitation neurologist requires an answer is whether, given destruction of one group of abstracting neurons, another group of neurons may take on that function as a result of learning, training, drugs, insight into the problem or by any other means. If, then, a group of neurons can take on a new function, what happens to their previous function? Until neurophysiologists provide some insight into these problems it seems that rehabilitation must stick to the task of encouraging the development of alternative strategies in patients who have suffered cortical damage.

There are large areas of neurological rehabilitation where necessity demands attention but where the neurophysiologist can offer little or no help. Perhaps the most pressing area is that of aphasia, where the only advance since Broca and Wernicke has been the demonstration of an anatomical asymmetry of the hemispheres. Psychological and linguistic studies have proceeded apace, but perhaps it has been the lack of an animal model which has retarded the study of the brain in relation to speech. Evoked potential and EEG techniques are being applied to the subject, but there are serious methodological problems to be overcome (Wanner *et al.*, 1977).

WHITHER NEUROPHYSIOLOGY?

The answer to the question of whether to involve neurophysiologists in neurological rehabilitation is a self-evident affirmative. The prospect of attempting to advance rehabilitation without neurophysiology is gloomy indeed. There are certain areas in which rehabilitationists could actively involve neurophysiologists and vice versa. First there is the problem of monitoring long-term changes to establish in greater detail the natural history of diseases and the effects of treatment. Neurophysiological parameters are largely objective and many can be made numerical while some assess very specific changes relating to only one cell group. Many techniques already devised are relatively simple to apply from the point of view of the patient and the doctor.

Very practical assistance can be rendered to those using forms of electrical stimulation for treatment. Biocalibration of stimulators and the assessment and diagnosis of malfunction are essential for an electrical stimulation programme, and a neurophysiologist's familiarity with electrical matters enables him to play a useful part in such activities.

The course neurophysiology should take in the field of rehabilitation is not self-evident, but the directing force must be a spirit of enquiry into the detailed mechanisms underlying neurological deficit. There is a strong argument for directing one's efforts entirely towards studying animal models which, compared with human neurological disease, are compellingly simple and offer many advantages. The needs of society, individuals and humanitarian instincts, however, give human work a necessary attraction but can also detract from the basic scientific requirements of neurophysiology. The great intellectual challenge to neurophysiology in rehabilitation is to explain the clinical phenomena of neurological deficit within the framework provided by basic pre-clinical science. Such an exercise is destined to undergo an unexpected convolution whenever it is found that accepted animal models or frameworks are not entirely adequate and the rehabilitation neurophysiologist has to ask his colleagues in animal laboratories to re-examine their concepts. When a lively intellectual intercourse develops along these lines, understanding of the problems moves ahead apace with the inevitable revelation of useful strategies for treatment.

REFERENCES

ASHBY P., VERRIER M. & LIGHTFOOT E. (1974) Segmental reflex pathways in spinal shock and spinal spasticity in man. *Journal of Neurology, Neurosurgery and Psychiatry*, **37**, 1352–60.

BASBAUM, A.I. & FIELDS, H.L. (1978) Endogenous pain control mechanisms: review and hypothesis. *Annals of Neurology*, **4**, 451–62.

BERNSTEIN N. (1966) *The Co-ordination and Regulation of Movements*. Pergamon Press, Oxford.

BROWN T.G. (1914) On the nature of the fundamental activity of the nervous centres; together with an analysis of the conditioning of rhythmic activity in progression, and a theory of the evolution of function in the nervous system. *Journal of Physiology*, **48**, 18–46.

BULLER A.J., ECCLES J.C. & ECCLES R.M. (1960) Interactions between motoneurones and muscles in respect of their characteristic speeds of their responses. *Journal of Physiology, London,* **150,** 417–39.

BULLER A.J. & POPE R. (1977) Plasticity in mammalian skeletal muscle. *Philosophical Transactions of the Royal Society, London,* Series B, **278,** 295–305.

BUSSEL B. & PIERROT-DESEILLIGNY E. (1977) Inhibition of human motoneurones, probably of Renshaw origin, elicited by an orthodromic motor discharge. *Journal of Physiology,* **269,** 319–39.

CARLEN P.L., WERMAN R. & YAARI Y. (1980) Post-synaptic conductance increase associated with presynaptic inhibition in cat lumbar motoneurones. *Journal of Physiology,* **298,** 539–56.

DESMEDT J.E. (1977) Auditory evoked potentials in man: psychoparmacology correlates of evoked potentials. *Progress in Clinical Neurophysiology,* **2,** S. Karger, Basel.

DEVOR M. & GOVRIN-LIPPERMANN R. (1979a) Selective regeneration of sensory fibres following nerve crush injury. *Experimental Neurology,* **65,** 243–54.

DEVOR M. & GOVRIN-LIPPERMANN R. (1979b) Maturation of axonal sprouts after nerve crush. *Experimental Neurology,* **64,** 260–70.

DIMITRIJEVIC M.R., FAGANEL J., LEHMKUHL L.D. & SHERWOOD A.M. (1980) Motor control in man with spinal cord injury. In *Motor Control in Man: Suprasegmental and Segmental Mechanisms* (Ed. Desmedt J.E.). *Progress in Clinical Neurophysiology,* Vol. 8. Karger, Basel.

DIMITRIJEVIC M.R. & NATHAN P.W. (1967a) Studies of spasticity in man. 1. Some features of spasticity. *Brain,* **90,** 1–30.

DIMITRIJEVIC M.R. & NATHAN P.W. (1967b) Studies of spasticity in man. 2. Analysis of stretch reflexes in spasticity. *Brain,* **90,** 333–57.

DIMITRIJEVIC M.R. & NATHAN P.W. (1968) Studies of spasticity in man. 3. Analysis of reflex activity evoked by noxious cutaneous stimulation. *Brain,* **91,** 349–68.

DIMITRIJEVIC M.R. & NATHAN P.W. (1970) Studies of spasticity in man. 4. Changes in the flexion reflex with repetitive cutaneous stimulation in spinal man. *Brain,* **9,** 743–68.

DIMITRIJEVIC M.R. & NATHAN P.W. (1971) Studies of spasticity in man. 5. Dishabituation of the flexion reflex in spinal man. *Brain,* **94,** 77–90.

DIMITRIJEVIC M.R., NATHAN P.W. & SHERWOOD A.M. (1980) Clonus: the role of central mechanisms. *Journal of Neurology, Neurosurgery & Psychiatry,* **43,** 321–32.

DIMITRIJEVIC M.R., SPENCER W.A., TRONTELJ J.V. & DIMITRIJEVIC M. (1977) Reflex effects of vibration in patients with spinal cord lesions. *Neurology,* **27,** 1078–86.

DRACHMAN D.B. (1974) The role of acetylcholine as a neurotropic transmitter. *Annals of the New York Academy of Sciences,* **288,** 161–76.

EL-NEGAMY E. & SEDGWICK E.M. (1978) Properties of a spinal somatosensory evoked potential recorded in man. *Journal of Neurology, Neurosurgery and Psychiatry,* **41,** 762–8.

EVARTS E.V. (1974) Sensorimotor cortex activity associated with movements triggered by visual as compared to somaesthetic inputs. In *The Neurosciences, Third Study Program* (Eds. Schmitt & Worden), pp. 327–37. MIT Press, Cambridge, Mass.

FRANK K. (1959) Basic mechanisms of synaptic transmission in the central nervous system. Institution of Radio Engineers. *Medical Electronics,* ME-**6,** 85–8.

HAGBARTH K.E., WALLIN G. & LÖFSTEDT L. (1975a) Muscle spindle activity in man during voluntary fast alternating movements. *Journal of Neurology, Neurosurgery and Psychiatry,* **38,** 625–35.

HAGBARTH, K.E., WALLIN G., LÖFSTEDT L. & AQUILONIUS S.M. (1975b) Muscle spindle activity in alternating tremor of parkinsonism and in clonus. *Journal of Neurology, Neurosurgery and Psychiatry,* **38,** 636–41.

HAGBARTH K.E. & YOUNG R.R. (1979) Participation of the stretch reflex in human physiological tremor. *Brain,* **102,** 509–26.

HAMMOND P.H., MERTON P.A. & SUTTON G.G. (1956) Nervous gradation of muscular contraction. *British Medical Bulletin,* **12,** 214–18.

HANNINGTON-KIFF J.G. (1974) Intravenous regional sympathetic block with guanethidine. *Lancet,* **i,** 1019–20.

HENNEMAN E., SOMJEN G. & CARPENTER D.O. (1965) Functional significance of cell size in spinal motoneurones. *Journal of Neurophysiology,* **28,** 560–80.

HOFFMANN P. (1918) Uber die Beziehungen der Schnenreflexe zur willkurlichen Bewegung und zum Tonus. *Zeitschrift Biologie*, **68**, 351–570.

HOLMES G. (1922) The Croonian Lectures on the clinical symptoms of cerebellar diseases and their interpretation. *Lancet*, **100** (1), 1177–82; 1231–7; (2) 59–65; 111–15.

HUGHES J., SMITH T.W., KOSTERLITZ M.W., FOTHERGILL L.A., MORGAN B.A. & MORRIS H.R. (1975) Identification of two related pentapeptides from the brain with potent opiate agonist activity. *Nature, London*, **258**, 577–9.

HULTBORN H. & PIERROT-DESEILLIGNY E. (1979) Changes in recurrent inhibition during voluntary soleus contractions in man studied by an H reflex technique. *Journal of Physiology*, **297**, 229–251.

JANKOWSKA E. & TANAKA R. (1974) Neuronal mechanism of the disynaptic inhibition evoked in primate spinal motoneurones from the corticospinal tract. *Brain Research*, **75**, 163–6.

KNUTSSON E. & RICHARDS C. (1979) Different types of disturbed motor control in gait of hemiplegia patients. *Brain*, **102**, 405–30.

KORNHUBER H.H. (1971) Motor functions of cerebellum and basal ganglia. *Kybernetik*, **8**, 157–62.

KORNHUBER H.H. (1974) Cerebral cortex, cerebellum and basal ganglia: an introduction to their motor functions. In *The Neurosciences. Third Study Program* (Eds. Schmitt F.O. & Worden F.G.), pp. 267–80. MIT Press, Cambridge, Mass.

LEE R.G. & TATTON W.G. (1978) Long loop reflexes in man: clinical applications. In *Cerebral Motor Control in Man: Long Loop Mechanisms* (Ed. Desmedt J.E.). Vol. 4, pp. 320–33. Kager, Basel.

McCOMAS A.J. (1977) *Neuromuscular Function and Disorders*. Butterworths, London.

McDONALD W.I. (1977) Pathophysiology of conduction in central nerve fibres. In *Visual Evoked Potentials in Man* (Ed. Desmedt J.E.), pp. 427–37. Oxford University Press.

MARSDEN C.D., MERTON P.A. & MORTON H.B. (1972) Servo action in human voluntary movement. *Nature, London*, **238**, 140–3.

MARSDEN C.D., MERTON P.A. & MORTON H.B. (1973) Is the human stretch reflex cortical rather than spinal? *Lancet*, **i**, 759–61.

MATTHEWS W.B. (1970) The clinical implications of the H reflex and other electrically induced reflexes. In *Modern Trends in Neurology* (Ed. Williams D.), Vol. 5, pp. 241–53. Butterworths, London.

MATTHEWS W.B. & SMALL D.G. (1979) Serial recording of visual and somatosensory evoked potentials in M.S. patients. *Journal of the Neurological Sciences*, **40**, 11–21.

MELZACK R. & WALL P.D. (1965) Pain mechanisms: a new theory. *Science*, **150**, 971–9.

MILLER & SCOTT P.D. (1977) The spinal locomotor generator. *Experimental Brain Research*, **30**, 387–403.

MILNER-BROWN H.S., STEIN R.B. & YEMM R. (1973a) Contractile properties of human motor units during voluntary isometric contractions. *Journal of Physiology*, **228**, 285–306.

MILNER-BROWN H.S., STEIN R.B. & YEMM R. (1973b) The orderly recruitment of human motor units during voluntary isometric contractions. *Journal of Physiology*, **230**, 359–70.

MILNER-BROWN H.S., STEIN R.B. & LEE R.G. (1974a) Pattern of recruiting human motor units in neuropathies and motor neurone disease. *Journal of Neurology, Neurosurgery and Psychiatry*, **37**, 665–9.

MILNER-BROWN H.S., STEIN R.B. & LEE R.G. (1974b) Contractile and electrical properties of human motor units in neuropathies and motor neurone disease. *Journal of Neurology, Neurosurgery and Psychiatry*, **37**, 670–6.

MIZUNO Y., TANAKA R. & YANAGISAWA N. (1971) Reciprocal group I inhibition on triceps surae motoneurones in man. *Journal of Neurophysiology*, **34**, 1010–17.

MOUNTCASTLE V.B. (1975) The view from within: pathways to the study of perception. *The Johns Hopkins Medical Journal*, **136**, 109–31.

MOUNTCASTLE V.B. (1978) Brain mechanisms for directed attention. *Journal of the Royal Society of Medicine*, **71**, 14–28.

OYAMA T., JIN T., YAMAYA R., LING N. & GUILLEMIN R. (1980) Profound analgesic effects of β-endorphin in man. *Lancet*, **i**, 122–4.

PHILLIPS C.G. & PORTER R. (1977) *Corticospinal Neurones; their Role in Movement*. Academic Press, London.

PIERROT-DESEILLIGNY E., KATZ R. & MORIN C. (1979) Evidence for 1b inhibition in human subjects. *Brain Research*, **166**, 176–9.

RASMINSKY M. (1978) Physiology of conduction in demyelinated axons. In *Physiology and Pathobiology of Axons* (Ed. Waxman S.G.), pp. 361–76. Raven Press, New York.

ROBINSON K. & RUDGE P. (1978) The stability of the auditory evoked potentials in normal man and patients with multiple sclerosis. *Journal of the Neurological Sciences*, **36**, 147–56.

RUSHWORTH G. (1960) Spasticity and rigidity: an experimental study and review. *Journal of Neurology, Neurosurgery and Psychiatry*, **23**, 99–118.

SCHAUF C.L. & DAVIS F.A. (1974) Impulse conduction in multiple sclerosis: a theoretical basis for modification by temperature and pharmacological agents. *Journal of Neurology, Neurosurgery and Psychiatry*, **12**, 152–61.

SEDGWICK E.M., ILLIS L.S., TALLIS R.C., THORNTON A.R.D., ABRAHAM P., EL-NEGAMY E., DOCHERTY T.B., SOAR J.S., SPENCER S.C. & TAYLOR F.M. (1980) Evoked potentials and contingent negative variation during treatment of multiple sclerosis with spinal cord stimulation. *Journal of Neurology, Neurosurgery and Psychiatry*, **43**, 15–24.

SHAW J.C., O'CONNOR K.P. & ONGLEY C. (1977) The EEG as a measure of cerebral functional organization. *British Journal of Psychiatry*, **130**, 260–4.

SHIK M.L. & ORLOVSKY G.N. (1976) Neurophysiology of locomotor automation. *Physiological Reviews*, **56**, 465–501.

SIMOYAMA M. & TANAKA R. (1974) Reciprocal 1a inhibition at the onset of voluntary movements in man. *Brain Research*, **82**, 334–7.

SOMJEN G., LOTHMAN E., DUNN P., DUNAWAY T. & CORDINGLEY G. (1978) Microphysiology of spinal seizures. In *Abnormal Neuronal Discharges* (Eds. Chalazonitis N. & Boisson M.). Raven Press, New York.

STÅLBERG E. & EKSTEDT J. (1973) Single fibre EMG and microphysiology of the motor unit in normal and diseased man. In *New Developments in Electromyography and Clinical Neurophysiology*. Vol. 1 (Ed. Desmedt J.E.), pp. 113–29. S. Karger, Basel.

TANAKA R. (1972) Activation of reciprocal Ia inhibitory pathway during voluntary motor performance in man. *Brain Research*, **43**, 649–52.

TANAKA R. (1974) Reciprocal Ia inhibition during voluntary movements in man. *Experimental Brain Research*, **21**, 529–40.

TWITCHELL T.E. (1951) Restoration of motor function following hemiplegia in man. *Brain*, **74**, 443–80.

VALLBO A.B., HAGBARTH K.E., TOREBJÖRK H.E. & WALLIN B.G. (1979) Somatosensory, proprioceptive and sympathetic activity in human peripheral nerves. *Physiological Reviews*, **39**, 919–57.

WALL P.D. (1978) The gate control theory of pain mechanisms. A re-examination and re-statement. *Brain*, **101**, 1–18.

WALL P.D. & GUTNIK M. (1974) Ongoing activity in peripheral nerves; the physiology and pharmacology of impulses originating from a neuroma. *Experimental Neurology*, **43**, 580–93.

WALL P.D., SCADDING J.W. & TOMKIEWICZ M.M. (1978) The production and prevention of experimental anaesthesia dolorosa. *Pain*, **6**, 175–82.

WANNER E., TEYLER T.J. & THOMPSON R.F. (1977) The psychobiology of speech and language—an overview. In *Language and Hemispheric Specialization in Man: Cerebral ERPS* (Ed. Desmedt J.E.). *Progress in Clinical Neurophysiology*, Vol. 3, pp. 1–27. Karger, Basel.

WEXLER B.E. (1980) Cerebral laterality and psychiatry: a review of the literature. *American Journal of Psychiatry*, **137**, 279–91.

YANAGISAWA N., TANAKA R. & ITO Z. (1976) Reciprocal Ia inhibition in spastic hemiplegia of man. *Brain*, **99**, 555–74.

PART II
THE NEUROLOGICAL PATIENT: REHABILITATION

This part deals with specific neurological problems: head injury, stroke, spinal injury, the neuropathic bladder, peripheral nerve disorders, pain and neuro-muscular disease. Important themes recur in these chapters even though the clinical problems are very different. First there is the natural history of patients with neurological deficit, which is of fundamental importance for planning services and for prevention of complications by anticipating their likely develop-ment. Next there is the need for careful assessment, both at the start and at intervals during rehabilitation. This allows the practitioner to set a realistic goal for the patient and the team of rehabilitation workers. Some assessments are very practical and express daily needs, others are rooted in basic physiological science, e.g. bladder and peripheral nerve injury. Where both approaches can be made the rehabilitation exercise seems to be more successful. Another theme is that of timing. Surgical intervention needs to be not only the correct procedure but applied at the right time. Less obviously, preventative follow-up, psycho-logical measures and introduction of aids such as wheelchairs must be timed to offer maximum advantage to the patient.

Recent advances have been made and the chapters on bladder, peripheral nerve and pain could not have been written a few years ago. The reader will become aware that with good organization of resources, one can improve considerably the lot of the patient with seemingly intractable neurological deficits.

Chapter 5
Rehabilitation of Head Injury

'When I use a word it means just what I choose it to mean, neither more and certainly nothing less.'
(Humpty Dumpty, *Alice's Adventures Through the Looking Glass*.
Lewis Carroll. Macmillan: London)

Reading the literature regarding the problems surrounding brain damage, whether from stroke or injury, it is apparent that the statement attributed to Humpty Dumpty applies to a great deal of the writing over the last 30 or 40 years. There is almost a separate definition of levels of severity, effectiveness of treatment, and outcome measures from each author. Only in relatively recent years has some attempt been made to make specific definitions, and even now these are far from being universally adopted.

In discussing patients who have sustained secondary brain damage, two major groups attract attention. The first are those who have been severely affected by a major injury, and who became totally dependent, disrupting their families, or occupying a permanent bed in hospital or nursing home. This group frequently make themselves conspicuous by behaviour which is difficult to tolerate by those who care for them. For the majority of these patients it is quite clear that from the outset they suffered a major head injury, so that at least the basic cause is apparent and they are able to gain attention, sympathy and care since the deficits and the reasons appear obvious. The provision of such care is expensive and time consuming, so there is much debate as to how much skill and time should be spent in efforts towards rehabilitation, and at what stage it should be given.

In the other group are those in whom the injury has been apparently trivial, but whose subsequent symptoms include giddiness, headache and inability to concentrate, where there seems to be no very good reason apparent to an observer. If the original trauma seemed trivial, then this latter group is known variously as the post-traumatic syndrome, post-concussional syndrome, or by other and less flattering names. The nature of this trivial lesion, whether it is organic or functional in origin, has been extensively debated (Symonds, 1962; Miller, 1961), but even now the debate is not finally resolved.

Establishing firm statistics about these groups of patients is difficult, because there are no complete figures kept. An estimate can be given based on the Hospital In-Patient Enquiry by the Department of Health and Social Security (DHSS). Although only an estimate, it suggests that approximately 140 000 patients are discharged from, or die in, hospitals in England and Wales each year, with head injury as the major diagnostic code (see Fig. 5.1 and Table 5.1). Of this group, 7000 are so severely handicapped that their work potential suffers,

123

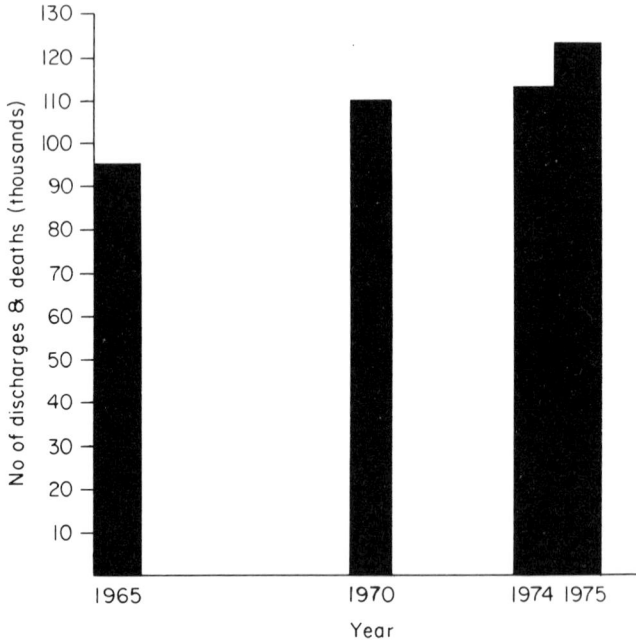

Fig. 5.1 Intracranial injury (not fracture). Estimated annual discharges and deaths from hospitals in England and Wales 1965-1975.

Table 5.1 Estimated total discharges and deaths in 1975, with mean duration of stay (in days) (MDS), nature of injury, and place of occurrence for intracranial injury (not fracture).

RTA*		Home		Other, unspecified		Total	
Est. no.	MDS	Est. no.	MDS	Est. no.	MDS	Est. no.	MDS
33 000	4.5	19 490	4.1	69 420	3.1	121 910	3.6
Concussion							
8 420	3.7	3 230	4.4	14 870	2.8	26 520	3.3
Total						148 430	

* Road traffic accident.

and several hundred of these rendered completely unfit for work again (London, 1967; Lewin, 1970). Jennett estimates that four or five times this number of patients attend their general practitioner with a head injury which it is felt is too trivial to seek hospital advice. No doubt there are many other patients who receive a head injury but do not even get as far as the practitioner's surgery. The overwhelming majority of those patients are seen, possibly admitted overnight for observation, and discharged without apparent sequelae. This amounts to a very substantial load of patients each year, and Jennett queries whether the routine of admission and observation of such patients is, in economic and medical terms, justifiable. He argues that it might be more profitable to the community as a whole to establish a regime whereby the casualty doctor makes a thorough examination, excludes fracture where this is feasible, and then, assuming that the clinical condition of the patient is satisfactory, sends the patient home instead of observing him in hospital. The friends or relatives are told the possible signs of deterioration, and given precise information as to how to get urgent admission should it seem to be indicated. Provided certain criteria are fulfilled, the chance of somebody developing an undiagnosed treatable secondary haematoma, or deteriorating otherwise clinically, appears remote. The other reason behind the recommendation is that even in those patients in whom there has been observed unconsciousness which is sustained on admission, or which improved to a point where consciousness has been obtained, the deterioration afterwards can be observed for quite long periods by the staff at the hospital without any appropriate action being taken until the optimum time has been passed (Jennett, 1977).

However, although there may be no major lesion sustained by the patient which calls for surgical intervention, it is not to say that patients do not suffer significant organic damage which may materially affect their future life. In spite of being recognized and treated at this stage, some of the patients may subsequently develop the post-concussional syndrome. Newcombe *et al.* (1979) have tried to establish whether minor head injuries admitted for observation demonstrate objective evidence of impairment of intellectual function, even if only for a short period. The results of this work indicate that there may frequently be minor problems which remain undetected unless specifically sought, and which may contribute to a vicious circle of impaired concentration, poor job performance and increasing anger and frustration at inability to cope with that which had previously seemed easy. It is important for these patients to see whether identification and treatment at an early stage would reduce the number of patients who subsequently become labelled 'post-traumatic syndrome' with all its consequences. Some feel that an aggressive policy of rehabilitation of such patients does, in fact, pay dividends, though confirmation by research is difficult.

Brain damage from stroke or injury has an acute, not to say dramatic, onset, and if survival is the outcome of the initial stages, subsequent recovery is likely to be slow, and the separation of the natural course from that assisted by the medical art is extremely difficult. Some contemporary neurophysiological work shows that there are possible mechanisms for recovery of brain function. This means everybody concerned with the patient's welfare, will have to understand these mechanisms and try to decide whether any are appropriate for exploitation as methods of treatment.

EPIDEMIOLOGY

The Hospital In-Patient Enquiry deals with a 10% sample of all discharges and deaths of patients who have been admitted to National Health Service hospitals in England and Wales. Since the figures refer to deaths and discharges, and not to individual patients, a patient being transferred from one hospital to another will appear in a sample twice. The Hospital In-Patient Enquiry carries a considerable amount of other useful information. Table 5.1 gives the annual discharges and deaths from hospital in England and Wales for 1965, 1970, 1974 and 1975, these being the most up-to-date figures. Table 5.1 looks at the 121 910 patients who were discharged in 1975 who had sustained intra-cranial injury without fracture, and analyses them, giving the mean duration of stay, in days, (MDS), where the injury took place and added to this the figures of patients discharged with the diagnosis of concussion.

It can be seen from Fig. 5.2 that there are two peaks of incidence of head injury: one between the ages of 15 and 19 years of age, and the other for the

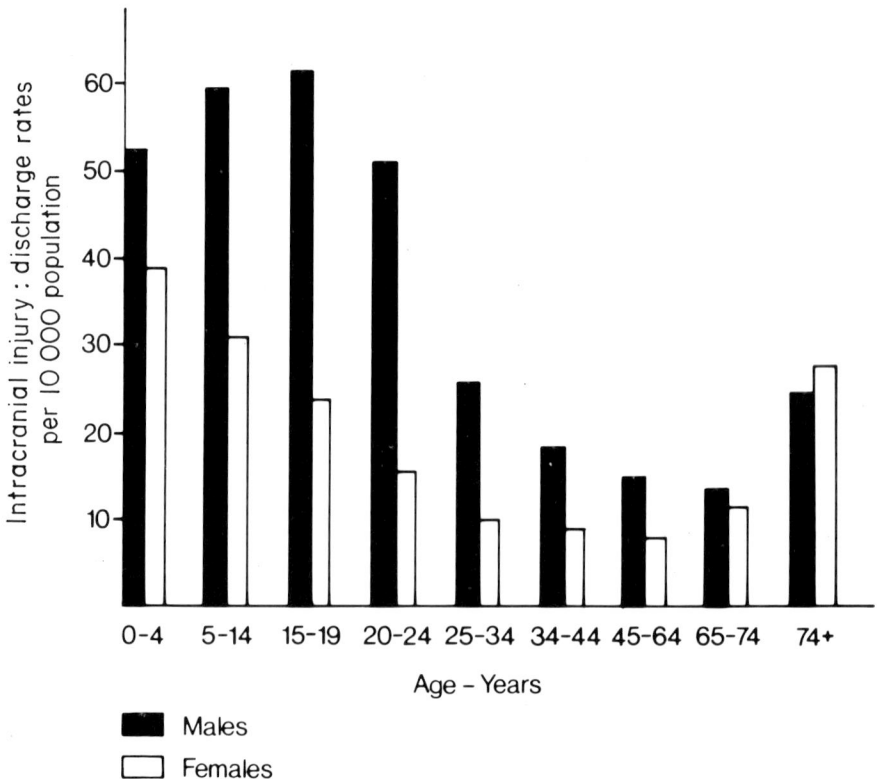

Fig. 5.2 Discharge rates per 10 000 population: sex, age group and diagnostic groups.

elderly over 75. The same table shows that young men are much more at risk than young women, and men of all ages are twice as likely to sustain head injury than women. The study also breaks down the numbers of children under 15 in greater detail, and Fig. 5.3 shows that for both sexes the vulnerable age is between 5 and 9. All these figures need to be treated with some caution, but in

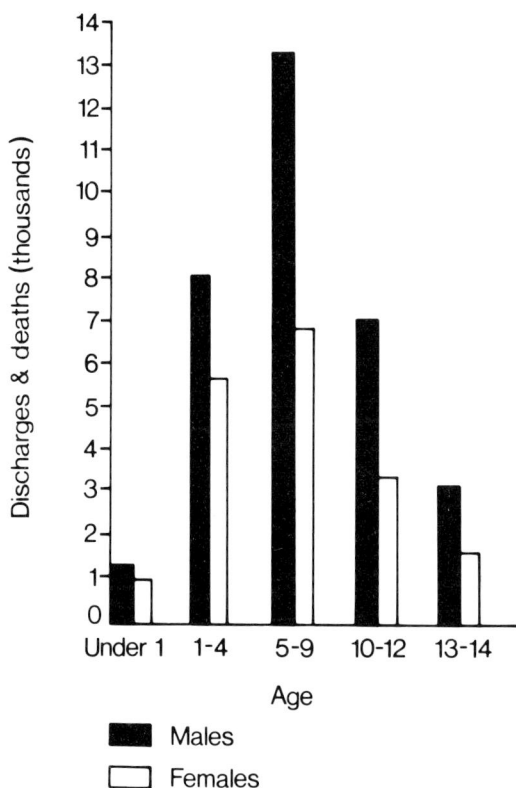

Fig. 5.3   Intracranial injury. Estimated total discharges and deaths of children under 15 years of age.

general Figs. 5.2 and 5.3 confirm what common sense indicates: that the majority of accidents are to young men, and that road traffic accident is the overwhelming single cause of these injuries. Field, in a report commissioned by the DHSS in 1976, has studied the figures with great care and analyses the available information in much greater depth, in addition to reviewing the literature and outlining active research projects (Field, 1976).

ASSESSMENT OF THE SEVERITY OF HEAD INJURY

For the last six years a prospective study has been undertaken on a cohort of patients who were admitted to the Joint Services Medical Rehabilitation Unit at Chessington and followed back into the community. The study was initiated because of difficulties the staff had in establishing whether they were contributing towards clinical recovery, or merely observing it. In order to compare groups of patients, it was important to establish first how severe the original injury had been. This proved difficult, because the only measure which had been in consistent use was the duration of either post-traumatic (anterograde) or retrograde amnesia, and the definition of these terms is not precise. Neither had a definition of coma been used consistently. Because of this lack of precision, it was indifferently recorded in the vast majority of cases. Jennett *et al.* (1976) have written of their experiences on the neurosurgical unit of the Southern General Hospital in Glasgow, and now have established that the duration and quality of coma is of major significance, not only in the clinical management during these stages but also in acting as a predictor of final outcome. For this study, therefore, we adopted their criteria and definitions, and our interpretation of these is given below.

POST-TRAUMATIC AMNESIA (PTA)

'The loss of memory from the time of the original injury to the time when continual day-to-day memory has been re-established.' This has been used as the standard measure of the severity of the accident and was placed firmly in the forefront since the paper by Russell and Smith (1961). Table 5.2 gives the

Table 5.2   Grading of the severity of head injury using PTA.

0	PTA	Nil
1	PTA less than 1 hour	Mild
2	PTA more than 1 hour, less than 1 day	Moderate
3	PTA more than 1 day, less than 1 week	Severe
4	PTA more that 1 week	Very severe

grading of severity of a head injury according to their criteria. PTA is of use in giving an impression of severity for those patients who have been relatively lightly injured and whose PTA is going to be in the order of hours or days rather than weeks or months, but when the duration of PTA is known it is a good predictor of final outcome, but it has two major snags. The first is that the end point in patients with moderate brain damage is very difficult to assess, and the second that for patients with severe brain damage it is unusable for prediction since it is wholly retrospective.

UNCONSCIOUSNESS

Unconsciousness lasts from the time of injury to the time when a patient can make a meaningful response which is better than 'yes' or 'no', but which takes into account the limits of speech which might be imposed by mechanical factors, e.g. tracheostomy. In theory the duration of coma should be easier to use once its definition is agreed, and the Glasgow workers, in collaboration with those in Groningen and New York, find it is possible to make accurate predictions and base clinical management on duration and depth of coma and the rate at which the patient surfaces (Jennett *et al.*, 1976; 1977). Both the figures from Glasgow and those from the study at Chessington suggest that the duration of coma is roughly a quarter of that of PTA, though by the time that unconsciousness has been present for two or three months the establishment of normal memory may never appear. The use of the duration of unconsciousness as a predictor is made more difficult where other factors have contributed to its duration, such as alcohol or operations for causes unrelated to the head injury.

RETROGRADE AMNESIA

This was defined as the loss of memory from some point in time before the accident up till the time it took place. It appeared to have had no value as a predictor but had occasional marginal relevance if grossly prolonged, when some question may be raised as to the reason behind this disproportionate symptom in that it might be manipulative. It is also sometimes used to measure severity in minor head injuries, such as on a football field.

Concussion. Definition of this term is loose, and its use was avoided.

ASSESSMENT OF THE SEVERITY OF BRAIN DAMAGE FOLLOWING HEAD INJURY

Assessment will only be useful if it is being done for a specific purpose and the assessment itself is capable of answering the questions asked of it. An enormous number of assessments are done, both informally through clinical examination and by ordinary patient/staff contact, and there are many more done formally which produce no valid information since no useful question was asked. For example, it is reasonable for an occupational therapist to assess a patient to see whether he is capable of self care at home, but it is irrelevant if the social conditions will prevent his return there. If time used in assessment, then, is to be profitable, the results of the assessment need to be relevant, repeatable, record-able and retrievable.

There are two widely separate groups of reasons for initiating formal assessments: the one being concerned with research and the other concerned with the practical aspects of the patient's care. In the former case, changes need to be observed precisely, and it must be accepted that some information that may be redundant will be obtained, which may turn out to have no practical value. Provided this sort of assessment is not confused with the second group, which is much more practically orientated, then there is little problem. But persuading therapists who are concerned with giving a service for the handicapped patient to do prolonged investigations which seem futile is difficult unless the project is thoroughly explained at the beginning and extra staff recruited with the aim of doing the assessments. The two aims, in the event, need not be incompatible, and a well-designed research assessment does eventually help therapists to produce better service assessments with greater precision.

REPEATABILITY

It should not matter which therapist has undertaken a particular assessment, provided they have been trained to do it. One recent study, in which the observer-error was minimized, was undertaken at Oxford by Lincoln and Leadbitter (1979) and shows their careful assessment of functional ability and the length to which the therapists went in order to determine, and reduce, observer-error. This particular study was done on patients recovering from stroke, but the development of similar techniques is possible with patients who have suffered traumatic brain damage.

RECORDABILITY

Subjective narrative reports are misleading and time-consuming, though never entirely dispensable. If the luxury of such aids as video-tape recording are unavailable, then the next best thing is either to devise or use available systems of scored assessments where answers to the question of ability are done by a straight yes/no choice. (Provision of such a questionnaire often seems more difficult than it is.) Dozens of questionnaires have been produced for activities of daily living which were reviewed by Donaldson *et al.* (1973). They came to the conclusion that it was confusing to offer more than a five-point scale of any given activity, because as the precision required increased, so did observer-error. This problem is simply solved by phrasing in a different way. In Fig. 5.4a a system is shown based on the therapist's choice, where the opportunity for error appears, as the therapist is forced to make one choice out of five. But if the question is asked in a different way, and displayed as Fig. 5.4b, the observer has an easier set of choices. If, in a subsequent assessment, change is shown, then information

Information can be recorded on a graded scale. Score 0–5.

A Joint position sense

Right Left

Metatarso-phalangeal joints

Scale of Grading

0 = Unaware of movement
1 = Aware at extremes only
2 = Aware of gross movement (> 60°)
3 = Aware of coarse movement (> 30°)
4 = Aware of fine movement (> 10°)
5 = Normal

or . . . .

As a series of True/False choices.

B Joint position sense
    The metatarso-phalangeal joint of the right foot has:

	True	False
No awareness of movement		
Awareness at extremes only		
Aware of gross movement (> 60°)		
Aware of coarse movement (> 30°)		
Aware of fine movement (> 10°)		
Normal		

Fig 5.4 Alternative methods of recording information.

has been recorded without too much stress for the therapist! Ideally, information is supplemented by video-tape recordings.

RETRIEVABILITY

From the information observed a huge stack of figures is easy to obtain, but to extract common sense is more difficult. However, with modern methods of information processing, data are storable on computer. At a more humble level, it is feasible to record the information and then produce a graphic summary, such as in Fig. 5.5, in which areas of handicap, or inability, are simply marked off in black. Reassessment later shows that a change has taken place, and in Fig. 5.6 that this change is confirmed over the next few weeks, and continued for the next few years (Fig. 5.7). For these particular figures to be significant, they do, of course, have to be compared with some other yardstick, and the question of relevant outcome measures is discussed towards the end of the chapter.

   When a suitable method of assessment has been adopted, it becomes easier to set up realistic aims of rehabilitation, and on occasions to be able to give accurate individual prognoses.

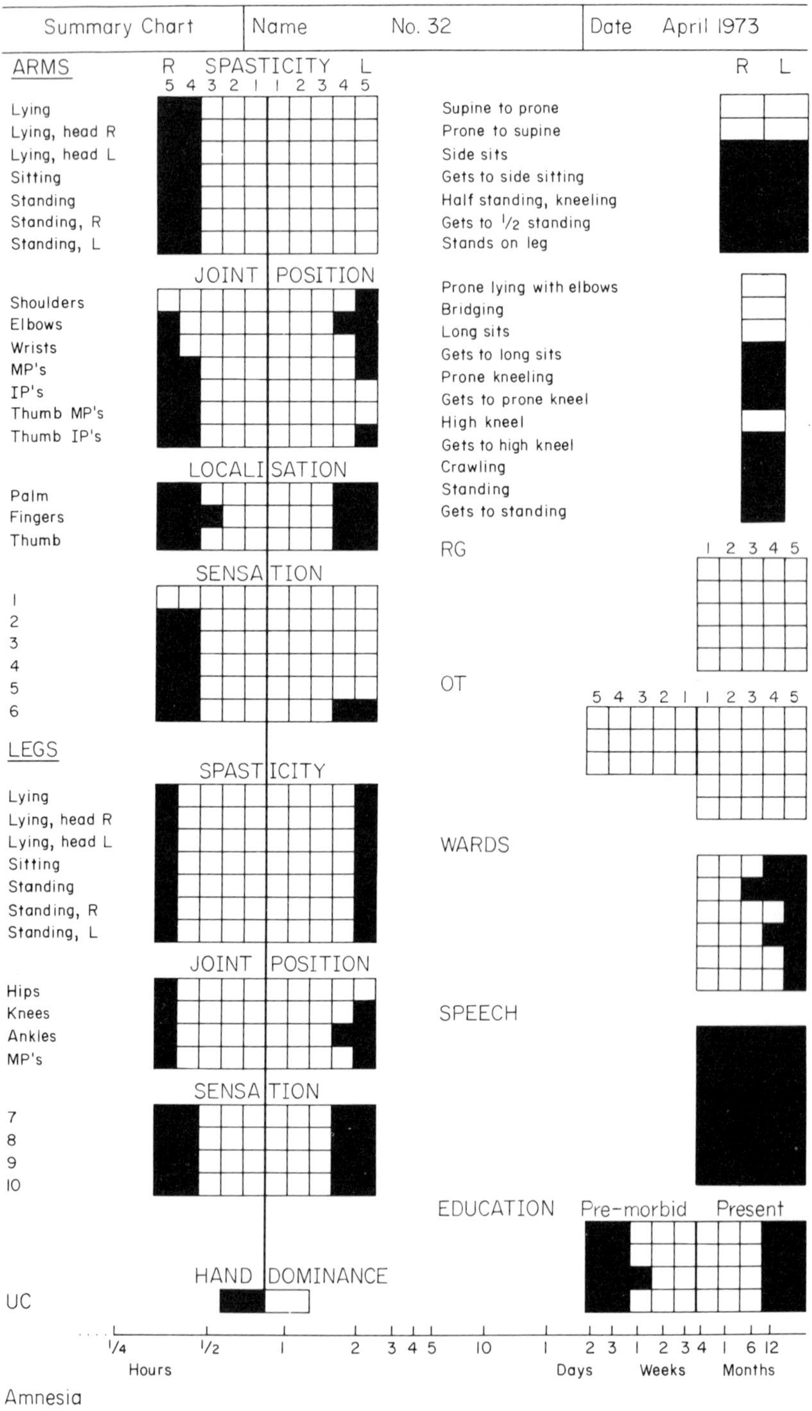

Fig. 5.5 Summary chart of one patient showing that recovery is recordable and takes place over many years.

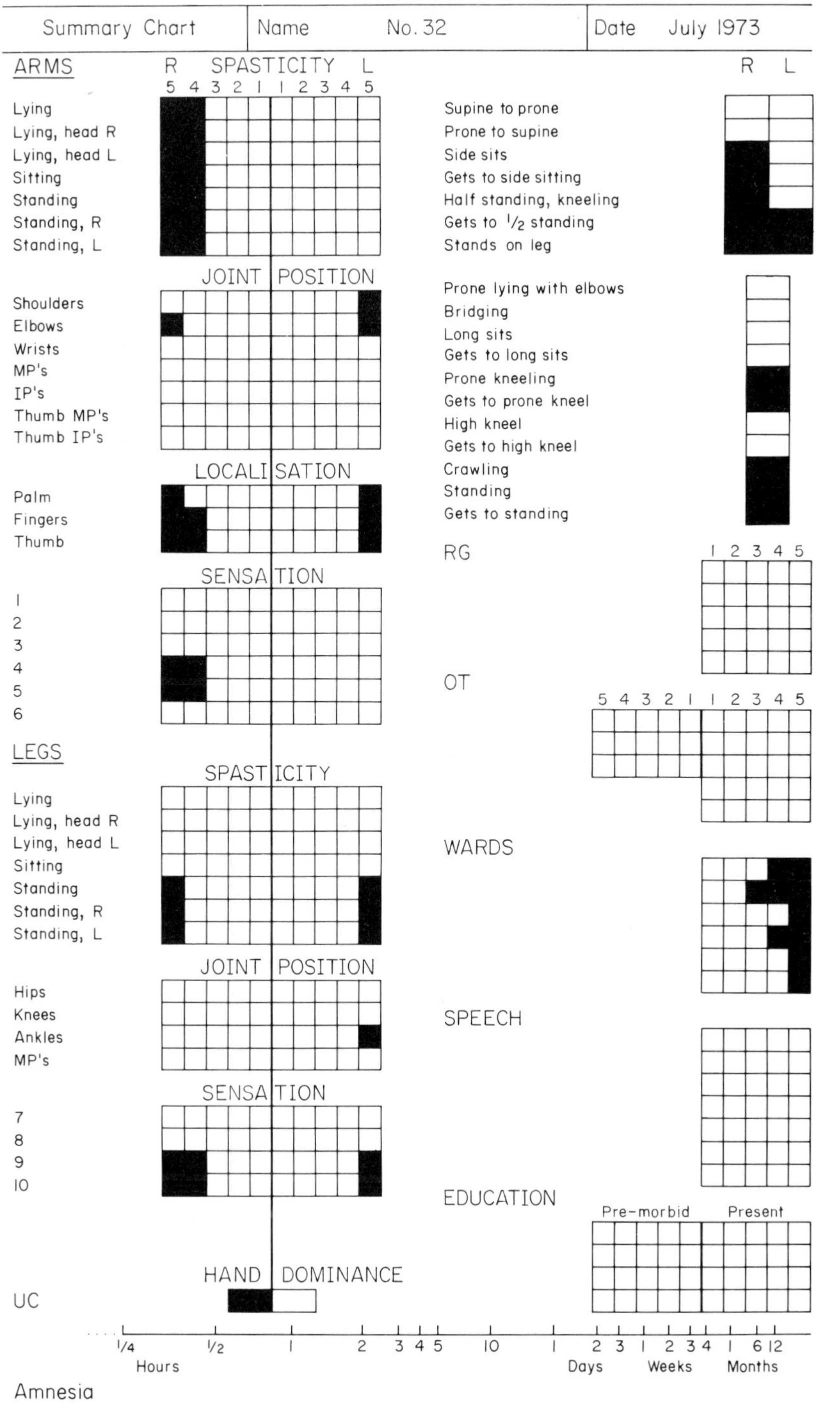

Fig. 5.6 Summary chart of one patient showing that recovery is recordable and takes place over many years.

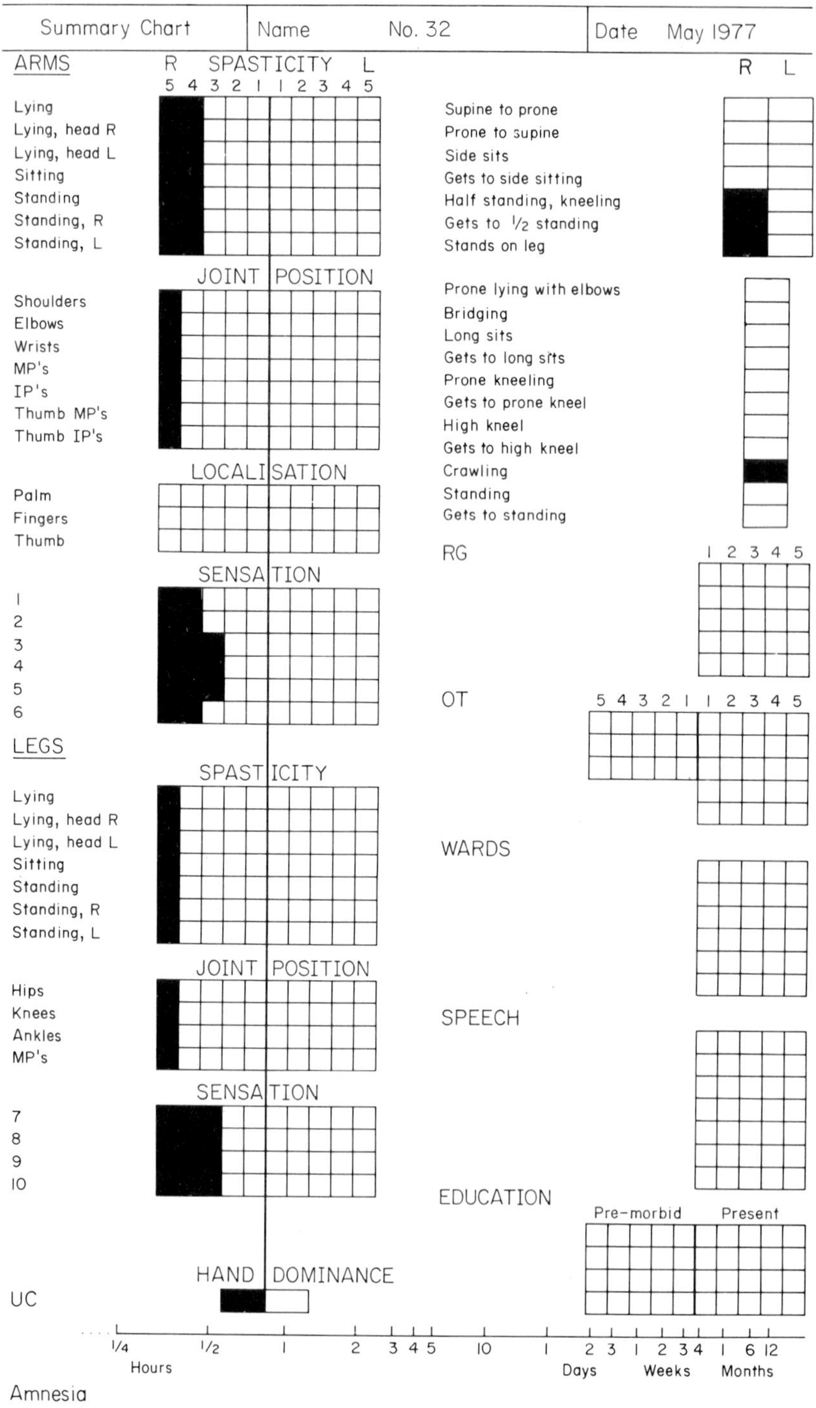

| Summary Chart | Name | No. 32 | Date | May 1977 |

ARMS   R   SPASTICITY   L   R   L
5 4 3 2 1 | 1 2 3 4 5

Lying
Lying, head R
Lying, head L
Sitting
Standing
Standing, R
Standing, L

Supine to prone
Prone to supine
Side sits
Gets to side sitting
Half standing, kneeling
Gets to ½ standing
Stands on leg

JOINT POSITION

Shoulders
Elbows
Wrists
MP's
IP's
Thumb MP's
Thumb IP's

Prone lying with elbows
Bridging
Long sits
Gets to long sits
Prone kneeling
Gets to prone kneel
High kneel
Gets to high kneel

LOCALISATION

Palm
Fingers
Thumb

Crawling
Standing
Gets to standing

RG   1 2 3 4 5

SENSATION

1
2
3
4
5
6

OT   5 4 3 2 1 1 2 3 4 5

LEGS

SPASTICITY

Lying
Lying, head R
Lying, head L
Sitting
Standing
Standing, R
Standing, L

WARDS

JOINT POSITION

Hips
Knees
Ankles
MP's

SPEECH

SENSATION

7
8
9
10

EDUCATION   Pre-morbid   Present

HAND DOMINANCE

UC

¼   ½   1   2   3 4 5   10   1   2 3   1   2 3 4   1   6 12
Hours   Days   Weeks   Months

Amnesia

Fig. 5.7 Summary chart of one patient showing that recovery is recordable and takes place over many years.

THE THERAPEUTIC TEAM

Lists of members of a team are always open to the danger that somebody crucial will be omitted, so although this is intended to be a list of all the relevant disciplines in a rehabilitation team, apologies are offered if any group remains unrepresented.

The list has been given in alphabetical order, in order to ensure that no hierarchy is implied, and perhaps this point should be taken up and clarified first. Up until the last few years, it has been universally assumed that the doctor will be the head of the rehabilitation team, but throughout the world there is now some challenge to this assumption. In some instances the challenge is made because senior members of remedial professions feel that their expertise is sufficient, so that the doctor's role should be confined to the diagnosis and clinical management, and that the work that takes place within the department run by the remedial profession itself should be a matter for the remedial therapists. In other circumstances, therapists or nurses take charge of teams where there is no doctor available and this is particularly common in developing countries. Either way, it means that the doctor involved with the rehabilitation process has to identify clearly the boundaries of his responsibilities and to ensure that excellent communications exist across them. In most countries of the world, it is the doctor who carries the responsibility for his patient, but if he is to fulfil this role usefully, then he has to be seen to be in charge and in touch with all the rest of the members of the rehabilitation team, and so establish his leadership, rather than take it for granted.

CLINICAL PSYCHOLOGISTS

This group usually have an academic background and have qualified with a university degree. A psychologist is one who is involved in the study of mind, and clearly following brain damage this aspect is crucial. In practical terms the clinical psychologist is expected to be able to make formal assessments of such qualities as memory, mood, intellect, comprehension and expression. All are of great moment both to the attendants and relatives of those who have suffered brain damage. In most departments the numbers of clinical psychologists are insufficient to do all the work that could be set before them, so that frequently they are left with the unhappy task of being asked to do assessments and then unable to give any form of therapeutic help as a result of the assessment they have made, and it is a rare unit where there is establishment large enough for the clinical psychologist to make a significant contribution to treatment. If such contributions are possible, then the setting of realistic goals, behaviour modification, introducing suitable incentives for patients (and sometimes for their relatives and the staff), can be considered. In many units there is no establishment for a clinical psychologist at all, and then their role may be partly taken over by speech therapists or occupational therapists.

DISABLEMENT RESETTLEMENT OFFICERS (DRO)

These officials are not members of the National Health Service in the United Kingdom but are responsible to the Department of Employment. Their help in providing support for people with brain damage, and indeed many other forms of injury, is invaluable. If it appears that there is likely to be a problem of employment, then the earlier that the good offices of the DRO can be invoked, the better. Even if it later becomes apparent that the patient may be able to get back his original job, suitable re-training courses can be arranged, and if a change of job appears inevitable, then the use of the Employment Medical Advisory Service can also be invoked through the DRO, and a wide range of assessment and training and help with employment can be given. This may amount to the provision of money for courses which are not available within United Kingdom Government Training Centres (Skill Centres). The advantage of recruiting the DRO early is that it will minimize, or eliminate, the delay between the patient leaving hospital or rehabilitation centre and the time he starts work. A long period of delay before starting work is very destructive to morale for the vast majority of those for whom work has previously been part of their ethic.

DOCTORS

It has already been suggested that the role of the doctor during the rehabilitation phase is equivocal, and is now undergoing change. There seems to be no alternative but that a doctor should be, and in most centres is, legally responsible for the general care and direction of the rehabilitation. Sometimes, however, which doctor has this task is not always clear. For example, during the acute stage, whilst the patient is in hospital, then the overall management is the responsibility of the neurosurgeon, general surgeon or consultant in whose department the patient is, but once the patient has left hospital and gone home, or is attending a rehabilitation centre, then the responsibility becomes divided. Furthermore, because of the original doctor's main role, which will involve him in much routine medical work, he usually has little time to take a direct interest in the rehabilitation after the acute stage. This responsibility is then delegated, formally or informally, either to junior medical staff, who quite frequently have little experience in the field, or to the therapists. The first system is unworkable, and if the second is to be adopted then it needs to be done formally so that, in the event of medical advice being required, the channel to get it is clear.

NURSES

The role of the nurse in rehabilitation is changing rapidly. Once the ward sister and nursing staff assumed much responsibility for the day-to-day management of the patient's care. Some years ago the ward sister would organize voluntary help or other forms of help to provide what we now ask an occupational therapist to do. Social enquiry, talking to relatives and the preparation for the patient's discharge, would also have been the nurses' responsibility. With proliferation of rehabilitation staff, this is now not always so. Where a clear allocation of responsibility has been agreed, problems are trivial, but where it is unresolved, duplication of effort and conflicting advice results. Conflict may occur at many levels, but the one of greatest importance is the link between the therapists and the nursing staff. Frequently the therapeutic staff may decide that a given form of system of physical treatment should be adopted (and there are many such available, all with their special advantages claimed). Possibly the individual system is significant, though this has yet to be proved, but there seems universal agreement that if one system of lifting is used by the therapists in the departments, and a totally different one used in the wards, it will cause uncertainty from the patient's and relatives' point of view. It is feasible, and occasionally practical, for the therapists to spend time ensuring that members of the nursing staff are aware of the current system. They can explain why particular techniques of lifting, sitting, posturing and feeding should be adopted. In a really dedicated unit, the therapists will come in late at night in order that the night staff shall then share this information as well. When the treatment programme becomes consistent, better results seem to be achieved, though as with many other problems in rehabilitation, establishing this to be statistically significant is difficult.

Frequently the reason given for the nurses to dress and feed a patient is that it is quicker to do the work for the patient than wait whilst unsuccessful attempts are made. So help is not given to the patients to perform the tasks themselves. If nurses are to play their full part in the rehabilitation effort, their establishment level must be such to allow enough time to be given with patients so that work initiated in departments is carried on through weekends and evenings, consistently, if more slowly.

OCCUPATIONAL THERAPISTS

The occupational therapist trains over a three-year period, and has a working knowledge of anatomy, physiology and medical conditions and some knowledge of craft work. Recently they seem to have specialized in assessment of activities of daily living (ADL), provision of aids, and, in some instances, into the assessment of basic psychological problems. The Association of Occupational Therapists is running courses to train OTs to administer some of the basic psychological tests which hitherto have been administered only by clinical psychologists. This is a constructive development since it is unrealistic to expect that all hospitals can establish clinical psychologists as part of the rehabilitation team in the foreseeable future. Because of the number of hospital departments in which occupational therapy is available, the therapists play a significant part in the rehabilitation of patients with brain damage, and are often called in to give the final assessment prior to attempting to discharge the patient home into the community. Some progressive departments are also assessing perceptual problems, and make active strides to retrain such deficits. Where this facility is available then it is ideally requested as early as possible in the rehabilitation of the patient.

PHYSIOTHERAPISTS

This profession has a three-year training course, at the end of which the physiotherapist is expected to have a working knowledge of general anatomy and physiology, with a detailed cover of the musculo-skeletal and nervous systems. Over the last few years this profession has also spent a great deal of time trying to develop assessments of physical ability, several papers having been published as a result of this work (Stichbury, 1975; Graham, 1975; Lincoln & Leadbitter, 1979). Both in the United Kingdom and overseas physiotherapy departments have been responsible for developing many different systems of physical rehabilitation—Bobath methods being just one such. In some of the systems under use, the neurophysiological basis has always seemed somewhat sketchy, but where the system being developed appears to have common sense behind it, there seems little reason why one given system should not be used. As to which is best, it seems that the conviction of the therapist that what he or she is doing is correct, is probably of more significance than the actual technique itself. Where a department decides on a specific technique, then it is imperative that all the other disciplines are aware of this decision and respect it. Frequently, the introduction of such a system necessitates close collaboration between the therapy departments; this in itself leads to what, in contemporary jargon, is called the integrated team approach.

RELATIVES

Some reasons why relatives should be included as part of the therapy team are sufficiently obvious to require mention but no elaboration. For somebody with severe brain damage, the people most likely to be left with the major responsibility and problem are the relatives, and a tremendous amount of cooperation and help must be given if they are to achieve this very difficult task with any prospect of success. The chance of success depends not only on the severity of the injury but on which relative it is who subsequently has to look after the victim. The prospects of a satisfactory return home appear greatest when the injured themselves are young and where the mother is still able to care. If only the father is available, then the chance of a successful return home is smaller. If the patients themselves are older, and the relatives are elderly, then returning a patient home is unstable, because with increasing frailty either the mother or father, or both, are unable to continue with the task. Then another solution has to be sought. It is also difficult to resettle an elderly patient with brain damage with their children for a long time as a very small disturbance in the domestic set-up will turn this into an unacceptable position. It may be possible with planned support, holiday relief and other forms of social and medical aid, that the problem for the caring relatives can be eased; so these aids should be used as early as possible to help the whole family.

Relatives can also be of major value much earlier. The presence of relatives beside the bed, constantly reassuring the patient as to who they are, where they are and what has happened, seems often to have a major positive benefit. Unfortunately, proof of this statement in statistical terms is impossible, but apocryphally, many brain-damaged survivors have been able to recall, with considerable precision, information that was being given them during the time when they appeared to be unconscious and uncommunicative. They recall this attention with deep gratitude and affection. On a completely common-sense basis, it appears a reasonable course of action, and in practical terms it is usually encouraged by all acute units where feasible. One group of relatives introduced, after the first two or three days on a ward, a visitors' book, where each relative or friend who came noted the date and the subject of any conversation that they may have had with the patient, and any observations that they made, particularly with reference to what was known about the patient from before the accident. Since this information is so rarely available, this book, charting the recovery of the patient from deep coma, provided a tremendous insight for the nursing and medical staff on the ward concerned. It seems a simple and useful way of gathering information and involving the relatives from a very early stage in the programme of rehabilitation. It also permitted much more communication between the nursing staff and the relatives than can normally be guaranteed.

REMEDIAL GYMNAST

This discipline has a great deal in common with physiotherapy: to the outside observer indeed, the similarities in task are more apparent than the differences. There are historical reasons why the two professions should have grown up separately, and other reasons why they are unable to merge. Numerically there are far fewer remedial gymnasts than physiotherapists and in general terms their work is designed more to the administration of physical exercise than to the application of electrically or other physically based treatments. However, with the move away from such treatments by the physiotherapists and the adoption by remedial gymnasts of the skills to give basic heat and ice therapy, the differences have become even fewer. In practice their recruitment and involvement in the team of a rehabilitation unit depend more on local history and staff availability than anything else, and the role in which they are used is similarly unpredictable. However, they are frequently employed in a manner which appears to the observer to be indistinguishable from the physiotherapist, though possibly in the later stages of work they may get themselves more involved with class work; even this generalization is open to dispute.

REHABILITATION ENGINEERS

Few units will have the services of such a professional, it being almost inevitable that at the present time they are confined to research units and university departments. However, if these specific services are not available and some item of equipment requires individually making, there are alternative sources available, and one such in the UK is REMAP; this association can be contacted at the Biological Engineering Society whose address will be given at the end of this chapter.

SPEECH THERAPISTS

Again this profession has developed over the last few years, but for wide areas of the UK the amount of staff available is only a token. Where this situation obtains, the most profitable role for the therapist is to assess at what level communication with the patient exists and how the relatives and nursing staff may capitalize upon what comprehension and expression there are. In the absence of both the speech therapist and a clinical psychologist, the responsibility for this particular function may devolve upon the occupational therapist, but rest somewhere it must, for establishment of any method of communication as early as possible with the brain-damaged survivor seems to be of crucial importance. As in stroke, it would appear that perception of hearing and seeing may precede recovery in expression by a considerable time. In theory, this information is widely known: in practice it is frequently forgotten, and the patient can easily become the equivalent of a pillow in the bed to be talked over, and around, but never to. In patients who recover after a long time, this is commented on, often in terms of strongest resentment. In later stages of recovery, when speech content may be relatively normal but its articulation slow and confusing, it is again of the utmost importance that the response of the therapeutic staff and the relatives should be to treat the patient as having a normal perception and comprehension, even if the evidence appears to point to the contrary. There is little to be lost by such a strategy, but everything to be gained.

TECHNICAL INSTRUCTORS

Technical instructors may supervise retraining, either for an original job, or assess and evaluate a suitable alternative. It is unlikely that these staff will be present in many hospitals, but they are represented in some rehabilitation centres. There needs to be close liaison between them and the occupational therapy department. In a few hospitals the instructors are actually part of such a department.

Although assessments carried out by technical instructors in hospital and rehabilitation centres have no statutory significance in subsequent placement through employment rehabilitation centres and skill centres, they allow people to be presented to industrial rehabilitation with a higher chance of success than if they are presented from the hospital or home without such preparation. In addition, a technical instructor can supervise work that may help to overcome resistance felt by some patients to the sort of craft or skill usually within the compass of occupational therapists. Occupational therapists recognize the problem of giving tasks which are significant and realistic, particularly to patients who have been previously employed on a technical or clerical basis, but have not the industrial expertise. The skills of a rehabilitation technical instructor, and the workshop facilities that he should have at his disposal, may make a significant contribution to overcoming this problem. At the Swiss Workers' Rehabilitation Unit at Bellikon near Berne, the facilities in the workshops are unparalleled, but if such a magnificence is unrepeatable in most places, the principle can be adopted.

SOCIAL WORK DEPARTMENT

Administratively social workers are no longer part of the health care team in the UK since they are almost always employed by the local authority, and subsequently seconded to work in hospitals or rehabilitation centres. Being a relatively new discipline the contribution that they have to make is still capable of being misunderstood. For example, nursing staff may feel that the contact with relatives and the counselling were originally part of their role and are not keen to feel that the responsibility for such counselling has passed out of their hands, although in the vast majority of cases they clearly have not the time to do it justice. Again, the social worker frequently makes the time to listen to problems of the patients and relatives and seems then to form a better contact than doctors or other staff involved. Again, the lack of time of the other disciplines is quoted as the reason that this relationship falls off, so it is imperative that somebody takes this responsibility, and it usually appears to devolve upon the social worker. Provided the case conferences are taken seriously and communication is good, no problem need arise, but the prime sufferer is the patient. Other professionals can see more clearly where their responsibility ends, but the social worker knows that he or she will be the person who, next to the relatives, will have the biggest responsibility for the longest period of time, once the patient has left hospital. They also frequently find themselves in the unenviable buffer-zone between relatives and medical staff. This can be very trying when the hospital or rehabilitation centre is trying to discharge a patient home and the social worker can see only too clearly the problems that are involved in this manoeuvre. The decision to return a patient to the community should be based on a consistent team approach and liaison with the available community services. A gradual transition, possibly by allowing the patient home at weekends only, or during the week, can encourage the relatives to take over in many cases, but it may often have to be supervised by the social work department which will also be responsible for ensuring that any statutory help is provided, and that the necessary adaptations to the home and work are undertaken and paid for.

VOLUNTARY ORGANIZATIONS

There are literally hundreds of organizations that may be involved in different parts of the country in the rehabilitation process. Some will act at the hospital level, such as the League of Friends, who are often able to provide some financial support or bits of apparatus which seem not to be forthcoming from the hospital service itself, such as page-turners, reading aids and so forth. It is also possible that these items may be provided through the Red Cross, and this organization also has loan fleets of wheelchairs and may be used in emergency to supplement the services of the ordinary method of supply of wheelchairs through artificial limb and appliance centres. Then organizations such as Cheshire Homes may eventually find themselves accepting long-term responsibility for the care of patients who cannot return to the community.

THE PATIENT

So far, two major aspects have been left unexplored. The first is the definition of rehabilitation itself, and the second the contribution that the patient has to make to the solution of his problems. Attempting to define rehabilitation is difficult: but perhaps the neatest definition, by an anonymous medical student, is 'the reintegration of a patient with his original environment'. As a definition, this could be said to include the entire range of medicine, but it does have the advantage that it draws attention to the process of restoration and invites attention to the original environment. This means paying careful attention to what the patient and his family were like before the accident.

Many who work with those who have suffered brain injury feel that the population is skewed and does not represent a true cross-section. It is quite possible that patients who suffer any injury come from specific sections of the population, even allowing for the already discussed age and sex differentials. It seems common sense that people who are aggressive are more likely to be hit by a bottle, that bad drivers are more likely to be involved in accidents and that drunken pedestrians are more likely than sober ones to be hit by cars. Much information on the timing of accidents is available from the Road Research Laboratory and confirms the clinical impression that they are not a random selection of the population.

In the Chessington study a great deal of time and care was taken to try to re-establish the circumstances of the patient before the accident took place, and it seemed that quite a fair prediction can be made of some aspects of the quality of recovery. If, before the accident, the patient was known to be a short-tempered, aggressive boor, and is so described, or was a work-shy, alcoholic lay-about, then the occurrence of severe head injury was unlikely to improve his personality. This could not always be assumed since one particularly aggressive young man was received home by his relatives with glee, for they found he was much less aggressive than before the accident. In general, it seemed that behaviour and motivation of a patient before the accident had an important bearing on the fortitude of his attempts afterwards to come back to normality, and since these unhappy groups of patients often come from the most deprived social groups, with poor family support and often bad environment, they represent the biggest challenge to any rehabilitation attempt.

PLANNING TREATMENT

Planning the rehabilitation of patients with severe brain damage depends first of all upon a precise knowledge, where possible, of the extent of the original injury, both in anatomical terms where this can be gained and, where not, by inference from the duration of observed unconsciousness, or the duration of PTA. It involves assessments of the physical and intellectual deficits and abilities of the patient at the start of a rehabilitation programme, and the deployment of as many therapists as are available for as much time as possible in a consistent fashion. The formal effort must be made with the help of relatives and friends to produce a stable and consistent pattern of treatment. The amount of new information provided should be assimilable. The aims of any week's programme should be capable of realization, and yet should not underestimate potential that may be there. The precise techniques used by individual departments seem less important than the general morale and spirit of the team which undertakes the rehabilitation, and the consistency by which any given series of techniques is applied.

SPECIFIC PROBLEMS

There are, however, some specific problems that occur in the course of recovery from brain damage and which may require special attention as they occur. This list has been compiled from an analysis of the patients who passed through Chessington between 1972 and 1974 and who could be said to have failed. For this argument it will be assumed that a failure in the rehabilitation process has occurred when the patient is unable to reintegrate in society. It may be because he cannot go home, or is unemployable, or dependent on others for day-to-day needs, including financial support. In the group under discussion, four major factors emerged: epilepsy, behavioural change, impairment of memory and concentration, and the post-traumatic syndrome.

EPILEPSY

Jennett, in an article on the medical aspects of head injury (Jennett, 1977), goes into some detail on the incidence of late epilepsy in cases with severe brain damage. He draws a distinction between the fits that may occur through the early stages of recovery from brain damage, and late epilepsy, occurring after the first week. In his series, this occurred in about 5% of the head-injury patients admitted to hospital, but nevertheless represented a total within the UK of about 5000 per annum. Four factors predisposed to the incidence of late epilepsy: these were post-traumatic amnesia which lasted for more than 24 hours, a dural tear, focal signs and the incidence of early epilepsy. In the Chessington cohort, 22 patients out of the 107 followed up had developed late epilepsy, and it had proved one of the single most handicapping features as far as return to employment was concerned.

Most workers in rehabilitation find that the use of routine anticonvulsants by referring hospitals is uneven, and many patients will be on anticonvulsants in quite high dosage as a matter of routine and be left on them for long periods of time, even though no fit has ever been recorded. It is worth while referring patients back to the hospital for review of anti-epileptic drugs if the patient appears never to have had a fit and the use of drugs has been prophylactic. As Jennett points out, anticonvulsants should be used in high-risk patients but not in those patients with minimal risk; prolonged use of anticonvulsants may hamper the rehabilitation effort. It must also be borne in mind that there are those patients whose epilepsy preceded the head injury rather than followed it. The former will of course require examination and follow-up from a different point of view from those with post-traumatic epilepsy.

BEHAVIOURAL PROBLEMS

It is easy to be led into semantic discussions as to what constitute behaviour problems and how they are defined. In practice they are only too recognizable and the vast majority of complaints about patients who have suffered brain damage are either because of aggression or sexuality. Aggression itself may either be verbal or physical, and although the latter is more terrifying, neither is easy to live with in the long term. It is crucial whenever possible that the patient is involved in the decisions that affect him and every attempt is made to keep him informed about what is taking place. Failure can lead to a very sharp deterioration of relations between the patient and his relatives, as well as the staff. Inconsistency of approach, where one set of workers perhaps encourages an informal, christian-name approach, and another section within the same hospital is more formal, will produce insecurity and conflict. Again, consistency is more important than the actual technique. It is also extremely important that the staff know how to respond to threats, either physical or verbal, and any sanctions that are threatened against a patient are capable of being followed through. This is one of the roles in which a clinical psychologist can offer advice to alleviate a lot of stress to staff, relatives and, frequently, other patients. The clinical psychologist may advise on behaviour modification programmes, such as the introduction of a token economy or other form of incentive which will provide positive responses for 'good' behaviour and a realistic negative one for 'bad'. It would seem preferable to adopt this approach before a pharmacological therapeutic one, though a wide range of drugs is available. If the bent of aggressive behaviour has been discovered in one department and commented on, then it is reasonable to raise this at the next group meeting to see whether a pattern of the aggression can be determined. It may be to only one person, or in only one department. If this is the case it is unwise to assume that the patient is always wrong. Staff, either wittingly, or unwittingly, are capable of giving cause for aggression.

Sexuality, unlike aggression, may either be seen as a problem because of an increase, in which case either the relatives or the staff may justifiably complain, or the sexuality may decrease, in which case the patient or the spouse may complain. Care has to be taken to respond sympathetically when a problem is presented, or to try to anticipate a problem and so reduce it. The other extreme of assuming a problem exists unstated has to be guarded against most carefully. One of the commonest causes for complaint is usually due to a lack of inhibition which may amount to promiscuity, with complete disregard for the feelings of other people. Frequently this is a transient phase during the process of recovery, so its appearance need not be a reason for panic. However, during this stage, if it is not possible to control the behaviour of women and they put themselves at risk of unwanted pregnancy, consideration should be given to the avoidance or termination of such a pregnancy. Masturbation also frequently causes staff, relatives or other patients to complain. Fortunately this is also normally transient, and a consistent approach by which the patient is discouraged from masturbating in public may be sufficient. More draconian measures such as the isolation of a patient, or the administration of heavy sedatives, are rarely required. Libido may be either increased or decreased after the head injury, but a frequent complaint from the spouse is that of intemperate demand associated with inconsiderate performance. If there is also distaste experienced at having to live with, and sleep with, a different personality from the one accustomed to, then it may readily be seen how this can amount to a very serious obstacle in resettlement. Occasionally it explains the fact that families will have patients back for the day, but are much more reluctant to keep them overnight. Sympathetic counselling can be offered, advice against unwanted pregnancy can be given, but the sad fact remains that the altered sexuality and personality of patients may lead to a total disruption of married life, or the complete breakdown of the marriage. Having said this, it needs to be borne in mind that the problems may not be those of the patient, but those of the relatives or staff. Care must be taken not to project their problems on to the patient, who will have quite enough of his own.

MEMORY AND CONCENTRATION

Many patients who have suffered moderate brain damage and whose physical recovery is excellent may be unable to return to work and hold a job down, although from casual experience of their talk and examination, few problems seem apparent. Bond and Brooks (1976) discuss this in more detail. Quite what qualities go to make up the ability to concentrate and to retain information is not yet known. Despite this it is possible to try and clarify some aspects of memory for the sake of the relatives and friends. It may be possible that some help can be gained from the expertise of the clinical psychologist, but unfortunately, in common with the medical profession, there is very considerable confusion as to what constitutes memory and how it may be defined. Since this confusion already exists, some definitions have to be attempted, without universal agreement. The first broad division that can be made is between the recall of information that was present before the accident took place, such as biographical details, information about job, family and general knowledge, and the problems of the acquisition of new information after the head injury. It is the second aspect which causes the greater confusion. There is agreement that there is a difference between short-term and long-term memory and that there are various strategies for getting information that is available in the short term into a long-term store. But it is uncertain at what point long-term memory takes over from short-term: various definitions have placed this at anything from a few seconds to several minutes, or even longer. Then again, it seems possible that the failure to acquire new information may not be failure of memory in the sense of recall, but a failure to perceive new information in the first instance. In addition,

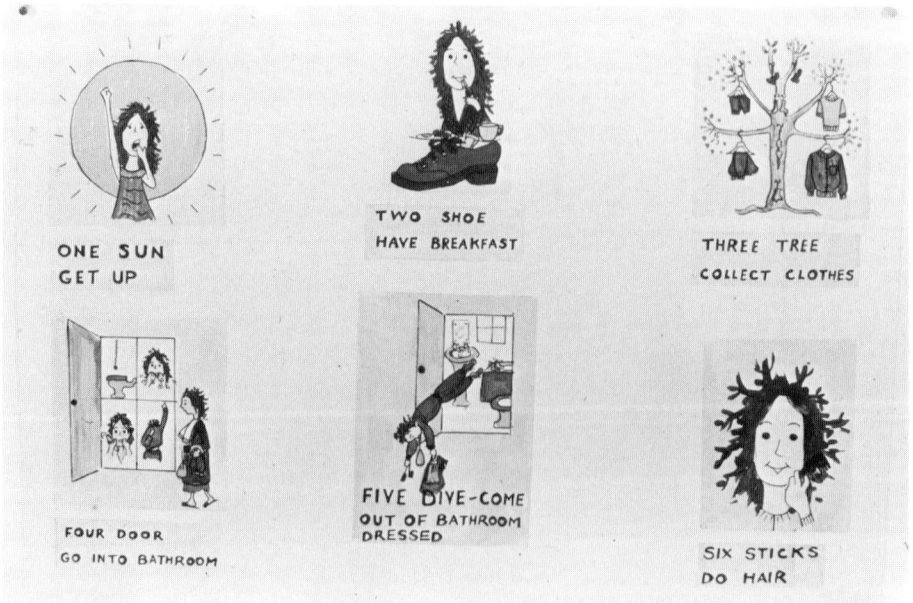

Fig. 5.8 Visual aid produced by the speech therapists to aid a patient who had severe sequencing problems after head injury.

perception of the different methods of giving information may be totally separate. For example, it is possible to talk about a cup of tea, write the words down, draw a picture, make the appropriate sounds or present it for drinking. Tremendous possibilities for research into the development of ability to perceive information are apparent. Fig. 5.8 shows a simple series of pictures and the mnemonics that were drawn for a patient who suffered, after brain damage, with inability to retain new information. Re-examining her years later, she had never forgotten the impact of these mnemonics and could still remember the therapists and the items of equipment by the pictures which were drawn for her. For her, it acted as the stepping stone from which she could then start to establish verbal memory. It seems appropriate, wherever possible, to use such bridges. At a simpler level, the use of diaries and slates contributes to independence. Perhaps even more important than the actual aids is the willingness to recognize that a problem exists. Then these simple aids can help, and continued rehearsal may lead to the eventual abandonment of the aid.

POST-TRAUMATIC SYNDROME

This is another minefield, both in diagnosis and in treatment. The classic description of the post-traumatic syndrome is a combination of symptoms such as concentration failure, poor memory, dizziness and headache. These symptoms are necessarily associated with momentary or no recorded unconsciousness to be truly classified as the post-traumatic syndrome, and it seems almost as though the incidence of this condition varies inversely to the duration of unconsciousness that has been observed. Certainly in the cohort that was examined, the only two patients who had symptoms suggestive of post-traumatic syndrome were those in whom the period of unconsciousness had been momentary and had been included in the series, later to be withdrawn for just this reason. Since so many of these symptoms are subjective, there has been much discussion as to whether the syndrome is a purely functional one, or even one in which symptoms are deliberately exaggerated and manipulated by the sufferer, and it may be that in some instances this is true. However, quite a lot of work has been done recently on the very mild brain injury, as judged by duration of unconsciousness and PTA. Bremner and Gillingham (1974), Jones (1974), and Newcombe *et al.* (1979) have all been searching for the objective evidence that even in the mild head injury there is some structural damage which may result in behavioural changes.

PROGNOSIS

Two aspects can be considered: the first is that of a general prognosis to be given on the basis of statistics that are known about patients in the past. This assumes that the severity of the injury can be equated between one patient and the next, and although this in some measure is possible, it is very difficult to generalize. However, the evidence of all cohorts of patients examined, together with common sense, would suggest that the longer the period of either unconsciousness or PTA is, then the more severe the subsequent handicap. This refers to groups and not individuals, so giving an individual prognosis is a greater risk as there are a substantial minority of patients who do not fit into the pattern, and who have prolonged periods of unconsciousness and make good recoveries, or negligible unconsciousness with disastrous social results. This suggests that another area of research could be into defining what constitutes a satisfactory social outcome measure. Up to now, even the most sophisticated series have used only relatively narrow bands of recovery (see Table 5.3). When trying to make a

Table 5.3   Outcome categories (After Jennet & Bond).

Classification	Outcome Categories
Carlsson *et al.*	Persisting coma; persisting dementia; mental restitution
Pazzaglia *et al.*	Prolonged coma; partially re-integrated; recovered
Heiskanen & Sipponen	Permanent invalid; recovery
Vigoroux *et al.*	Serious sequelae; nil/slight sequelae
Overgaard *et al.*	Apallic; severe deficit; good recovery
Vapalahti & Troupp	Vegetative existence; recovery

prediction for the individual, the only basis upon which we have to work seems to be the rate of recovery. Again, while this may appear to be stating the obvious, if the ability to predict at an early stage can be established, then a technique may be developed for evaluating the effectiveness of treatment.

Finally, the incidence of brain damage, both from road accident and stroke, has increased over the last years and figures from the Hospital In-Patient Enquiry confirm this. Some of the increase may be accounted for by the increase in the population, but another important factor is the improved techniques for resuscitation and life support during the acute stages following the incident. Although this means that fewer people die in the acute phase, it does mean that more people with severe handicap survive, for whom the availability of rehabilitation is sparse at the moment. Efforts are being made to evaluate rehabilitation, but it is difficult to isolate the effects of natural recovery from those induced by treatment. There are two extreme views taken: on the one hand it is said that there is no influence to be made by rehabilitation effort and that recovery takes place without outside interference: the other point of view is that an intensive and dramatic effort by staff, relatives and friends, perhaps for years, will pay dividends, but it is difficult to perform satisfactorily because of the enormous amount of time it takes. Some of the research methods which may help to elucidate these problems are just beginning to emerge. It is hoped that in future rehabilitation programmes can be developed on a rational basis so that the maximum amount of socially significant improvement can be obtained by the most rational use of the time of staff and relatives. It is also important to develop sympathetic alternative care for those unable to get back into society.

PROGNOSIS

Assessing the severity of a head injury and forecasting the future have to be done at several different stages of the recovery process, and the reasons for attempting the prognosis at each stage are different.

In the accident service itself, an initial trial is carried out, and this is designed to identify those patients who are beyond help and those who need no help, so that assistance can be given to those who will benefit from it and who need it. The Glasgow workers have concentrated on this aspect of prognosis and can make effective predictions as to the likelihood of recovery by using a small selection of effective indicators of outcome. This depends upon the assessment of the best verbal response, the best motor response and eye movements during the initial stages of recovery from brain damage. This information, fed into a computer, enables predictions for groups to be made, and also for individuals, though, as they point out, this is intended to be another method of supporting clinical judgement and not designed to replace it.

Once initial recovery has been assured, the next aspect of prognosis that has to be considered is the fitness of the patient to leave hospital, go home or take up his former occupation. For these, the sort of assessments that have been devised by doctors and therapists (Stichbury, 1975; Lincoln & Leadbitter, 1979) and many other workers give an indication of the state of the patient either as they leave hospital or as they start in a rehabilitation centre. Making a prognosis at this stage is much more difficult. Experience with the long-term follow-up of 103 brain-damaged survivors (Evans, *et al.* 1980) suggests that outcome can be measured for the majority of those with brain damage in terms of five outcome measures (see Table 5.4). Initial examination of the early assessments and relating them to final outcome reveal that the duration of unconsciousness seems

Table 5.4   Socially orientated outcome measures.

Outcome measures
Accommodation required
Aids needed
Employability compared with pre-accident ability
Financial independence
Personal independence

very significant, and all those patients who were observed to be unconscious for more than three months have remained totally dependent. Similarly, all those who were unconscious for less than a week have regained either initial or equivalent employment and are independent both financially and socially, and all are in work. The onset of epilepsy following head injury also has a severe impact on employability, if that is to be taken as the outcome measure, though whether this suggests that the epilepsy represents the severity of the underlying lesion or is a problem on its own has yet to be resolved. Its effect on independence, however, is drastic; only one of the fifteen who had epilepsy after the injury being in employment.

It is also necessary to provide information for relatives which is as accurate as possible, so that they may plan their lives and also help the patient to the maximum. Giving a prognosis in statistical terms such as have just been referred to is not too difficult, but relating this to the individual becomes much more uncertain. Whilst the extremes are reasonably clear, the group with handicap are those about whom the uncertainty is greatest and for whom the need for information is urgent. In addition to this difficulty, the other problem is the continual change that may take place within a patient. This may be best illustrated by a case example of a young man who was involved in an aircraft accident and rendered unconscious, with other multiple injuries, for several weeks. It was felt by the admitting hospital that he had no chance of survival and his wife was so informed. The patient, however, did not die, though by the time any form of consciousness was recovered, he had developed severe flexion contractures of knees, hips, elbows, and also the fractures which he had sustained at the time of the head injury were uniting in a poor position. At this stage, his wife was informed that he would never be able to walk, talk or go home. Over a year after the initial accident, the patient was admitted to a rehabilitation centre, and over the next three years continued to make progress to the point finally of being able to talk coherently, requiring operations both on his eyes and on his fractures and to relieve contractures, and his wife was then told that the patient would eventually be fit to go home. By this time his wife had become used to the idea, first of all that there was no prospect for life, then that there was no prospect of his going home, but finally she had to adjust to the idea that not only would her husband be at home but would probably also have an altered and impaired personality. This sad history is frequently seen and emphasizes the extreme care with which relatives must be informed of the future, and the stress placed on the fact that the situation is likely to be unstable for months or years, and that decisions regarding the future should only be taken as far as it is possible at that time to see.

FUTURE DEVELOPMENTS

Elsewhere in this book, Professor Bach-y-Rita, Dr Devor, Professor Weller and Dr Illis describe the underlying flexibility of the central nervous system to change, and this new approach to the neurophysiology of recovery presents an enormous challenge to those whose work is primarily concerned with neurological rehabilitation. The challenge consists in that it has to be established that an intensive rehabilitation programme involving periods of physiotherapy, occupational therapy, speech therapy, throughout the day, several days a week, can be justified in terms of its ultimate effectiveness. It is also necessary to establish whether one particular method of rehabilitation is better than another, and although many systems have been devised and claims made for each, there are no figures and no certainty with which to support these arguments. This lack is due to one fundamental deficiency in rehabilitation, and that is of accurate measurement. It is this that must occupy the attention in the future of those who concern themselves with rehabilitation, be it neurological or otherwise. Controlled trials of 'treatment' against 'no treatment', or one treatment against another, have ethical implications, and indeed until recently it seemed that there was very little point in such an exercise anyway. But the recognition of the plasticity of the nervous system, the presence of unused pathways capable of retraining, the recognition of the complexity of the synaptic system around the anterior horn cell, give a great deal of encouragement to those concerned with rehabilitation that there may be some neurophysiological basis for recovery which is far better than adaptation. Until accurate assessment, accurate prognosis and the ability to predict recovery can be firmly established, however, there can be no scientific foundation upon which to base a claim that rehabilitation works. Inwardly, one may have the conviction that it does so, but in the future, with increasing competition for funds, conviction alone will beinadequate.

REFERENCES

BOND M.R. & BROOKS D.N. (1976) Understanding the process of recovery as a basis for the investigation of rehabilitation for the brain injured. *Scandinavian Journal of Rehabilitation Medicine*, **8**, 127–33.

BREMNER D.J. & GILLINGHAM F.J. (1974) Patterns of convalescence after minor head injury. *Journal of the Royal College of Surgeons of Edinburgh*, **19**, 94–7.

DONALDSON S.W., CONLIN C.W. & GRESHAM G.E. (1973) A unified ADL evaluation form. *Archives of Physical Medicine and Rehabilitation*, **54**, 175–85.

EVANS C.D., DAVENPORT M.J., ROBINSON J.E. & STITCHBURY J. Report to the DHSS on the long term outcome of brain-damaged survivors. (In preparation.)

FIELD J.H. (1976) *A Study of the Epidemiology of Head Injury in England and Wales, with Particular Application to Rehabilitation.* Department of Health and Social Security (United Kingdom) Research Division.

GRAHAM O. (1975) Closed circuit television assessment of disability following severe head injury. *Physiotherapy*, **61**, 272–4.

JENNETT B. (1976) Assessment of the severity of head injury. *Journal of Neurology, Neurosurgery and Psychiatry*, **39**, 647–55.

JENNETT B. (1977) Traumatic epilepsy—the scale of the problem. *Medicine*, **35** (2), 2129–40.

JENNETT B., TEASDALE G., BRAAKMAN R., MINDERHOUD J., KNILL-JONES R. (1976) Predicting outcome in individual patients after severe head injury. *Lancet*, **i**, 1031–4.

JENNETT B., TEASDALE G., GALBRAITH S., PICKARD J., GRANT H., BRAAKMAN R., AVEZAAT C., MAAS A., MINDERHOUD J., VECHT C.J., HEIDEN J., SMALL R., CATON W. & KURZE T. (1977) Severe head injuries in three countries. *Journal of Neurology, Neurosurgery and Psychiatry*, **40**, 291-8.

JONES, R.K. (1974) Assessment of minimal head injuries: indications for in-hospital care. *Surgical Neurology*, **2**, 101-4.

LEWIN W. (1970) Rehabilitation needs of the brain-injured patient. *Proceedings of the Royal Society of Medicine*, **63**, 28-32.

LINCOLN N. & LEADBITTER D. (1979) Assessment of motor function in stroke patients. *Physiotherapy*, **65**, 48-51.

LONDON P.S. (1967) Some observations on the course of events after severe injury of the head (Hunterian Lecture). *Annals of the Royal College of Surgeons of England*, **41**, 460-79.

MILLER H. (1961) Accident neurosis (Milroy Lecture). *British Medical Journal*, **i**, 919-25.

NEWCOMBE F. (1979) In press.

NEWCOMBE F., MARSHALL J.C., CARRIVIC P. & HIORNS R.W. (1975) Recovery curves in acquired dyslexia. *Journal of Neurological Sciences*, **24**, 127-33.

RUSSELL W.R. & SMITH R. (1961) PTA in closed head injury. *Archives of Neurology*, **5**, 4-17.

STITCHBURY J.C. (1975) Assessment of disability following severe head injury. *Physiotherapy*, **61**, 268-72.

SYMONDS C. (1962) Concussion and its sequelae. *Lancet*, **i**, 1-15.

Specialized equipment designed to suit individual needs can be obtained from

Biological Engineering Society,
Royal College of Surgeons,
Lincoln's Inn Field,
LONDON.
WC2A 3PM

Chapter 6
Rehabilitation of Stroke

Stroke is one of the most important causes of disability and handicap. The subject has attracted considerable interest during the past few years, and a large literature is developing. This chapter deals with selected topical subjects. The incidence, prevalence and natural history of post-stroke disability are obviously of great importance to the planning of rehabilitation services. It is only in recent years that data have become available, and even now, reliable figures relating to the prevalence of post-stroke disability are sparse. Logistics of care are discussed in relation both to the district general hospital and to specialized stroke units. The importance of adequate and systematic assessment of disabled stroke patients, both for clinical and research purposes, is discussed. The setting up of randomized control trials of methods of management depends upon the availability of well-validated assessment 'tools'. There has been much recent interest in the problems of aphasic patients, and there have been some attempts to evaluate the effectiveness of speech therapy. For this reason, the subject is discussed in some detail. Lastly, it was felt important to discuss, albeit briefly, the psychosocial aspects of rehabilitation—a subject which is frequently neglected, but of great importance.

DEFINITION OF STROKE

A number of definitions of 'stroke' are currently in use. Marquardsen (1978) gives the recommended World Health Organization (WHO) definition—'rapidly developed signs of focal (or global) disturbance of cerebral function, leading to death or lasting more than 24 hours, with no apparent cause other than vascular'. A similar definition was given by WHO in 1971 and by the Royal College of Physicians' Working Group on Strokes (1974). Weddell (1974) undertook a study of medical care given to a total population of stroke patients. She used as her definition 'a focal neurological deficit lasting 24 hours or more, due to any underlying pathological cause of sufficient severity to necessitate medical or nursing care at home or in hospital'. Brocklehurst et al. (1978) used the definition 'any degree of hemiparesis of rapid onset with weakness of one or more limbs, lasting for longer than 24 hours'. The problem of definition and classification is discussed by Capildeo *et al.* (1978). Any clinical definition of the term 'stroke' is a compromise, but in general there does not seem to be any good reason to deviate from the WHO recommended definition.

Incidence

There have been few community-based studies on cerebrovascular disease. Hospital studies inevitably deal with selected patients and it is necessary to interpret data based on such material with caution.

The incidence of stroke has been documented in a number of studies, and it is generally accepted as being about 2 per 1000. The range was 1.65–2.45 in 6 studies surveyed by Marquardsen (1978). The precise figure will clearly depend upon the method of ascertainment, the definitions of disease (as mentioned above), and the size and age structure of the population base. The incidence rises markedly with age. The rate for persons aged between 35 and 44 is 0.25 per 1000 persons per year. The rate for persons aged between 75 and 85 is about 20 per 1000 persons (Sahs *et al.*, 1979). It is clear that the majority of strokes occur in older patients—probably about 75 per cent occurring in persons aged 65 or over. The incidence rate for males exceeds that for females, but the sex difference is modest compared with that observed in ischaemic heart disease (Marquardsen, 1978).

Data relating to the incidence of disabled stroke survivors are sparse. Curiously, virtually none of the published population studies give information on this point. Our own, unpublished, data indicate that by three weeks after the stroke, approximately one-third of patients will have died, and a further one-third will be left with a neurological deficit which usually includes a hemiplegia.

In most European countries the mortality rates for cerebrovascular disease are about 100 per 100 000 population (Marquardsen, 1978). Cerebrovascular disease accounted for 75 445 deaths in England and Wales in 1976—12.6% of all deaths (HMSO, 1978). It was the third commonest cause of death.

Prevalence

When planning rehabilitation facilities, it is necessary to be able to estimate the number of handicapped people existing in a population at any given time. It must be noted, however, that not all stroke survivors are disabled. Prevalence is a function of incidence, mortality, and rate of recovery.

Amelia Harris and co-workers (1971) estimated that there were 130 000 people in Great Britain disabled as a result of cerebrovascular disease. This gives a prevalence of roughly 2.4 per 1000 (assuming a population of Great Britain of 55 million). Whisnant (1976) surveyed some of the data from the Rochester, Minnesota, Study. He calculated the age-adjusted prevalence rate for stroke at between 5.33 and 6.70 per 1000 population. However, prevalence increases markedly with age—being 3.3–4.7 per 1000 in the age group 45–54, rising to 57.8–81.8 over the age of 75. At least 70% of the survivors in the Rochester Study were aged 65 or more; 29% were said to be functioning normally, but 54% had some degree of neurological deficit.

Petlund (1970) studied the prevalence of the Aust Agder county of Norway. He found an overall prevalence of 4.4 per 1000 population. The prevalence of disabled stroke patients was 2.7 per 1000.

It seems, therefore, that the overall prevalence rate of stroke survivors is between 4.4 and 6.7 per 1000; 50–60% of the survivors will be disabled. Table 6.1 gives rough incidence and prevalence rates for the average general practice in the UK of 2500 and for a population of 250 000—served by the 'average' district general hospital.

Table 6.1 Incidence and prevalence of stroke.

	Per 1000	Per 'average' United Kingdom general practice of 2500 persons	Per United Kingdom 'average' health district of 250 000 persons
New stroke cases per year	2	5	500
*New stroke cases surviving 3 weeks with a disability	1	2–3	170–250
†Prevalence	4.4–6.7	11–17	1100–1670
†Prevalence of disabled stroke survivors	2.2–3.3	6–8	550–825

*Assuming that one-half to one-third of stroke patients will survive three weeks with a disability. (Based on our own unpublished series.)
† Based on Petlund (1970) and Whisnant (1976).

ASSESSMENT

Most, but not all, survivors of an acute stroke have a hemiplegia. Other neurological deficits such as dysphasia, spatial disorientation, and disturbances of posture are of equal, and frequently greater, importance. They result in loss of communicative ability, immobility, and dependence upon others for self-care activities. Assessment involves the identification and, if possible, quantification of these problems, and is now recognized as being important both for the efficient day-to-day management of patients, and research. The overall objectives of assessment may be summarized as follows:

1. to describe objectively a patient's functional status at a given time
2. to detect change in a patient's condition by undertaking sequential reassessments

3.   to provide a basis for future action—for example, discharge from hospital or change of therapy
4.   to educate medical and paramedical staff
5.   for research

There are three particular reasons for devising reliable assessment 'tools':

1.   for epidemiological purposes—so that the incidence and prevalence of conditions causing neurological disability, particularly stroke, can be determined
2.   to give information about the speed and duration of recovery
3.   to enable the value of different intervention procedures to be assessed. Examples include the comparison of intensive with non-intensive physiotherapy, or the comparison of hospital management with home care. In addition, assessment procedures may be used to assess the usefulness of particular forms of therapy such as biofeedback.

Neurological and general notes do not usually contain much information about function. Indeed, in some instances it is impossible to ascertain, by reading the notes, whether the patient can stand or walk. Information relating to everyday activities, such as feeding, dressing and bathing, is often totally absent. It is, however, possible to use a simple assessment *proforma* to display information about the patient's functional status on different occasions. The form currently being used in the Bristol Neurological /Stroke Rehabilitation Unit is shown in Fig. 6.1. This form has been used for two years and has been found to be useful and acceptable to the junior staff, who are usually required to 'fill in' the relevant information. Such a form, which can be used equally well for other disabling conditions such as multiple sclerosis, has an important educational purpose—helping young doctors to understand the significance of functional assessment when giving the patient and his family advice on how to cope with the problems of disability.

For research purposes it is necessary to use properly validated assessment 'tools'. These must be sensitive to change, but must also give results which are repeatable, and give good inter- and intra-observer correlation. Some of the test procedures being used are discussed below.

Activities of Daily Living (ADL)

One of the most important group of outcome measures concerns the ability to perform self-care activities such as feeding, dressing and toileting. Mobility is frequently included in the ADL grouping. Many ADL scales have been devised, of which some of the best known are those of Katz *et al.* (1963), Kenny (Shoening *et al.*, 1965) and Barthel (Mahoney & Barthel, 1965). The Pulses Profile has been used recently by some workers (Granger *et al.*, 1979). The subject was reviewed by Donaldson *et al.*, (1973) who surveyed 25 published scales which were used by authors between 1950 and 1970. Unfortunately, many published scales do

FUNCTIONAL ASSESSMENT FOR NEUROLOGICAL PATIENTS

CLINICAL INFORMATION

Diagnosis . . . .

Date or year of onset . . . .

Dates of further episodes . . . .

. . . .

Addressograph label

DAILY ACTIVITIES

	Date	Date	Date	Date	Date
Feeding					
Toilet					
Washing					
Bathing					
Dressing					
Preparation of meals					
Totals					

MOBILITY

Transferring bed-chair					
Walking indoors					
Stairs					
Walking outdoors					
Wheelchair use					
Totals					
Time taken to walk 10 metres					

CODE
(for above
questions)

2 – Independent: no help needed

1 – Partially dependent: help of one person needed

0 – Dependent: cannot contribute significantly
to the performance

N.K. – Information not available or not known

N.A. – Not applicable

CONTINENCE   (please tick)

		Yes/No	Yes/No	Yes/No	Yes/No	Yes/No
Bladder	*Catheter*					
	Day					
	Night					
Bowels						

Fig. 6.1

COMMUNICATION

VISION: Acuity   R . . . .   L . . . .

	Date	Date	Date	Date	Date
	. . . .	. . . .	. . . .	. . . .	. . . .
	Adq. Not	Adq. Not	Adq. Not	Adq. Not	Adq. Not
Reading					
Distant					
HEARING: Both ears					
SPEECH					
COMPREHENSION:					
READING:					
WRITING					

Comments

(Please
tick)

MENTAL STATUS

Specify: (e.g., confused, demented, anxious, depressed, unrealistic, realistic, hopeful, etc.)

Comment					
Camden Score					

ADDITIONAL MEDICAL PROBLEMS AFFECTING INDEPENDENCE

Pressure sores					
Pain					
Painful spasms					
Contractures					
Amputation					
Dyspnoea					
Angina					
Spasticity					
Arthritis					
Other					

(Please tick)

Fig. 6.1 (*cont.*)

SOCIAL FACTORS

Date . . . .

```
┌─────────────────────────────────┐
│                                 │
│        Addressograph label      │
│                                 │
└─────────────────────────────────┘
```

(Please answer, delete or tick
as appropriate)

MARITAL STATUS: Married/single/widowed/divorced

MAIN CARER: . . . . Relationship: . . . .
          Age: . . . . Fit/unfit   If unfit, specify problem below:
. . . .
. . . .

NUMBER OF FAMILY AT HOME (excluding patient) Adults: . . . .
                                              Children: . . . .

HOUSING: House/flat/sheltered housing/hostal/council/private/rented

TOILET: Upstairs/downstairs/both

AIDS AND ADAPTATIONS IN USE

  Specify . . . .
           . . . .

SERVICES BEING SUPPLIED:

	Yes	No
Meals on wheels		
Home Help		
Day Centre			(Please tick)

EMPLOYMENT:

  Nature of present or last job

	Yes	No
Full time		
Part time		
If normally in employment, date when last worked		

TRANSPORT: Car driver/regular car passenger/bus passenger

MAIN PROBLEMS IN APPROXIMATE ORDER OF IMPORTANCE
(Medical, Social and Other)

1. . . . .
2. . . . .
3. . . . .
4. . . . .
5. . . . .
6. . . . .

Fig. 6.1 (*cont.*)

not give precise information about the methods used in undertaking the assessment. The problem is discussed in detail by Sheikh *et al.* (1979). These authors reviewed the various problems involved in developing the Northwick Park Scheme. For instance, good agreement was found between what the patient could do in hospital and what he could do at home. However, there was some evidence to suggest that patients do not always undertake certain activities although they *can* do so. The point has been made by Andrews *et al.* (1979) in a study aptly entitled, 'He can but does he?' The value of ADL scales has been discussed in detail by Nichols (1976). Unfortunately, there is still no overall agreement about which system of assessment is desirable, and new scales are still being introduced.

Quality of Life

ADL scales give an idea of the patient's level of independence in self-care activities. They do not give information relating to how the patient participates in everyday activities—inside and outside the home.

Sarno *et al.* (1973) presented a detailed functional life scale. This scale was later simplified, validated and published as Level of Rehabilitation Scale—LORS (Carey & Posavac, 1978). The scale includes 47 items which are divided into 5 groups—ADL, cognition (e.g. reading and writing), home activities (e.g. preparing food, use of the telephone, etc.), outside activities (e.g. shopping and use of public transport), and social interaction (going to work or school and visiting friends). The authors claim that the scale, which depends upon an interview with a person who knows the patient well, can usually be completed in 15 minutes. The results are expressed as a percentage of normal function.

It is remarkable that there is so little published work relating to the quality of life of disabled persons. Hopefully, this situation will change with the advent of the new scales described above, and we shall no longer be content to judge the efficacy of rehabilitation programmes on the basis of ADL ratings.

Neuropsychological Problems

Adams and Hurwitz (1963) have pointed out the importance of a number of deficits which are not always recognized and which are also difficult to classify and quantify. These include such problems as impaired learning ability, disturbed awareness of self or space, disordered integrated action, and emotional disorders. Various attempts have been made to quantify the various perceptual and intellectual abnormalities which occur in elderly patients (Adams, 1974; Denham & Jeffreys, 1972; Hodgkinson, 1972; Isaacs & Marks, 1973). The identification of these complex and often subtle problems can perhaps best be achieved by examining the patient with a series of simple tests outlined by Isaacs

(1971). However, the area needs further exploration—hopefully with neuro-psychologists and doctors working in close collaboration.

Gross Motor Activity

The problem of assessing deficits of motor control is well recognized. Fugl-Meyer *et al.* (1975) attempted an assessment of upper and lower limb function, and was able to construct curves of recovery on the basis of information obtained. Bobath (1978) and Brunnstrom (1970) have also published detailed assessments. However, many of the published scales are too long for practical use and others have not been shown to be either reliable or valid. The problem was discussed by Lincoln and Leadbitter (1979) who devised and validated an assessment of physical recovery from hemiplegia following stroke. A method for assessing recovery in the upper limb has been recently developed by de Souza *et al.* (1980). The development of electronic devices to monitor movement in space is now making it possible to describe recovery in more precise terms. An example is that of the polarized light goniometer (Mitchelson, 1979).

Objective and quantifiable assessments are, of course, required in many fields other than those mentioned above. However, it is worth noting that we are not yet able to quantify routinely such common neurological problems as spasticity, position sense, or ataxia. The patient's ability to walk is rarely properly assessed in remedial departments despite the fact that speed, safety and pulse rate are the only essential variables. The importance of evaluating the usefulness, or other-wise, of therapeutic procedures is obvious. Evaluation cannot be undertaken without reliable assessment methods which can, and will, be used by remedial and medical staff. Complicated equipment is not usually required.

OUTCOME

Mortality

Marquardsen (1969) has pointed out that, whereas no sharp distinction can be made between immediate and later mortality after cerebrovascular accident (CVA), the shape of the survival curve indicates that the majority of early deaths have occurred within three weeks of the stroke. Most publications give early mortality at either three or four weeks from the ictus. Marquardsen (1969) found that 50.5% of men and 44.8% of women in his retrospective hospital series had died by three weeks. Early mortality figures derived from community studies vary widely—33% (Marquardsen, 1978), 44.7% (Whisnant *et al.*, 1971), 47.4% (Weddell, 1974), 56.6% (Eisenberg, 1964) and 57% (Acheson & Fairbairn, 1971). The prognosis is determined mainly by the age of the patient and the type, size and anatomical site of the lesion. About 75% of cerebral haemorrhages but only 25–30% of ischaemic strokes are fatal (Marquardsen, 1978).

The survival prospects of those patients still alive at the end of the first month are of particular interest to those involved in the planning of services for the disabled. The number of four-week survivors who will die within the first year ranges between 27% and 35% (Eisenberg *et al.*, 1964; Acheson & Fairbairn, 1971; Marquardsen, 1976; Brocklehurst *et al.*, 1978); 56–63% will be dead by three years (Eisenberg *et al.*, 1964; Brocklehurst *et al.*, 1978) and 66% by five years (Eisenberg *et al.*, 1964).

Marquardsen (1969) followed 407 three-week survivors for between 10 and 23 years. Throughout the observation period, the mortality was much higher than that of the general population of similar age. The observed three-year mortality rate of 46% in contrast to an expected mortality rate of only 12%. A median survival time was 3.5 years as opposed to 10 years in the corresponding general population. The annual rate at which survivors decreased remained approximately constant for at least 10 years after the stroke—being 16% for males and 18% for females. Younger patients survived longer than older patients. The main causes of death in this series were recurrent strokes 23%, myocardial infarction 10%, and heart failure or broncho-pneumonia 30%.

It is apparent that the age at which the stroke occurs is an important prognostic factor. Marquardsen found that in the males below the age of 60 the number of survivors decreased at an annual rate of about 10%, whereas in the group aged 70–79 the rate was 25%. The corresponding median survival time was 6.5 years and 2.2 years respectively. Marquardsen found that one of the most important prognostic factors was the ultimate functional capacity achieved by patients during their stay in hospital. Thus, for instance, a strikingly bad prognosis was found in the most severely disabled patients. Four-fifths had died within two years of the stroke. The mean expectation of life in this category was 1.5 years.

Risk of a Further Stroke

The problem was considered in detail by Marquardsen (1969), who made the following observations:

1.   The annual risk of having a further stroke appears to be independent of the length of time which has elapsed since the primary stroke. The average annual recurrence rate was 8% for males and 9% for females.

2.   The time interval between the primary stroke and the first recurrence ranged from a few weeks to 17 years (average 3.7 years).

3.   The risk of having a further stroke is not significantly greater during the first 12 months after the initial stroke—8.6% for males and 12.2% for females.

4.   Marquardsen calculated that 50% of the survivors would have a second attack within eight years and 75% within 16.5 years. It is clear, however, that many patients will die from a different disease before having a further stroke.

Functional Outcome

It is only in recent years that the functional outcome following stroke has been documented. Even now, there are very few properly conducted population studies. A major difficulty concerns the lack of standardized assessment techniques. The problem was discussed by the Royal College of Physicians' Working Group on Strokes (1974).

Five community-based series give information relating to the outcome for patients who have survived the first three to four weeks (Wallace, 1967; Marquardsen, 1969; Petlund, 1970; Matsumoto *et al.*, 1973; Gresham *et al.*, 1975) (see Table 6.2). The papers show a considerable degree of agreement, although the results given by Petlund shows some divergence from the others—possibly because this was a prevalence rather than an incidence study: 29-36% of those working before the stroke were working, or able to work, afterwards; 20-27% could not walk unaided; 31-52% were dependent in some aspect of self-care activity; 12-21% of stroke survivors will require long-term institutional care—in a hospital or nursing home. Overall, the results of these community studies indicate that about 50% of stroke survivors will achieve a full, or almost full, functional recovery. Marquardsen (1969) reviewed the literature relating to hospitalized stroke survivors, and found that 50-70% were able to walk unaided and 20-30% had to be transferred to institutions. The proportion who could go back to work was highly dependent upon the age structure of the series, varying from 1% to 25%. The average duration of hospital stay of stroke survivors was 52 days for males and 73 days for females.

Prediction of Outcome

Marquardsen (1969) found that there were a number of clinical manifestations which were associated with an unfavourable functional prognosis. Of the adverse factors already present at the time of admission, the most important were: age over 70, severe motor impairment, impairment of consciousness of more than a few hours' duration, conjugate occular deviation, and conceptual disorders. During the subsequent course the following factors were indicative of a poor recovery: lack of improvement of motor function, persistent confusion or apathy, urinary or bowel incontinence, and extracerebral complications.

The importance of mental confusion, memory loss, depression, and cognitive and visuo-spatial disorders has been emphasized by many authors (Adams, 1974). However, Isaacs *et al.*, (1973) found that language and perceptual disorders did not necessarily present an insuperable barrier to recovery, since with an appropriate treatment programme many patients with these disabilities regained functional independence and were able to return home.

Marquardsen found that right-sided cerebral lesions carried a less favourable prognosis than left-sided lesions. Patients with lesions confined to the brain stem did better than those with hemisphere abnormalities.

Table 6.2 Final status of survivors—5 community studies.

	Chronic care or needing total nursing care	Working (this applies only to those who were working before the stroke)	Dependent in some self-care activities	Dependent in walking	Comments
Wallace, 1967	12.5%		34%		Important study but patients were only followed up for three months
Marquardsen, 1969	21% (11% bedridden)	36%	52%	27%	This is the most detailed published study
Petlund, 1970	14.2% total nursing care; 33% in an institution	54%	36%	26%	This was a prevalence study and includes some acute stroke cases
Matsumoto et al., 1973	4% required total care	36% working or able to work			Important study but gives very little information regarding the functional status of survivors
Gresham et al., 1975	16%	29%	31%	20%	Variable follow-up period—six months to 33 years

Rate of Recovery

Reliable data relating to the rate of recovery depend upon the availability of well-validated and sensitive measures of outcome. Twitchell (1951) described the course of motor recovery following stroke. This classic paper gives details of the physiological sequence of recovery in the limbs. All those who gained complete recovery of upper limb function had some voluntary hand movement by 15 days.

An important recent contribution is that of Brocklehurst *et al.* (1978) who studied 139 patients who had suffered a recent stroke and survived two weeks. These workers studied 7 parameters of recovery, including mobility, ADL, and mental confusion. Most recovery occurred within eight weeks. However, 12% showed improvement in their walking score beyond eight weeks and 28% showed improvement in their ADL score beyond this time. The study indicates that, apart from some patients with minimal disability, little further recovery could be expected beyond six months from the date of the stroke. The findings suggest that a major investment in physical therapy beyond six months is likely to be wasteful.

THE HOSPITAL

In 1971, the WHO Report on Cerebrovascular Disease recommended that every patient with an acute stroke should be admitted to hospital for accurate diagnosis and optimum care. However, in the UK general practitioners traditionally find it difficult to get their stroke patients into hospital, particularly if elderly (Warren *et al.*, 1967). Hospital physicians, for their part, are often reluctant to accept a stroke patient into a hospital bed because of the risk that the bed will become 'blocked'. Hospitals are the most expensive resources involved, and it is clearly desirable to establish the optimal relationship between home and hospital care (Report of Royal College of Physicians' Working Party on Strokes, 1974; Mulley & Arie, 1978).

Cochrane (1970) found that 60% of clinical strokes in South Wales did not go to hospital. Langton-Hewer (1976) found that 40% of stroke patients in Bristol were admitted within one week. Brocklehurst *et al.* (1978) in Manchester found that 40% of patients were admitted on the same day as the stroke, and a further 24% were admitted within the next two weeks.

Patients are admitted to hospital for four main reasons: diagnostic, therapeutic, nursing and social. Investigation was not a major reason for admission in the Manchester Study (Brocklehurst *et al.*, 1978). Of 135 cases of acute stroke — angiograms were undertaken on 2, LP's on 4, and EEG's on 6. Admission appears to have been primarily for nursing care and social reasons. This is borne out by the reason given for admission by the general practitioner — 89% showing a social reason. However, even here there were some apparent paradoxes in the admission pattern. For instance, of those admitted by two weeks 17% could walk unaided, but of those not admitted by two weeks 33% could not stand unaided and 25% could not turn over in bed without assistance.

The term 'stroke' is inexact and tends to indicate that a diagnosis has been made, whereas in fact it has not. Many diseases may cause the stroke syndrome, including such diverse conditions as meningitis, bacterial endocarditis, myocardial infarction, head injury, hypoglycaemia, neurosyphilis, polyarteritis, subdural haematoma, subarachnoid haemorrhage, and cerebral tumour. The distinction between cerebral haemorrhage and infarction is of fundamental importance and can now be made with accuracy using a Computerized Tomography (CT) scanner.

A proportion of stroke patients can be helped by active treatment and some examples have been given above. In addition, there is the large question of the management of the stroke in evolution. A detailed discussion is outside the scope of this chapter, but hopefully enough has been said to indicate that diagnostic and therapeutic nihilism is not always the most appropriate response of the doctor faced with a patient who has just had 'a stroke'.

There have been no recent studies of the effectiveness of acute stroke units. Two studies (Kennedy *et al.*, 1970; Drake *et al.*, 1973), both taken before the advent of neurodiagnostic techniques such as CT scanning, indicated that such units were not effective in reducing the mortality rate, although the complication rate may be reduced. Further studies are needed.

STROKE UNITS

The report of the Royal College of Physicians' sub-committee on stroke rehabilitation published in 1974 suggested that some departments might consider setting up stroke units. The report stated that 'any scheme designed to establish pilot stroke units must include a method of assessing their value. It is not enough to show that the patients did well; patients must be shown to have done better than they would have done if treated by other means.'

The unit at Lightburn Hospital in Glasgow (Isaacs, 1977) was one of the first stroke units to be establshed in the UK. Others have been set up in Edinburgh, Northwick Park, Greenwich, Sheffield, Dover and Bristol. Blower (1979) gave two main reasons for the setting up of the Greenwich Unit. First, that the care of patients with stroke is poor in most hospitals, and secondly, that the most effective way of improving stroke rehabilitation would be to collect patients together. Important secondary advantages include the education and training of remedial staff and the opportunity offered for research on a group of disabled patients whose status is well documented. Attempts at evaluation are being made at a number of centres in the UK. There was some evidence that patients with severe impairment improved more in a specialized unit than elsewhere (McCann & Culbertson, 1976), but the results of other evaluation studies are needed before the point can be proved one way or the other. The Edinburgh group is currently undertaking a randomized trial to test the hypothesis that a stroke rehabilitation unit can discharge a higher proportion of acute strokes back home functionally independent compared with a general medical ward (Garraway & Akhtar, 1977; Smith, 1979). Attempts are also being made in the USA to evaluate stroke units (McCann & Culbertson, 1976; Carey & Posavac, 1978; Feigenson *et al.*, 1979).

The relevance of stroke units and the principles of management employed therein has important implications for the way in which chronic disability should be managed in the district general hospital. (Blower & Ali, 1979) found that less than 10% of stroke survivors ever got to a residential rehabilitation centre. It thus seems likely that the majority of hospitalized stroke patients will continue to be managed in general wards.

The Bristol Stroke Unit was set up in 1975. It does not have beds attached to it, but draws patients from the locality and will also accept in-patients referred by physicians and others. The majority of published accounts of stroke units do not contain details of how a unit is organized. For this reason, some of the principles which have been applied in the Bristol Stroke Unit are given below:

OBJECTIVE ASSESSMENT AT REGULAR INTERVALS

Data relevant to the patient's neurological, functional and social status are recorded in retrievable form. Records are mainly 'problem-orientated'.

TEAM APPROACH

Medical, social work, nursing and remedial staff act as a coordinated team. This involves regular meetings to discuss treatment planning and progress.

STAFFING

Three important points should be made:
(a) It is essential to have the active involvement of the consultant, who should preferably be the team leader.
(b) The social worker will be concerned with the psychosocial and socioeconomic effects of the stroke. She should have her office in the unit.
(c) The roles of the staff members necessarily become blurred. Each skill group must be expected to be capable of dealing in a competent manner with the principal problems encountered by the patient. In the USA, the concept of a 'rehabilitation therapist' is emerging (Feigenson & McCarthy, 1977).

PROGRAMME OF MANAGEMENT FOR THE PATIENT

Each patient is given a weekly written programme, so that he knows precisely what he should be doing at different times of the week.

ESTABLISHMENT OF CONTACTS

Great importance is attached to the maintenance of contacts with the local authority services and personnel—including the home nursing service. Every effort is made to ensure that the requisite services such as home help and meals on wheels are provided. Attempts are also made to ensure that before the patient goes home necessary adaptations and aids have been made and provided—e.g. ramps, handrail on the stairs, commode, etc.

FOLLOW-UP

All patients are 'followed up' at regular intervals for two years. This has the advantage of allowing problems and complications to be identified and managed promptly. If necessary, the patient can be given a further course of treatment. Both patients and relatives appear to find comfort in being able to remain in contact with rehabilitation staff through the difficult period of adjustment to disability.

COMPLICATIONS

Complications of the original stroke, such as painful frozen shoulder, severe depression and severe spasticity, occur with some frequency. They should be identified and treated at an early stage.

MAXIMIZING PERFORMANCE

Efforts are made to ensure that the patient achieves his maximum potential. He is positively encouraged to develop hobbies and social contacts. This can be done partly through a volunteer support group—over 70 volunteers are currently working with patients who have been through the Bristol unit.

PSYCHOLOGICAL AND SOCIAL SUPPORT

Efforts have been made to manage the psychological and social problems which occur following a stroke. This has involved discussion with the patient and the family. Meetings for patients and relatives are held at which problems are discussed (see later).

The possible benefits of an integrated system of care should be looked for not only in terms of duration of stay in hospital, but also in the quality of life and general level of 'happiness'. Benefit might be looked for in terms of greater independence, more social and hobby activities, a greater number of younger patients returning to work, fewer physical complications, fewer secondary admissions to hospital and possibly fewer psychological problems. As already mentioned, the benefits of the type of approach mentioned above have yet to be 'proved'. Finally, it is worth noting that the principles involved in the rehabilitation of stroke patients are similar to those involved in dealing with other disabling conditions, such as multiple sclerosis, Parkinson's disease and motoneuron disease.

COMMUNITY CARE

Little has been written about the care of stroke patients in the community, despite the fact that 40-60% of such patients do not enter hospital. There have been no published studies in the UK comparing community with hospital care. Opit (1977) undertook an investigation of the costs of domiciliary care for 139 elderly sick patients. The data suggested that there was little economic advantage in home care for this group. It is clear that the relationship between the two services does need to be examined (Report of the Royal College of Physicians' Committee, 1974; Mulley & Arie, 1978).

APHASIA

Size of the Problem

There is little information in the literature relating to the incidence and prevalence of post-stroke aphasia. Hopkins (1975) made some estimates of the number of patients involved after reviewing the paper by Matsumoto *et al* (1973). A prevalence rate of 52 dysphasic survivors of stroke per 100 000 population was calculated, assuming that 9.3% of all survivors were dysphasic at six months from the date of the stroke. This figure does not, however, take into account the many patients who are dysphasic at first and recover by six months. If bedridden dysphasic patients are subtracted, it seems likely that in the UK, with a population of 55 million, there are about 26 000 dysphasic survivors of stroke.

There is no 'hard' information about the incidence of dysphasia in post-stroke survivors. None the less, an intelligent guess can be made if it is assumed that in Great Britain about 30 000 patients will be alive three weeks after a stroke with a substantial disability which usually includes a hemiplegia; 15 000 of these are likely to have a right hemiplegia. If two-thirds of this group are aphasic, there will be about 10 000 new aphasic patients each year. Hopkins estimated that the number of new dysphasic patients surviving six months was about 5200—the reduced number presumably being due to death of some patients, and recovery of the aphasia in others.

Table 6.3 gives the estimated incidence of dysphasia per 100 000 population, for a population of a quarter of a million (the average health district) and per 2500 (the average general practice).

Table 6.3 Estimated incidence and prevalence of dysphasia. Based on Matsumoto (1973) and Hopkins (1975).

	Per 100 000 persons	Per district general hospital population (250 000 persons)	Per average general practice (2500 persons)
Incidence (new cases each year)	20	50	0.5
Prevalence (number of cases existing at one time)	52	130	1.3

It will be seen that aphasia represents a numerically small problem and that the average general practitioner is not likely to see many aphasic patients. The small number of cases generated within the average health district indicates that therapeutic trials, which depend upon large numbers of cases, will need to be based on many centres. Paradoxically, however, there are insufficient therapists to provide more than a very small amount of therapy for each patient (Hopkins, 1975).

Natural History of Aphasia

It is recognized that most patients show some degree of spontaneous recovery. Important contributions to this subject include those of Culton (1969), Kenin and Swisher (1972) and Kertesz and McCabe (1977).

Most improvement occurs during the first three months, but demonstrable recovery can occur up to six months post-stroke, and possibly longer (Sands *et al.*, 1969). Recovery rates are higher for post-traumatic cases than for stroke patients, global aphasia has a poor prognosis and younger patients usually recover better than older ones. There is disagreement as to the relative outlooks of comprehension and expressive language (Kertesz & McCabe, 1977).

Effectiveness of Speech Therapy

The rationale of speech therapy remains unclear, but must be investigated if resources are to be rationally used (Leading Article, *British Medical Journal*, 1977). The problem of undertaking studies in this field has been reviewed by Darley (1972), Hopkins (1975) and Sarno (1976). Factors requiring consideration include:

1. the small number of cases likely to be available for study
2. the effect of spontaneous recovery

3. the difficulty of specifying the amount and details of treatment given
4. the impossibly large number of variables, including sex, age, site of lesion and type and severity of aphasia.

Firm evidence for the efficacy of speech therapy can only be obtained by controlled trials involving random assignment of patients to treatment and non-treatment groups. Ethical considerations currently preclude the total with-holding of therapy, and for this reason the control group is usually given either a non-specific general encouragement or is managed by untrained volunteers (see below).

Sarno (1976) reviewed the literature and could only find six studies in English which had addressed themselves specifically to recovery with rehabilitation in post-stroke aphasic patients. The only attempt at a control trial was that of Sarno *et al.* (1970). This study can be criticized on the grounds that it was non-random, only 31 patients were involved, only patients with severe aphasia were studied, and there was no attempt to match the patients for certain important variables such as site and size of the lesion.

The problems faced by aphasic patients and their families are considerable and the resources of speech therapy departments are limited. Furthermore, little is known about the most effective way of deploying the skills of professional speech therapists. As a result of this disparity, which was pointed out by Hopkins (1975), Griffith (1975) has pioneered the use of volunteer helpers. Many volunteer schemes based on her methods now exist in the UK, using non-professional helpers for aphasic subjects. The efficacy of such schemes has not yet been determined, although there is some evidence that social confidence does increase (Lesser & Watt, 1978).

Two recent UK studies (Meikle *et al.*, 1979; David *et al.*, 1979) compared the results of treatment by trained speech therapists with those obtained by volunteers. The first study showed no important differences between the two groups. However, the total number of patients in this study was only 31. The Bristol group have recently published details of their feasibility study (David *et al.*, 1979). Patients were allocated randomly to either individual speech therapy or to an equal amount of intervention from untrained volunteers. Their progress was closely followed for 12 weeks of treatment then subsequently until the end of one year. After some minor changes in protocol, this study is now continuing as a large multi-centre project involving about 20 centres.

Measurement of Change

Reliable and well-validated test procedures are required for describing both the natural history of aphasia and the possible efficacy of therapy. Several such procedures are in everyday use—the most frequently used is probably the Minnesota Test for differential diagnosis of aphasia (Schuell, 1965). The Porch Index of communicative ability (Porch, 1967) is another detailed test which is becoming increasingly popular, as it enables the assessor to record such important items as the latency of response and the ability to use substitute words, self-corrections, and the use of gesture with minimal cues.

The functional communication profile (Sarno & Sands, 1970) is being used increasingly as a short test which can be completed in 15–20 minutes. This is based on a structured conversation between examiner and patient and provides quantification in percentage terms of the patient's ability to function in a variety of language activities of daily life, including speech, understanding and writing.

Types of Therapy

It has been said that there are probably as many methods of aphasia therapy as there are aphasic patients. This overstatement reflects the many theories about language recovery in aphasia. The subject has been reviewed by Darley (1972) and Sarno (1976). The short space available does not allow a detailed discussion. Some of the techniques currently being used are listed below. It should be noted that there is considerable overlap between them.

GENERAL STIMULATION

The patient is encouraged to speak, whatever the content. Great importance is attached to taking note of the patient's interests and premorbid personality. Some workers made use of filmstrip to stimulate the patient's interest.

PROGRAMMED INSTRUCTION (Sarno *et al.*, 1970)

This views language rehabilitation as an educative process and applies operant conditioning methods drawn from learning theory and principles drawn from psycholinguistic analysis. Some workers use the language laboratory in much the same way as when used for teaching normal people foreign languages.

MELODIC INTONATION (Albert *et al.*, 1973)

This makes use of an assumed residual melody through a series of carefully graduated steps in which the patient, in unison with the therapist, intones a melody with meaningful words or phrases.

VISUAL COMMUNICATION THERAPY (Velletri-Glass *et al.*, 1973)

This system derives from the observation that severe aphasics usually use the visual system without difficulty. Patients are taught to recognize symbols drawn on cards to represent words, and then to manipulate these in order to make appropriate responses.

Other experimental techniques include exposure to hyperbaric oxygen, drugs, psychotherapy and hypnosis.

PSYCHOSOCIAL ASPECTS OF STROKE REHABILITATION

'When a patient suffers a cerebrovascular accident, a problem is created with both medical and social aspects, the latter not infrequently outweighing the former' (Collins *et al.*, 1960). The stroke may be seen as representing a threat to the integrity of the family and may have a catastrophic effect both upon the patient himself and on his close relatives. Common reactions include shock, disbelief, guilt, anxiety, unreasonable hope and depression. It is important that these reactions should be recognized by all therapeutic staff. The problems are too big to be left to the social worker alone.

Despite the evident importance of psychosocial factors in the management of brain-damaged patients, the subject receives little attention in practice or in published articles. The rehabilitation of the disabled stroke survivor still tends to be thought of only in terms of conventional, and readily understood, physiotherapy, occupational therapy and speech therapy. In our experience, it is important to identify and confront the psychosocial problems noted above, and unless this is done there will be much unresolved conflict and unhappiness. As a result, the patient may fail to achieve his full potential—the aim of every rehabilitation programme.

Some of the psychological and social problems of stroke patients have been discussed in articles by Espmark (1973) and by Waite (1975). Waite identified three different phases: crisis, adjustment and restoration. Our experiences (Holbrook, 1979) are broadly in keeping with those of Waite. Waite discussed the reactions of both the patient and the family, and emphasized the role of the social worker in helping in the adjustment process. The reactions are not stereotyped, are variable in timing and are affected by a number of factors, including whether or not the patient is admitted to hospital and the pre-morbid personality of the patient and his spouse.

PHASE 1. CRISIS PHASE

This covers the first few days following the stroke. Much will depend upon the severity of the stroke and whether or not it is seen as a threat to life. Support at this time is usually needed mainly by the patient's family, who are likely to react initially with acute anxiety. They may be unable to think and act sensibly. For patients managed at home, there will be immediate problems related to getting in and out of bed, continence, and general nursing care. The remedial staff have an important function in trying to reduce anxiety and tension, by quiet explanation and encouragement, and also by helping with practical problems.

When the patient's awareness of the crisis evolves, it is accompanied by the anxiety, and sometimes denial and anger, which the family have already been experiencing. The fact that most strokes occur suddenly may lead the patient to think that recovery will be equally rapid. He requires a clear definition, frequently repeated, of the medical problem as soon as he is thought to be capable of comprehending what is said to him. An obvious additional difficulty arises if the patient is dysphasic, or has major perceptual problems resulting from the stroke.

This covers the next three to four months following the stroke. Active therapy of some sort is usually given. The patient is likely to feel dismayed and possibly ashamed at the changes which have suddenly occurred. He may try to deny their existence, or alternatively, may 'give up', making no effort to cooperate with the remedial staff. He is described as 'lacking in motivation'. The patient may be unable to take any part in financial and family decisions and, as a result, he may feel excluded—losing self-image and self-esteem. Implicit demands by the family that he assume the role of a sick person increase the dilemma and lead to increasing depression. Paradoxically, however, some patients experience euphoria and unrealistic hopes about the future, when they are being given substantial amounts of therapy in the remedial departments.

The remedial staff can help by identifying the patient's feelings and sympathetically helping him to understand, express and ultimately control them. Only when these feelings have been worked through, can the patient be helped to start to think constructively about the future.

Ultimately, other problems will have to be faced, including those concerning reintegration within the family, the re-establishment of social contacts, transport (the patient may be unable to drive), hobbies, sexual activity, and employment.

It is at this point that physical therapy is usually terminated. Many patients and their families become intensely depressed, and may express feelings of isolation, anger that so little has been achieved, and rejection.

Support should continue to be provided for many months after the patient has been discharged from in-patient care. It appears important to avoid discharging the patient prematurely from the remedial departments so that he and his family are not left to fend for themselves before they have been able to come to terms with the situation. If they are, permanent depression and lack of social and other contacts may ensue. Regretably, such a situation is only too likely to arise in practice (Isaacs *et al.*, 1976; Mackay & Nias, 1979).

Practical Ways in which the Patient and his Family can be helped

The importance of family involvement has been emphasized in many articles (Editorial, 1974; Dzau & Boehme, 1978). Little can be achieved unless the patient and his family are willing to collaborate.

The remedial staff should ideally always be available and willing to discuss the patient's problems. This can be done during treatment in all the remedial departments. Some patients and their relatives do seem to benefit by special sessions set aside for individual counselling. Group activities have also been found to be helpful.

GROUP DISCUSSIONS FOR PATIENTS (ORADEI & WAITE, 1974)

Interaction amongst disabled patients can provide a community in which the disabled patient is able to achieve some degree of social acceptance and identification. Patients can compare their disabilities and can be confronted with the realities of their problems. They no longer feel so peculiar, and realize that they are not unique.

RELATIVE GROUPS (Wells, 1974; Mykyta *et al.*, 1976)

Relatives also appear to find it helpful to be able to meet the remedial staff to discuss problems. Matters discussed include information about strokes, advice on how to cope with the stricken relative, help with understanding their own reactions, and information about services and provisions for the disabled.

Following discharge from active treatment, remedial staff can participate in the patient's and the family's adjustment by providing continuous assessment and support through telephone and direct contacts. Advice is likely to be required on such matters as transport, finance, employment, and opportunities for socialization.

Some units have established stroke clubs (Isaacs, 1977). The Chest, Heart and Stroke Association has supported the formation of stroke clubs throughout the UK—there are now 260 clubs in existence. There is also a network of speech groups (Griffith, 1975). Other patients have joined PHAB clubs. A variety of hobbies and other activities are open to younger stroke patients. Examples include gardening, golf and even archery (Guttman, 1976; Hale, 1979). These activities can all be used to implement the general principle that disabled patients should not, if possible, be allowed to remain socially isolated.

REFERENCES

ACHESON R.M. & FAIRBAIRN A.S. (1971) Record linkage in studies of cerebrovascular disease in Oxford, England. *Stroke*, **2**, 48–57.

ADAMS, G.F. (1974) *Cerebrovascular disability and the ageing brain.* Churchill Livingstone, Edinburgh.

ADAMS G.F. & HURWITZ L.J. (1963) Mental barriers to recovery from strokes. *Lancet*, **ii**, 533–7.

ALBERT M., SPARKS R. & HELM N. (1973) Melodic intonation therapy for aphasia. *Archives of Neurology*, **29**, 130–1.

ANDREWS K. & STEWART J. (1979) Stroke recovery: he can but does he? *Rheumatology and Rehabilitation*, **18**, 43–8.

BLOWER P. & ALI S. (1979) A stroke unit in a District General Hospital: the Greenwich experience. *British Medical Journal*, **ii**, 644–6.

BOBATH B. (1978) *Adult Hemiplegia: Evaluation and Treatment*, 2e. William Heinemann Medical Books Ltd, London.

BROCKLEHURST J.C., ANDREWS K., MORRIS P.E., RICHARDS B. & LAYCOCK P.J. (1978) Medical, Social and Psychological Aspects of Stroke—Final Report. University of Manchester.

BRUNNSTROM S. (1970) *Movement Therapy in Hemiplegia: a Neurophysiological Approach*. Harper and Row, New York.

CAPILDEO R., HABERMAN S. & ROSE F.C. (1978) The definition and classification of stroke. *Quarterly Journal of Medicine*, New Series XL, vii, **186**, 177–96.

CAREY R.G. & POSAVAC E.J. (1978) Program evaluation of a physical medicine and rehabilitation unit: a new approach. *Archives of Physical Medicine and Rehabilitation*, **59**, 330–7.

COCHRANE A.L. (1970) Burden of cerebrovascular disease. *British Medical Journal*, **iii**, 165.

COLLINS P., MARSHALL J. & SHAW D. (1960) Social rehabilitation following cerebrovascular accidents. *Gerontologica Clinica*, **2**, 246–56.

CULTON G. (1969) Spontaneous recovery from aphasia. *Journal of Speech and Hearing Research*, **12**, 825–32.

DARLEY F.C. (1972) The efficacy of language rehabilitation in aphasia. *Journal of Speech and Hearing Disorders*, **37**, 3–21.

DAVID R.M., ENDERBY P. & BAINTON D. (1979) Progress report on an evaluation of speech therapy for aphasia. *British Journal of Disorders of Communication*, **14**, 85–8.

DENHAM M.J. & JEFFERYS P.M. (1972) Routine mental testing in the elderly. *Modern Geriatrics*, **2**, 275–9.

DONALDSON M.A., WAGNER C.C. & GRESHAM G.E. (1973) A unified A.D.L. evaluation form. *Archives of Physical Medicine and Rehabilitation*, **54**, 175–9.

DRAKE E.W., HAMILTON M.J., CARLSSON M. & BLUMENKRANTZ J. (1973) Acute stroke management and patient outcome: the value of neurovascular care units. *Stroke*, **4**, 6, 933–45.

DZAU R.E. & BOEHME A.R. (1978) Stroke rehabilitation: a family team education programme. *Archives of Physical Medicine and Rehabilitation*, **59**, 236–9.

EDITORIAL (1974) Stroke and the family. *British Medical Journal*. **iv**, 122.

EISENBERG H., MORRISON J.T., SULLIVAN P. & FOOTE F.M. (1964) Cerebrovascular accidents— incidence and survival rates in a defined population, Middlesex County, Connecticut. *Journal of the American Medical Association*, **189**, 883–8.

ESPMARK S. (1973) Stroke before 50. A follow-up study of vocational and psychological adjustment. *Scandinavian Journal of Rehabilitation Medicine*, Suppl. 2.

FEIGENSON J.S. (1979) Stroke rehabilitation: effectiveness, benefits and cost: some practical considerations. *Stroke*, **10**, 1–4.

FEIGENSEN J.S., GITLOW H.S. & GREENBERG S.D. (1979) The disability orientated rehabilitation unit—a major factor influencing stroke outcome. *Stroke*, **10**, 5–8.

FEIGENSON J.S. & MCCARTHY M.L. (1977) Guidelines for establishing a stroke rehabilitation unit. *New York State Journal of Medicine*, 1430–4.

FUGL-MEYER A.R., JAASKO L., LEYMAN I., OLSSON S. & STEGLIND S. (1975) The post-stroke hemiplegic patient: 1. A Method for evaluation of physical performance. *Scandinavian Journal of Rehabilitation Medicine*, **7**, 13–31.

GARRAWAY M. & AKHTAR A.J. (1977) Theory and practice of stroke rehabilitation. In *Recent Advances in Geriatric Medicine* (Ed. Isaacs B.), Churchill Livingstone, Edinburgh.

GRANGER C.B., ALBRECHT G.L. & HAMILTON B.B. (1979) Outcome of comprehensive medical rehabilitation: measurement by Pulses Profile and the Barthel Index. *Archives of Physical Medicine and Rehabilitation*, **60**, 145–53.

GRESHAM G.E., FITZPATRICK T.E., WOLF P.A., MCNAMARA P.M., KANNEL W.B. & DAWBER T.R. (1975) Residual disability in survivors of stroke—the Framingham Study. *New England Journal of Medicine*, **293**, 954–6.

GRIFFITH V.E. (1975) Volunteer scheme for dysphasia and allied problems in stroke patients. *British Medical Journal*, **iii**, 633–5.

GUTTMAN SIR L. (1976) *Textbook of Sport for the Disabled*. H.M. & M Publishers, Aylesbury, England.

HALE G. (1979) *The Source Book for the Disabled*. Paddington Press Ltd, New York and London.

HARRIS A.I., COX E. & SMITH C.H.W. (1971) *Handicapped and Impaired in Great Britain: Part I*. Office of Population Censuses and Surveys. HMSO, London.

HMSO (1978) *Mortality Statistics*. Office of Population Censuses and Surveys, Series DH1, No. 4.

HODGINSON H.M. (1972) Evaluation of a mental test score for assessment of mental impairment in the elderly. *Age and Ageing*, **1**, 233–8.

HOLBROOK M. (1979) Social work with stroke patients in a multi-disciplinary rehabilitation unit. Submitted as part of a personal Social Services Fellowship, Bristol University.

HOPKINS A. (1975) The need for speech therapy for dysphasia following stroke. *Health Trends*, **7**, 58–60.

ISAACS B. (1971) Identification of disability in the stroke patient. *Modern Geriatrics*, **1**, 390–402.

ISAACS B. (1977) Five year experience of a stroke unit. *Health Bulletin*, **35**, 94–8.

ISAACS B. & MARKS R. (1973) Determinants of outcome of stroke rehabilitation. *Age and Ageing*, **2**, 139–49.

ISAACS B., NEVILLE Y. & RUSHFORD I. (1976) The stricken: the social consequences of stroke. *Age and Ageing*, **5**, 188–92.

KATZ S., FORD, A.B., MOSKOWITZ R.W., JACKSON B.A. & JAFFE M.W. (1963) Studies of illness in the aged: the index of A.D.L., a standardised measure of biological and psychosocial function. *Journal of the American Medical Association*, **185**, 914–19.

KENIN M. & SWISHER P.L. (1972) A study of pattern of recovery in aphasia. *Cortex*, **8**, 56–68.

KENNEDY F.B., POZEN T.J., GABELMAN E.H., TUTHILL J.E. & ZAENTZ S.D. (1970) Stroke intensive care—an appraisal. *American Heart Journal*, **80**, 188–96.

KERTESZ A. & MCCABE P. (1977) Recovery patterns and prognosis in aphasia. *Brain*, **100**, 1–18.

LANGTON-HEWER R. (1976) Stroke rehabilitation in stroke. *Proceedings of the 9th Pfizer International Symposium* (Eds. Gillingham F.J., Mawdsley C. & Williams A.L.). Churchill Livingstone, Edinburgh.

LEADING ARTICLE (1977) Recovery patterns and prognosis in aphasia. *British Medical Journal*, **ii**, 848–9.

LESSER R. & WATT M. (1978) Untrained community help in the rehabilitation of stroke sufferers with language disorder. *British Medical Journal*, **ii**, 1045–8.

LINCOLN N. & LEADBITTER D. (1979) Assessment of motor function in stroke patients. *Physiotherapy*, **65**, 48–51.

MACKAY A. & NIAS B.C. (1979) Strokes in the young and middle-aged: consequences to the family and to society. *Journal of the Royal College of Physicians of London*, **13**, 2, 106–12.

MAHONEY F.I. & BARTHEL D.W. (1965) Functional evaluation: the Barthel Index. *Maryland State Medical Journal*, **14**, 61–5.

MARQUARDSEN J. (1969) *The Natural History of Acute Cerebrovascular Disease*. Munksgaard, Copenhagen.

MARQUARDSEN J. (1976) An epidemiological study of stroke in a Danish urban community. In *Stroke* (Eds. Gillingham F.J., Mawdsley C. & Williams A.E.). Churchill Livingstone, Edinburgh.

MARQUARDSEN J. (1978) The epidemiology of cerebrovascular disease. *Acta Neurologica Scandanavica*, Suppl. **67**, 57–75.

MATSUMOTO N., WHISNANT J.P., KURLAND C.T. & OKAZAKI H. (1973) Natural history of stroke in Rochester, Minnesota. *Stroke*, **4**, 20–9.

MCCANN B.C. & CULBERTSON R.A. (1976) Comparison of two systems for stroke rehabilitation in a general hospital. *Journal of the American Geriatrics Society*, **24**, 211–16.

MEIKLE M., WECHSLER E., TUPPER A., BENENSON M., BUTLER J., MULHALL D. & STERN G. (1979) Comparative trial of volunteer and professional treatments of dysphasia after stroke. *British Medical Journal*, **ii**, 87–9

MITCHELSON D.C. (1979) Bioengineering in motor function assessment and therapy. In *Progress in Stroke Research* (Eds. Greenhalgh R.M. & Rose F.C.). Pitman Medical, Tunbridge Wells.

MULLEY G. & ARIE T. (1978) Treating stroke: home or hospital? *British Medical Journal*, **ii**, 1321–2.

MYKYTA L.J., BOWLING J.H., NELSON D.A. & LLOYD E.J. (1976) Caring for relatives of stroke patients. *Age and Ageing*, **5**, 87.

NICHOLS P.J.R. (1976) A.D.L. Indices of any values. *Occupational Therapy*, **39**, 160–3.

OPIT L.J. (1977) Domiciliary care for the elderly sick—economy or neglect? *British Medical Journal*, **i**, 30–3.

ORADEI D.M. & WAITE N. (1974) Group psychotherapy with stroke patients during the immediate recovery phase. *American Journal of Orthopsychiatry*, **44**, 386–95.

PETLUND C.F. (1970) *Prevalence and Invalidity from Stroke in Aust Agder County of Norway*. Norwegian Monographs on Medical Science, Oslo.

PORCH B. (1967) *The Porch Index of communicative ability*.

Report of Royal College of Physicians' Working Group on Strokes (1974) Consultant Psychologists, Palo Alto. London.

SAHS A.C., HARTMAN E.C. & ARONSON S.M. (1979) *Stroke: Cause, Prevention, Treatment and Rehabilitation*. Castle House Publications Ltd, London.

SANDS E., SARNO M.T. & SHANKWEILER D. (1969) Long-term assessment of language function in aphasia due to stroke. *Archives of Physical Medicine and Rehabilitation*, **50**, 202–6.

SARNO M.T. (1976) The status of research in recovery from aphasia. In *Recovery in Aphasics Neurolinguistics* (Eds. Lebrun Y. & Hoops R.), pp. 13–30. Swets & Zeitlinger, Amsterdam.

SARNO M.T. & SANDS E. (1970) An objective method for the evaluation of speech therapy in aphasia. *Archives of Physical Medicine and Rehabilitation*, **51**, 49–54.

SARNO J.E., SARNO M.T. & LEVITA E. (1973) The functional life scale. *Archives of Physical Medicine and Rehabilitation*, **54**, 214–20.

SARNO M.T., SILVERMAN M. & SANDS E. (1970) Speech therapy and language recovery in severe aphasia. *Journal of Speech and Hearing Research*, **13**, 607–23.

SCHUELL H. (1965) *Differential Diagnosis of Aphasia with the Minnesota Test*. University of Minnesota Press, Minneapolis.

SHEIKH K., SMITH D.S., MEADE T.W., GOLDENBERG E., BRENNAN P.J. & KINSELLA G. (1979) Repeatability and validity of a modified activities of daily living (A.D.L.) Index in studies of chronic disability. *International Rehabilitation Medicine*, **1**, 51–8.

SHOENING H.A., ANDEREGG L. & BERGSTROMM D. (1965) Numerical scoring of self care status of patients. *Archives of Physical Medicine and Rehabilitation*, **46**, 689–97.

SMITH M.E. (1979) The Edinburgh Stroke Rehabilitation Study. *British Journal of Occupational Therapy*, **42**, 6, 139–41.

SOUZA L.H. DE, LANGTON-HEWER R. & MILLER S. (1980) Assessment of recovery of arm control in hemiplegic stroke patients. 1. Arm function tests. *International Rehabilitation Medicine* **2**; 1, 3–9.

TWITCHELL T.E. (1951) The restoration of motor function following hemiplegia in man. *Brain*, **47**, 443–80.

VELLETRI-GLASS A., GASSANIGA M. & PREMACK D. (1973) Artificial language training in global aphasics. *Neuropsychologica*, **11**, 95–103.

WAITE N.S. (1975) Social problems and the social work role. In *Stroke and its Rehabilitation* (Ed. Licht S.), pp. 417–34. Waverly Press, Baltimore, Maryland.

WALLACE D.C. (1967) A study of the natural history of cerebral vascular disease. *Medical Journal of Australia*, **1**, 90–5.

WARREN M.D., COOPER J. & WARREN J.L. (1967) Problems of emergency admissions to London hospitals. *British Journal of Preventive and Social Medicine*, **21**, 141–9.

WEDDELL J.M. (1974) Rehabilitation after stroke—a medicosocial problem. *Skandia International*

Symposium on Rehabilitation—After Central Nervous System Trauma (Eds. Bostrom H., Larsson T. & Ljungstedt N.). Nordiska Bokhandelns Forlag, Stockholm.

WELLS R. (1974) Family stroke education. *Stroke*, **5**, 393–6.

WHISNANT J.P. (1976) A population study of stroke and T.I.A. Rochester, Minnesota. In *Stroke* (Eds Gillingham F.J., Mawdsley C. & Williams A.E.). Churchill Livingstone, Edinburgh.

WHISNANT J.P., FITZGIBBONS J.P., KURLAND L.T. & SAYRE G.P. (1971) Natural history of stroke in Rochester, Minnesota, 1945 through 1954. *Stroke*, **2**, 11–21.

WORLD HEALTH ORGANIZATION (1971) Report of WHO Meeting. *Cerebrovascular Diseases: Prevention, Treatment and Rehabilitation.* WHO, Geneva.

Chapter 7

Natural History and Rehabilitation in Spinal Cord Damage

TERMINOLOGY

The term 'paraplegia' indicates motor and sensory paralysis of the lower limbs with involvement of bladder, bowel and male sexual function. The word 'tetraplegia' (quadriplegia) implies a higher spinal cord lesion causing partial or complete paralysis of the upper limbs in addition to paralysis of the chest, trunk, abdomen and lower limbs as well as impairment of the bladder and bowel and male sexual function. When applied to the description of an individual patient the word 'complete' implies total loss of all motor and sensory function. The word 'incomplete' implies any lesser degree. For assessment of prognosis and follow-up the classification introduced by Frankel *et al.* (1969) is used:

1. *Complete* (A). This means that the lesion is found to be complete both motor and sensory below the segmental level named.
2. *Sensory incompleteness only* (B). This implies that there is some sensation present below the level of the lesion but that the motor paralysis is complete below that level. This applies to sensory sparing as well as sacral sparing.
3. *Motor useless* (C). This implies that there is some motor power present below the lesion but it is of no practical use to the patient.
4. *Motor useful* (D). This implies that there is useful motor power below the level of the lesion. Patients in this group can move the lower limbs and many can walk with or without aids.
5. *Recovery* (E). This implies that the patient is free of neurological symptoms, i.e. no weakness, no sensory loss, no sphincter disturbance. Abnormal reflexes may be present.

To indicate the exact level of a lesion, the last normal segment is used, i.e. tetraplegia complete below C6 segment means that C6 segment is intact and C7 and the distal spinal cord is not in connection with the brain.

This chapter is confined to spinal cord lesions of acute onset and of a non-progressive nature. It is based on experience at the National Spinal Injuries Centre, Stoke Mandeville Hospital, and does not include multiple sclerosis, malignant tumours involving the spinal cord, or other progressive neurological diseases.

CAUSES OF SPINAL CORD LESION

In the UK the majority of non-progressive acute spinal cord lesions are due to trauma, the main causes being road accidents, industrial accidents, domestic accidents and sporting accidents. Most of these are due to fracture dislocations or severe fractures of the vertebral column and the major cause in relationship to the level of bony injury is shown in Table 7.1, which is the result of an analysis

Table 7.1   The level of bone injury to the spine in 682 patients

Vertebral injury	Cervical	T1–10	T11, 12; L1	Lumbar	Total
Road accidents					
Car (and lorry);					
driver	46	20	24	3	93
passenger	42	23	21	3	89
Motor cycle:					
driver	36	50	12	1	99
pillion	1	6	5	2	14
Bicycle	12	5	7	0	24
Pedestrian	11	2	8	0	21
					340
Aeroplane	1	1	6	0	8
Work					
Fall down	16	31	62	4	113
Dropped upon	2	8	12	3	25
Crushed	2	3	19	2	26
Hit	4	0	12	0	16
Other	1	0	0	0	1
					181
Domestic					
Fall	28	18	15	1	62
Dropped upon	0	1	0	0	1
Crushed	0	1	1	0	2
Hit	1	1	1	0	3
Other	1	2	1	0	4
					72
Sport					
Diving	41	0	1	0	42
Riding	0	4	3	1	8
Rugby football	5	0	0	0	5
Gymnastics	5	0	0	0	5
Other	4	1	4	2	11
					71
Assault	0	1	1	0	2
Attempted suicide	0	4	3	1	8
					10
Total	259	182	218	23	682

of 682 such patients admitted to Stoke Mandeville Hospital within 14 days of injury. The cause of the accident in different countries varies. In certain parts of Africa the commonest cause is falling from coconut trees. Penetrating injuries are much more common in other countries. In North and South America gunshot wounds are much more common and in South Africa stab wounds are frequent.

Stoke Mandeville Hospital also treats patients with non-traumatic spinal cord lesions whose onset and stability mimic that of traumatic cases, the commonest being transverse myelitis, benign tumours, vascular disturbances of the spinal cord (anterior spinal artery thrombosis, spinal strokes, arterio-venous malformation, and decompression sickness), abscesses compressing the spinal cord, either pyogenic or tuberculous.

NATURAL HISTORY

Following a physical transection of the spinal cord there is complete and permanent paralysis of voluntary motor power below the affected segment with complete and permanent loss of somatic sensory function and there is severe impairment of bladder, bowel and male sexual function as well as visceral and autonomic function. The evolution in time of each of these functions is briefly described below.

Motor Function

Though there can be no recovery from a complete transection the initial paralysis is usually somewhat higher than the final paralysis. On the second or third day after an acute transection the level of paralysis commonly rises by one segment. Over the next weeks this returns to the original level, then finally may end up one segment lower than the original physiological lesion; this pattern of events is of significance if the lesion is in the cervical region. Paralysis is at first of the flaccid type. Tendon reflexes and plantar responses may be present in the first hours after injury, then there is a period of spinal shock during which these reflexes are apparently abolished. The period of spinal shock varies from days to weeks and is usually shorter in younger patients and those with higher spinal cord transections. In general the period of spinal shock as assessed by the tone of the paralysed muscles and the absence of tendon reflexes and plantar responses is roughly related to the period of spinal shock as assessed by the evolution of bladder, bowel and vascular functions, but this correlation is not accurate in individual patients. Following the period of spinal shock, tone in the paralysed muscles returns and subsequently becomes abnormally high and varying degrees of 'spasticity' develop.

In cases where distal spinal cord is destroyed by the trauma or where all the spinal roots are destroyed, particularly in fracture dislocations of the lumbar spine, there is a permanent flaccid paralysis.

Sensory Function

Following complete transection of the spinal cord the changes in level by a segment or so described for motor function are also seen in the sensory level.

Bladder Function

Following spinal cord injury there is usually a period of severe disturbance of bladder function which may be classified as follows:

1. *Complete retention.* This is almost invariable in adult Europeans, but West Indians and European children may not have a period of complete retention.
2. *Passive incontinence* due to overflow from the distended bladder.
3. *Periodic micturition*
(a) By reflex activity of the automatic bladder,

or

(b) By expressing the urine by using the muscles of the abdominal wall, or pressing on the lower abdomen with the hand.

The time scale for the development of an automatic bladder or an expressive bladder is extremely variable and tends to be shorter in patients with high spinal cord lesions and in younger people, particularly in children. The average time for starting periodic micturition was found to be 4.3 weeks and the average time until catheterization could be stopped 8.8 weeks (Frankel, 1974).

If the bladder was left entirely to itself it is possible that many patients would die of renal failure in the first weeks. Some form of catheterization is almost invariably used in patients with complete spinal cord lesions and the various methods are described later in this chapter.

Bowel Function

THE SMALL INTESTINE

Immediately following a high spinal cord transection there may be a period of ileus, particularly on the second or third day. This can give rise to gross abdominal distension and dilated stomach, particularly if the patient is given excessive fluids early on or allowed to eat solid food in the first few days. It is particularly dangerous in patients with tetraplegia, as their ventilation may already be seriously impaired. Following these early days small intestinal function appears to return to normal, as judged by normal absorption of food and the normal transit time of a barium meal. The ileus is likely to recur throughout the patient's subsequent life if he is given an anaesthetic, even for relatively minor procedures such as dental extraction.

LARGE INTESTINAL AND RECTAL FUNCTION

Immediately following a complete spinal cord transection rectal tone is low and faeces tend to accumulate in the sigmoid colon. During this period laxatives and digital evacuations are required. Subsequently, patients with upper motoneuron lesions tend to develop reflex defaecation while those with lower motoneuron lesions do not. In both cases there is permanent loss of bowel sensation and control.

Sexual Function

Patients with high spinal cord lesions tend to have an initial priapism. Subsequently patients with complete spinal cord lesions above T12 often have reflex erections and no psychically induced erections; most such patients are incapable of having seminal emissions. Patients with complete cauda equina lesions below T12 segment may be capable of having psychically induced erections and/or having seminal emissions.

Vascular Changes

The resting blood pressure in patients with high spinal cord lesions is low. Problems of postural hypotension and autonomic dysreflexia are dealt with subsequently. The degree of 'hypotension' is related to the level of the spinal cord transection as shown in Figs. 7.1a and 7.1b.

NATURAL HISTORY IN COMPLETELY UNTREATED PATIENTS

Tetraplegics

A tetraplegic patient is breathing entirely with his diaphragm and accessory muscles of respiration and is, therefore, unable to cough effectively. It is, therefore, usual for such a patient to drown in his own secretions within the first 12 days after injury. If, as is likely, he also develops an ileus and dilated stomach, he may die sooner of inhalation of vomit.

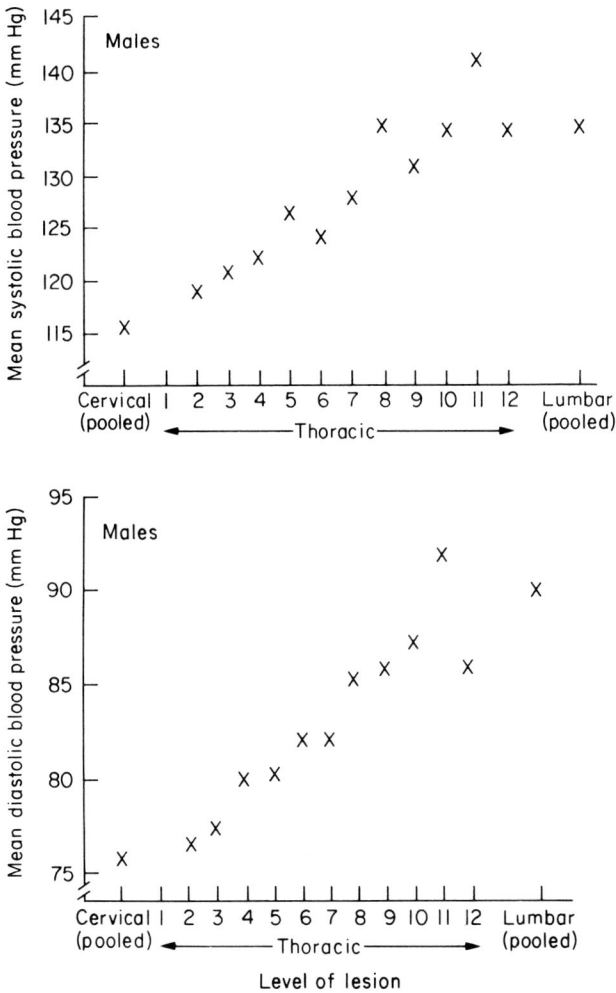

Fig. 7.1a   Mean systolic blood pressure/level of spinal cord lesion.
Fig. 7.1b   Mean diastolic blood pressure/level of spinal cord lesion.

Paraplegics

Paraplegics and any surviving tetraplegics are likely to develop severe penetrating pressure sores, contractures and severe urinary tract complications. If they are given no prophylaxis against these and no treatment when they develop, they are likely to die of the pressure sores within a few months, usually due to osteomyelitis and septicaemia; if for any reason they survive longer than this, they are likely to die of severe urinary tract complications within two years. The full natural history of this disorder is of course only rarely seen in civilized countries; however, as soon as the level of care and supervision of a paraplegic patient falls below an excellent standard, various aspects of this natural history manifest themselves remorselessly.

The alterations in human physiology, and their natural consequences as described above, are the background against which these patients must be rehabilitated. As there is at present no 'treatment' for the spinal cord lesion itself, our rehabilitation must be based on utilizing all remaining intact functions and on a detailed understanding of the altered physiology of the patient.

PROGNOSIS OF SPINAL CORD FUNCTION

The prognosis varies with the type of injury and my experience is limited to closed spinal cord injuries. Where the initial spinal cord lesion is physiologically incomplete the prognosis for some improvement or recovery is good. Even where the initial examination reveals a physiologically complete lesion, a certain number of patients make a partial or substantial recovery. Table 7.2 shows a change in neurological status in 218 patients with tetraplegia (from Frankel *et al.*, 1969). The first letter in each square for grade shows each patient's status on admission

Table 7.2   In each square of the grid are two letters of the alphabet, the first related to the neurological lesion on admission and the second to the neurological lesion on discharge. The numbers of patients are indicated. (Reproduced by permission of the Editor of *Paraplegia*.)

Cervical injuries

A/A	A B	A C	A D	A E
81	21	10	11	0
B A	B B	B C	B D	B E
3	9	2	14	5
C A	C B	C C	C D	C E
0	1	4	11	5
D A	D B	D C	D D	D E
0	0	0	30	11
E A	E B	E C	E D	E E
0	0	0	0	0

to Stoke Mandeville Hospital and the second figure shows his status on discharge. This indicates that even when there is a complete lesion initially there is a small chance of some or substantial recovery. If the lesion remains physiologically complete for 14 days then the prospect of any significant recovery is extremely slight. In patients who do eventually make a substantial recovery the onset of useful motor function in the lower limbs may be delayed for many weeks. I have seen several patients who, though they had sensory sparing, had complete motor paralysis at six weeks, who subsequently made a substantial recovery sometimes good enough to walk without the aid of sticks. For the rest of this chapter I describe the management and expected course for patients with complete permanent lesions. For most purposes management of patients with incomplete lesions is easier and the complications are less severe. The only exception to this is that patients with slightly incomplete lesions may have a far greater spasticity than those with complete lesions, and patients with substantially incomplete lesions often have greater difficulty in adjusting psychologically to their residual disability than those who are far more severely and completely paralysed.

We have no evidence of any treatment that affects the recovery of spinal cord function and it is the author's opinion that in the present stage of knowledge all that our management of the vertebral column can achieve is to avoid any further damage of the spinal cord.

MANAGEMENT AND REHABILITATION—EARLY STAGES

This phase of management covers the period that the patient spends in bed during the stabilization of the fracture or fracture dislocation. It usually varies from six to twelve weeks, although some patients may require more than twelve weeks in bed and some patients who have no substantial skeletal problems may be mobilized within a few days of the onset of their paralysis.

The phase of bed rest consists of postural management of the spinal column injury, which at Stoke Mandeville is achieved by posturing the patient on a Stoke Mandeville/Egerton turning bed in a position appropriate to the injury (Fig. 7.2). The patient is turned on this turning bed three-hourly to prevent pressure sores and, in addition, there is a daily inspection of all his pressure points. As long as the patient is admitted to a spinal injuries centre in the early stages, pressure sores are totally avoidable.

Position

If a paralysed or partly paralysed muscle is overstretched for long periods of time, recovery will be impaired; the patient must therefore be nursed in a posture which keeps muscles in a neutral position. This is particularly important where

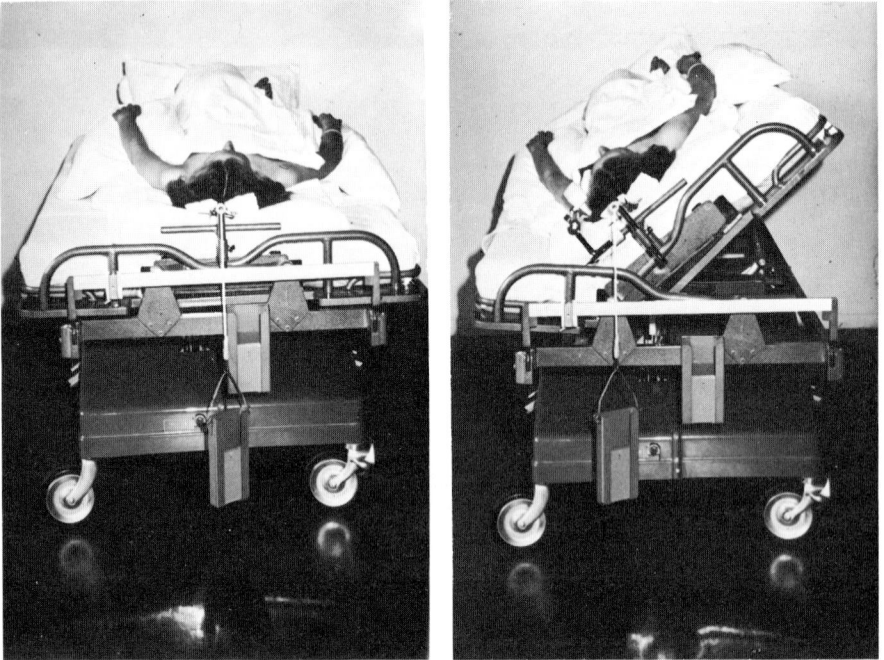

Fig. 7.2   Stoke Mandeville turning bed.

the opposing muscle is unparalysed or less paralysed. For example a patient with traumatic tetraplegia complete below the C6 segment will have active power in his deltoids, biceps and extensor carpi radialis longus and will tend to adopt a posture of abduction and internal rotation of the shoulders, flexion of the elbows, and extension, with radial deviation, at the wrists. Not only will this cause contractures, but any partial recovery which might be hoped for in the triceps will be prevented. In such cases where opposing muscles are unparalysed, the patient's position may have to be corrected frequently because he is able to flex the elbows actively but cannot extend them again.

Care of Joints and Soft Tissues

When paralysed limbs and joints are allowed to remain in the same position for prolonged periods, soft tissue contractures will develop extremely rapidly unless specific measures are taken to prevent them. The tendency to form contractures is most pronounced in the early weeks after the onset of paralysis and during that time a full range of passive movement must be given to every joint at least twice daily, seven days a week. As long as such care is started on the first day of the paralysis it is possible to perform a complete range of movements gently without the use of any undue force. Use of powerful passive movements may be necessary in a previously neglected patient but should be avoided whenever possible as it may cause damage to the soft tissues and over-vigorous physiotherapy may play some part in the production of para-articular ossification.

During the period of bed rest rehabilitation of the bladder and bowel will have started but not yet be under the patient's own management. During this period the patient will learn of the prognosis of his lesion. If the lesion is still complete after two weeks the physician will be virtually certain of the prognosis. The exact timing of when the patient is told this prognosis varies with different physicians and of course with different patients. It is the author's practice to wait until the patient asks for his prognosis for at least the first few weeks. Very often the patient refrains from asking and then the subject must be carefully approached. If the patient is being treated in a spinal injuries centre he will already be aware of the presence of wheelchair-bound patients around him and is very likely to make his own enquiries from other patients or trained or untrained staff before wanting to discuss it with the doctor. The majority of patients with complete lesions do understand and to some degree accept the permanence of their lesion by the time the ten weeks have passed. The amount of professional help, support and counselling that is given to patients on this aspect varies from centre to centre and doubtless the patient community is itself the main source of information and support. It is common to see severe reactive depression or denial of permanence of the injury. These are usually temporary phases, but if they become prolonged they interfere with the process of physical and social rehabilitation and drug treatment seems to be useless. It has not been established whether any form of psychotherapy or sophisticated counselling has any beneficial effect. The presence of a trained psychologist and counsellors in a spinal injuries team certainly speeds up the identification of those patients with the greatest problems.

During the acute phases and during the period of bed rest, it is of course natural that the patient's relatives and friends visit as frequently as possible. The staff at the centre take this opportunity of getting to know them and enlisting their cooperation in future planning.

Towards the end of the period of bed rest strict immobilization of the spine is stopped and a period of mobilization and back or neck strengthening exercises in bed is started. In most cases normally innervated muscles traverse the spinal fracture site; during the period of immobilization there is relative atrophy of these muscles and they can be strengthened by systematic exercises with the patient lying down so that his spinal fracture is more adequately stabilized when he starts to sit up.

Period of Mobilization

SITTING UP

In patients with high spinal cord lesions the normal reflex arc controlling the blood pressure in the sitting or standing position is largely abolished when the spinal cord lesion is above the level of the sympathetic outflow. By an arbitrary method of training described below it is usually possible to maintain an adequate blood pressure in these patients:

1.   Sit the patient up very slowly in a winding bed.
2.   When he can tolerate the sitting position repeat the process several times each day.
3.   All patients should eventually tolerate the sitting position for prolonged periods without any loss of consciousness.

The mechanisms by which this training is successful are not fully explained but are due in part to activation of the renin–angiotensin system and the ability of the patient to perfuse his brain adequately with low blood pressue. The use of abdominal binders or cuffs around the calves and administration of 25 mg of ephedrine before raising the patient from horizontal may help to achieve circulatory readjustment in this phase.

In the early stages in the wheelchair pitting oedema of the ankles is relatively common. This should be managed by limiting the number of hours which the patient spends sitting up, elevating the legs while in bed and occasionally by the use of well-fitting elastic stockings.

The Active Phase of Rehabilitation

Once the patient can tolerate the sitting position in a wheelchair the more active phase of his rehabilitation starts. This is a combined operation between the physician, nurses, physiotherapists, occupational therapists and social workers. Different members of this team are relatively more important at certain phases and for certain activities, thus the nurses will lead in training the patient in the prevention of pressure sores and management of bladder and bowels, in some centres they also teach patients in dressing. Physiotherapists are responsible for the care of the joints and teach transfers, standing and ambulation. The occupational therapist will largely concentrate on the training of the upper limbs and on dressing for tetraplegics.

The actual techniques of physiotherapy and occupational therapy are unremarkable and are deployed as appropriate to the condition of the patient. An excellent account of the different techniques are available in Bromley (1975).

The general principle on which our physical rehabilitation is based is to both strengthen and increase the skill of the remaining intact musculature.

By the time the patient is ready to leave the spinal injuries centre he should be approaching the optimum level of independence for his particular cord transection. Obviously the degree of independence achieved and the length of time taken also depend on the patient's age and motivation. The expected goals that can be achieved by typical representative cord lesions are shown in the tables for patients with complete lesions below C3, C4, C5, C6, C7, C8, T7, T10, T12, L3 and L4. These tables also show any special personal equipment that the patients may use.

Table 7.3   C3. Lowest muscles: sternomastoid; trapezius—part; diaphragm—part.

Independent	Assisted	Dependent

Talking
Swallowing
	Breathing—*ventilator*, part or full time
	Coughing ⎫
	Writing ⎬ *mouth stick or POSSUM*
	Typing ⎪
	Telephoning ⎭
	Environmental controls—*POSSUM*
	Electric wheelchair
		Drinking
		Feeding
		Turning
		Lifting
		Washing
		Shaving
		Dressing
		Bowels
		Urinal
		Transfers—
		  sometimes *hoist*
		Car—*special*
		  safety belt

C4. Lowest muscles: trapezius; rhomboid; diaphragm—part.

Independent	Assisted	Dependent

Talking
Swallowing
Breathing
	Coughing
	Writing—*mouth stick*
	Typing—*electric continuous paper*
	Telephoning—*POSSUM and other
	  adaptation*
	Environmental controls—*POSSUM*
	Shaving—*electric razor on stand*
	Electric wheelchair
	Drinking
		Feeding
		Turning
		Lifting
		Washing
		Dressing
		Bowels
		Urinal
		Transfers—
		  sometimes *hoist*
		Car—*special*
		  safety belt

Table 7.4   C5. Lowest muscles: deltoids; biceps; diaphragm.

Independent	Assisted	Dependent

Talking
Drinking—*Thermos mug*
Teeth Cleaning—*strap to hold brush*
Swallowing
Hair brushing—*strap to hold brush*
Breathing
Make-up—some
Push self-propelled *wheelchair*
  on flat surface
Writing—*pen holder*
Typing—*electric typewriter*
Telephoning—*POSSUM* or *adaptation*
 	
Shaving—*electric shaver*
	Coughing
	Feeding
	
	Transfers
	Turning
	Lifting
	Washing
	
	Dressing
	Transfers—
	  sometimes *hoist*
		Bowels
		Urinal
		
		Car

Table 7.5 C6. Lowest muscles: brachioradialis; extensor carpi radialis longus; triceps—sometimes.

Independent	Assisted	Dependent
As C5 plus:		
Typing—*standard typewriter*	Coughing	Bowels
Feeding	Turning	Urinal
Teeth cleaning		
Hair brushing		
Hair washing		
Washing		
Lifting		Car—*most*
Dressing—some	Dressing—some	
Cooking		
Kitchen work		
Writing—some—no aid		
Transfers—some using *sliding board*	Transfers—some, *hoist* or manual	
Push *wheelchair* up incline 1 in 12	Standing—in *standing frame*	
Car—some, *hand controlled car, automatic gearbox*		

Table 7.6 C7. Lowest muscles: triceps; wrist flexors.

Independent	Assisted	Dependent
As C6 plus:		
Turning (most)	Coughing	Bowels (most)
Washing (some)	Turning (few)	Urinal (most)
Dressing (most)	Washing (some)	Car (some)
Wheelchair—'back wheel balance' (some)	Dressing (few)	
Bowels (few)—*suppository insertor*	Transfers (few)— *hoist* or manual	
Urinal (few) apply and empty	Standing—in *standing frame*	
Transfers (most)—some use *sliding board*		
Family shopping—assisted		
Car (some)—*hand controlled, automatic gearbox*		

Table 7.7   C8. Lowest muscles: finger extensors; finger flexors.

Independent	Assisted	Dependent
As C7 plus:		
Turning	Coughing with respiratory infection	
Washing	Ambulate with *calipers* in parallel bars (not usually attempted)	
Dressing		
Transfers		
Full control of *wheelchair*—can mount 6″ kerb		
Car—*hand controls, automatic gearbox*		
Bowels		
Urinal		
Standing—in *standing frame*		

Table 7.8   T7. Lowest muscles: intercostals.

Fully independent for all personal needs in a suitable environment.
Never stand (some) may develop more severe demineralization of bones and fracture easily.
Stand in *frame* (some).
Ambulate with *long calipers* in *bars* (some), with *rollator* (some), with *elbow crutches* (some). Negotiate stairs (few). Most patients spend all day in a *wheelchair* and ambulate for exercise or special occasions.

Table 7.9   T12, L3 and L4.

T12. Lowest muscles: abdominals

As T7 but more patients ambulate with *elbow crutches*; however, the majority spend most of the day in a *wheelchair*.

L3. Lowest muscles: quadriceps; adductors

Walk with *long calipers* and *elbow crutches*, occasional *wheelchair* use.

L4. Lowest muscles: quadriceps; hamstrings

Walk with *short calipers* and *sticks*.

Skin Care

It is most important that patients fully understand the mechanisms by which their lack of sensation can cause pressure sores. If they do not have a full understanding of this subject, they may take inappropriate action when something goes wrong. They are taught to lift themselves at ten-minute intervals while in the wheelchair and to turn themselves at three-hourly intervals while in bed. Patients with high tetraplegia are unable to lift themselves and they either have to be lifted by someone else (at hourly or two-hourly intervals) or sit on a gel cushion or a ripple cushion. The recently introduced Roho cushion is very expensive but is the most effective means of pressure equalization that we have tried. Its use should be reserved for those with very high spinal cord lesions and those who have had recurrent problems with their ischial regions.

The patients and attendants are taught to inspect all their pressure areas daily and if there is the slightest redness or bruising they must keep off that point entirely until the condition has resolved.

Although the patients are taught to lift themselves at ten-minute intervals, certain patients, by trial and error, can extend this period gradually to once every half an hour. Likewise, for safety we prefer three-hourly turning while the patient is in bed. Certain patients can lie in one position for longer than this, particularly if a large cell ripple mattress is used. It is often possible for the patient to lie on his side for three hours then turn on to his back and remain there for the rest of the night—approximately another six hours. If the patient becomes ill for any reason and has a fever he is taught that more frequent turning is temporarily necessary under those conditions.

The patient's entire future is dependent upon his ability to prevent pressure sores. The importance of prophylaxis and the inevitability of pressure sores in the absence of adequate prophylaxis is repeatedly pointed out to the patient and the vast majority of patients absorb this information and act accordingly. A small proportion of patients (approximately 5%) develop recurrent pressure sores after their discharge from hospital, and this small proportion of patients makes up a substantial part of the workload of our readmission wards.

Bladder Care

The natural history of the untreated bladder in patients with spinal cord lesions was described earlier in this chapter. The major problem in the early stages of rehabilitation is protecting the patient's urinary tract from damage and chronic infection during the phase of complete or partial retention of urine. In European adults this almost invariably means some form of catheterization, either urethral or suprapubic. Nowadays urethral catheterization, either with an indwelling catheter or by intermittent catheterization, is almost always practised.

Foley catheters are the most commonly used indwelling catheters. These should be of small size (16 French gauge) and should be inserted aseptically, and in male patients the penis must lie in an upwards direction. If the penis is allowed to lie between the legs with an indwelling catheter in position there is severe pressure on the urethral wall at the peno-scrotal junction and the urethral diverticulum, and sometimes a fistula at that site will occur. While the urine remains sterile continuous closed drainage is recommended. Once the urine becomes infected (usually within a few days) the patients should have daily bladder washouts.

A Gibbon catheter may be used in the first instance and with a small Gibbon catheter size 10 Fg or 12 Fg the urine may remain sterile for several weeks, particularly if the patient has a high fluid output. Once the urine does become infected these small catheters almost invariably block and it is necessary to change to a Foley catheter.

Whether a Foley catheter or a Gibbon catheter is used, eventually a period of bladder training must be undertaken and this is usually attempted between eight and ten weeks after the injury.

INTERMITTENT CATHETERIZATION

At Stoke Mandeville Hospital the favoured method of management in the early weeks is by intermittent catheterization using a non-touch technique. This has been fully described elsewhere (Guttmann & Frankel, 1966; Frankel, 1974). Basically, the patients are catheterized three times in every 24 hours. Catheterization is performed with a soft flexible Jacques type catheter. Each catheterization is performed by a doctor assisted by a nurse or an orderly. It is essential for this method of management that the fluid intake is controlled so that at each catheterization not more than 700 ml of urine is in the bladder. It is also essential that all the urine is removed from the bladder on each occasion and as the bladder is atonic in the early stages this needs suprapubic pressure while the catheter is slowly withdrawn. If during this period a sub-clinical urinary infection occurs it is promptly treated with systemic antibiotic. If a severe urinary infection supervenes with rigors and high fever then the method is temporarily abandoned and an indwelling catheter is used until the acute infection is over (usually in three or four days).

Three times a day catheterization is continued until the patients are passing urine reliably between catheterization, then the midday catheterization is omitted and fluid intake increased. As soon as the residual urine is less than 200 ml catheterization is reduced to once daily. When the residual urine is less than 100 ml catheterization is finished. It is soon after catheterization is stopped that any residual infection which may have been acquired during the period of catheterization is likely to be troublesome, and at this stage careful bacteriological control and the appropriate antibiotic treatment are very important. The majority of patients have sterile urine at the end of their treatment, but in many cases sub-clinical or clinical infections may recur in the later stages. Some patients require bladder neck or extensive sphincter surgery.

After such treatment at Stoke Mandeville Hospital, almost all male patients leave hospital catheter-free. If they have a complete spinal cord lesion they will almost certainly be using a urinal device and we favour the condom-type urinal where the condom is glued to the penis with condom glue. These condoms are satisfactory for the majority of patients except those who have a retracting penis and those who are allergic to either the condom or the glue. These allergy problems have been well described by Bransbury (1979).

About 75% of our female patients leave hospital catheter-free and attempt to keep dry by regular visits to the lavatory where they stimulate their bladder in whatever manner works for them. Unfortunately most female patients with complete cord lesions sometimes are wet in between such times and have to wear absorbent pads and waterproof pants. The management of the female's urinary incontinence is one of the weakest points in present-day rehabilitation of para-plegics. Because of the extreme inconvenience of urinary incontinence in females it is very tempting to use a long-term indwelling catheter. While this may give good control of incontinence it inevitably gives rise to chronic bladder infection. In addition, after a certain length of time, either months or years, many such patients develop severe damage to the urethra and their Foley catheter then drops out. They then, therefore, end up with all the disadvantages of the indwelling catheter, particularly infection, and are finally incontinent again. The only measure then available to them is to divert their ureters into an ilial conduit. This is a major procedure but is often found to be satisfactory by the patient.

Bowel Training

During the first few weeks after injury laxatives and digital evacuations will almost certainly be required; these digital evacuations should be preceded by glycerin suppositories and should be performed carefully and gently; if undue violence or stretching occurs during the phase of spinal shock the anus may be over-stretched and the onset of 'automatic defaecation' may be delayed or prevented.

After the stage of spinal shock attempts are made to teach the patient 'planned defaecation'. The reservoir for faeces is the sigmoid colon and not the rectum. The rectum should be empty except immediately before defaecation. The ability of the sigmoid colon to act as a reservoir seems to be unimpaired in the para-plegic; it is the awareness of faeces passing into the rectum and the ability to assist or prevent their further passage which is lacking. As the last line of defence against faecal incontinence is permanently lost, our efforts must be directed to preserving the remaining function, i.e. the holding function of the colon. This can be done by completely emptying the sigmoid colon by appropriate stimulation at regular intervals and by ensuring that the rectum is also completely emptied.

At a later stage a mild laxative is taken on alternate evenings—senna is as good as anything. The smallest dose which has been found to be effective is used; the best time to take the laxative is determined in each case by trial and error. The laxative should 'load the gun and take off the safety catch, but should not pull the trigger'. The final stimulus should be one which can be accurately timed and in most cases glycerin suppositories are suitable—they stimulate and lubricate; the time between insertion and evacuation of the colon is usually 10–20 minutes. Dulcolax (bisacodyl) suppositories are sometimes more effective but may take one to two hours to act. Other accessory methods of stimulation may also be used, the most important being the utilization of the gastro-colic reflex, abdominal straining or abdominal massage and rectal stimulation with the finger.

In patients with upper motoneuron lesions when the rectum is filled from above it usually empties itself reflexly and completely, and in such patients digital evacuations are rarely required if the patient waits long enough.

In patients with lower motoneuron lesions the sigmoid colon will still empty itself into the rectum when stimulated. Although the patient may be able to expel some faeces from his rectum by straining, in most cases some faeces are left in the rectum. As the anal sphincters are lax there is then faecal leakage, so most of these patients need to remove some faeces digitally.

Having emptied the colon and rectum completely, the rectum should remain empty until the colon is stimulated again two days later. This is only a general plan. Every patient needs individual advice and much depends on previous bowel habit, neurological lesion and degree of motility. There are a number of things which can disturb this method of management, the most important of which is constipation. The method I have described depends on the delivery of a moderate amount of formed stool—neither too hard nor too soft—to the rectum. If a considerable length of colon is loaded with hard faeces liquid faeces may be forced past the stale faeces and cause spurious diarrhoea in paraplegics. In such cases a faecal softener such as Dioctyl can be given followed by larger doses of laxatives and by enemas.

The second cause of failure may be due to a change of diet or activity. Patients confined to bed may need larger doses of laxative. This is probably due to inactivity rather than inability to sit on the lavatory. We attempt to teach most patients to have their bowels open on a lavatory with a padded seat, but this is largely for social convenience. I do not think that the sitting position is of great importance to the act of defaecation, lying on the side with legs flexed is also effective.

The results of adequate bowel training are most gratifying. It prevents ill health due to constipation and avoids social embarrassment. The success of the method is shown by the fact that although the necessity to interfere with his own bowel function is at first distasteful and embarrassing to a new patient, very few patients who attend for check-up report any serious difficulty, and the colleagues

and friends of most paraplegics are unaware that these patients have any dysfunction of their bowels.

Skeletal Complications

In the early stages paraplegics are prone to develop contractures (described
earlier) and para-articular ossification. In later stages they are prone to suffer
from pathological fractures and Charcot joints.

PARA-ARTICULAR OSSIFICATION

A small proportion (approximately 5% in our experience) of paralysed patients
develop para-articular ossification. This starts as a hard swelling, usually within
a muscle, and gradually develops into ectopic new bone. It occurs most commonly around the hip joint, but may develop in the lower end of the quadriceps
or may occur around the elbow joint or the shoulder joint. If it is allowed to
progress it may form a complete extra-articular ankylosis. The joint itself is
never directly involved.

   While this condition may undoubtedly start at the site of a haematoma, the
majority of paraplegics who develop haematomas do not develop para-articular
ossification and why it occurs in some patients is unexplained. Once the condition is suspected an X-ray should be taken. Although in the first week or two it
may show only a soft tissue swelling, it then becomes radio-opaque over the next
few weeks. Gentle passive movements usually prevent the development of a
complete extra-articular ankylosis. These movements must be continued twice
a day, seven days a week, until the disease process becomes inactive. The degree
of activity can be judged on clinical and radiological grounds and by the alkaline
phosphatase which is substantially raised during the active phase. Patients who
have had para-articular ossification at one site are liable to develop it at other
sites, either spontaneously or in response to soft tissue injuries.

PATHOLOGICAL FRACTURES

All paralysed patients develop substantial demineralization of their lower limbs
and this process continues for one or two years after the onset of their paralysis.
Subsequently the patients may fracture their lower limbs, either by falling from
their wheelchair, or from some relatively minor trauma, for example when
attempting to put on their socks. The fractures usually heal rapidly. We attempt
to reduce the demineralization of the skeleton by regular weight-bearing. In
patients with low lesions this is done by standing and walking with the aid of
calipers; in patients with higher lesions regular use of a standing frame is
recommended. We have not yet been able to prove conclusively that regular
standing lessens demineralization or lessens the frequency of pathological
fractures.

CHARCOT JOINTS

These are liable to occur over a number of years whenever there is a discrepancy between motor and sensory function around a particular joint. The knee joint and ankle joint of patients with cauda equina lesions are particularly vulnerable if the patients walk with inadequate calipers. Charcot joints of the spine below the original fracture are quite common as a radiological phenomenon, but are usually of little clinical significance.

Spasticity

Some degree of spasticity is expected to develop in all patients where there is some remaining viable isolated spinal cord. Patients with complete lesions do not usually have such intense spasticity as those who have incomplete lesions. However, in some patients with complete lesions the spasticity is disabling in that it prevents certain activities being carried out without assistance. Spasticity as such should only be treated if it is inhibiting the patient's independence; a certain degree of spasticity and spontaneous movement is helpful to the patient's circulation and skin and if the patients are taught to understand this effect they will learn to accept spasticity as being beneficial and not evil or frightening.

If the spasticity is disabling the following techniques may be used in attempts to treat it.

POSITIONING AND PHYSIOTHERAPY

Careful positioning as described above will tend to cause a balanced and acceptable form of spasticity. Physiotherapy in the form of regular passive movements and standing are beneficial. Hydrotherapy in a warm pool (33°C) for periods of up to half an hour often causes temporary relief of spasticity which enables the patient to become more active. Cooling a muscle with ice or cold water can also give temporary localized relief of spasticity, but this cannot be used for the whole of the lower part of the body as it would induce hypothermia.

DRUG TREATMENT

In general drugs are only to be used on a temporary basis until other measures can produce some improvement.

Diazepam in doses ranging from 6 mg to 40 mg per day in divided doses has a definite effect on spasticity (Corbett *et al.*, 1972) but, unfortunately, it causes marked drowsiness and is unsuitable for patients who wish to drive cars.

Baclofen, 15–45 mg in divided doses, has also been used for spasticity, but the author has had less success with this drug. It also causes drowsiness and on occasions mental disturbance and hallucinations both during its administration and when it is stopped.

Dantrolene sodium, starting with doses of 25 mg t.d.s. and gradually working up to 100 mg q.d.s., very often has an effect on spasticity; this drug works directly on the muscle fibres and in effective doses may increase the patient's weakness. However, many patients find they can compensate for greater weakness and gain benefit from the drug. The drug sometimes gives rise to a feeling of drunkenness, probably due to an effect on the muscles of speech, but most patients can overcome this side effect with time.

PERIPHERAL SURGICAL PROCEDURES

Peripheral operations on tendons, in particular division of contracted hamstring tendons and lengthening of the Achilles tendons, may be beneficial. Obturator neurectomy is a relatively simple method of permanently abolishing adductor spasticity in the legs. Tenotomy of the adductors is often followed by wound infections, as is any operation in the groins of paraplegics. Division of the iliopsoas either below the inguinal ligament or intra-abdominally is sometimes beneficial.

Surgical anterior rhizotomy gives permanent relief of spasticity, but because of the number of roots that require treatment it is a major procedure and is rarely carried out. Likewise posterior rhizotomy is now rarely used and does not necessarily give permanent relief of spasticity.

INJECTIONS

Injections of 6% phenol in water into motor points is successful in the right hands. Intrathecal alcohol abolishes spasticity completely but unfortunately causes further impairment of bladder and bowel function and increases the patient's liability to develop pressure sores. Intrathecal phenol can be given in a more controlled and localized manner, but the beneficial effects are rarely permanent.

PAIN

The majority of paraplegic patients are pain-free. However, up to 10% of patients with closed injuries may suffer chronically disabling pains and the proportion is much higher when the spinal cord injury is due to a gunshot wound. Although the pains are of many different types they can be broadly divided into three categories: phantoms, root pains, hyperpathic pains.

Phantoms

These are analogous with the phantoms of amputees. The phantom sensations are not necessarily painful but are usually described as unpleasant. They usually manifest themselves well below the level of the cord transection, often in the feet, rectum or genitalia. Within a closed community like a spinal injuries centre there are occasionally epidemics of particular types of phantom pain. There have been occasions when in one ward there were four patients with penile phantoms. They usually respond to explanation of the nature of the phenomenon. Very often the patient can be persuaded to think of the phantom as pleasant rather than unpleasant. Drug treatment with large doses of Tegretol and an antidepressant is sometimes successful.

Root Pains

These are severe pains occurring in the segmental distribution, within anaesthetic segments one or two segments below the last intact segment. In patients with gunshot wounds they may start very soon after the injury; in patients with closed injuries they rarely start less than two months after injury. Patients who have complications such as pressure sores, which delay their mobilization for many months, are much more prone to these pains. We do not know the cause of the pains, or whether there is any abnormal 'electrical' activity in the stump of the cord. They are extremely difficult to manage and sometimes even major procedures such as cordectomy a segment or two above the lesion, or surgical or chemical division of the spinothalamic tract, may produce no improvement. The most helpful measures are of a general nature, i.e. early, active mobilization, and a full programme of rehabilitation including physiotherapy, occupational therapy and sport. Mild analgesics are usually useless and strong analgesics are addictive. Tegretol and an antidepressant may give partial relief. The majority of patients can learn to tolerate the pains if they are well settled at home and in full-time employment. In a very small proportion of cases the rest of their life is a misery because of the pains. These patients typically provoke hostility and resentment in the medical and nursing staff as well as the other patients. The reason for this is not clear; possibly it is because we cannot stand the repetition of details and symptoms that we are powerless to alter, possibly some of these patients do have a different personality, and often in their pre-paraplegic history there is evidence of them having suffered from chronic painful conditions. I have no personal experience of electrical stimulation of the spinal cord to control these pains, but it is probably no more helpful than any other powerful placebo.

Hyperpathic Pains

Some patients, particularly cervical patients, have hyperpathia or hyperalgesia in partially innervated segments of the border of their lesions. This is not usually a permanent phenomenon, but it can be very distressing, so the patient cannot bear to be touched even by the lightest bed-clothes on that part. Occasionally regular freezing of the affected part with an iced spray or crushed ice gives relief.

AUTONOMIC DYSREFLEXIA

The phenomenon has been extensively studied in recent years and has been reviewed by Frankel and Mathias (1976). It is a most interesting phenomenon which occurs in patients with high spinal cord lesions. In response to certain stimuli, the most important of which are bladder contraction, rectal contraction, ejaculation and skeletal muscle spasms, there is an intense vaso-constriction below the level of the spinal cord lesion. This results in a rapid marked degree of hypertension with compensatory bradycardia (the vagus nerves are intact in these cases). Associated with this there is usually sweating of the face and neck, a mottled erythema of the trunk to just above the groin, dilatation of the pupils and in severe cases a throbbing headache. Blood pressure can rise to extreme heights—for example from 100/60 to 260/150 mm HG (13.5/8–35/20 kPa) within a few heart beats of the onset of the stimulus—and very occasionally these acute episodes of hypertension cause cerebral haemorrhage. Autonomic dysreflexia is a non-specific warning of what would normally be a painful condition below the level of the lesion. The best treatment is to remove the cause, i.e. emptying a full bladder. In an emergency the blood pressure may be reduced by the use of ganglion-blocking agents, or by amyl nitrate or glyceryl trinitrate.

SPECIAL EQUIPMENT

Almost all paraplegics require a wheelchair and at Stoke Mandeville Hospital we favour folding self-propelling wheelchairs of the Zimmer/Everest and Jennings type. The vast majority of adult patients can be suited by either a standard wheelchair or a junior wheelchair, and a small number by a slim adult chair. For the majority of patients we recommend a four inch Sorbo cushion; only those who cannot lift themselves are provided with a gel, ripple or Roho cushion. A small number of patients who have used them for many years prefer to have the driving wheels at the front of their chair, but the vast majority have 24 inch driving wheels at the back with seven or eight inch castors at the front.

Electric chairs

Patients who are unable to push a wheelchair are provided with an electrically propelled one. The most suitable currently available is the Vessa Kerb Climber, which has a good proportional drive control unit. The Zimmer Power Drive has a slightly better seating position, but the control unit does not have proportional control and has a rather jerky mechanism.

Cars

Most paraplegics can get in and out of a car unaided, fold up their wheelchair and pull it into the car behind them or next to them. They can drive a hand-controlled car, preferably with an automatic gearbox. Many of our young male patients enjoy changing gear although the number of actions involved in de-clutching and changing gear is considerable. Surprisingly many tetraplegics, even those with complete C6 lesions, have learnt to drive cars and some have even passed the test of the Institute of Advanced Motorists!

The wheelchair and the hand-controlled car form the basis of the paraplegic's independence.

Calipers

For patients with lesions above L3, long calipers (not ischial bearing) with lockable knee joints and built-in foot-raising device (usually back stops) are used. For patients with good strength in their quadriceps and no power in their hamstrings we prescribe a long caliper with an open knee joint but with a posterior sling to prevent hyperextension.

SPORT

Sport for paraplegics was introduced by Sir Ludwig Guttman at Stoke Mande-ville soon after the Second World War. At that time darts, table tennis, archery, swimming and wheelchair polo were played although the last sport was too dangerous and was replaced by wheelchair basketball. Many other sports have since been added, in particular wheelchair racing, fencing, weight lifting, bowls and various field events.

It is our present practice to try to interest all new paraplegics and tetraplegics in some of the sports that are within their capacity. This is beneficial not only for the physical exercise, but it is sometimes the first 'fun' for a newly paralysed patient. It also aids their self-confidence and their reintegration into society.

Most patients do not continue with active sport at a later stage, but a few of them become interested in competitive sports and become extremely proficient and participate in regional, national, international and Olympic competitions. Apart from giving those chosen few some very enjoyable international trips, the International Stoke Mandeville Games and Olympics have had a profound influence on the attitude of society towards the disabled throughout the world. Indeed, when the Para-Olympics were held in Japan in 1964, the Japanese set up a spinal injuries centre two years in advance of these games so that they would have some paraplegics who could compete! The Stoke Mandeville Stadium for the Paralysed and Other Disabled is the world centre for all disabled sport and an 'Olympic Village' in memory of Sir Ludwig Guttman is at present being built.

REFERENCES

BRANSBURY A.J. (1979) Allergy to rubber condom urinals and medical adhesives in male spinal injury patients. *Contact Dermatitis*, **5**, 317–23.

BROMLEY I. (1975) *Tetraplegia and Paraplegia*. Churchill Livingstone, Edinburgh.

CORBETT M., FRANKEL H.L. & MICHAELIS L. (1972) A double blind, cross-over trial of valium in the treatment of spasticity. *Paraplegia*, **10**, 19–22.

FORD J.R. & DUCKWORTH B. (1974) *Physical Management for the Quadriplegic Patient*. F. A. Davis, Philadelphia.

FRANKEL H.L. (1974) Intermittent catheterisation. *Urologic Clinics of North America*, **1**, 115–24.

FRANKEL H.L., HANCOCK D.O., HYSLOP G., MELZACK J., MICHAELIS L.S., UNGAR G.H., VERNON J.D.S. & WALSH J.J. (1969) The value of postural reduction in the initial management of closed injuries of the spine and with paraplegia and tetraplegia, part one. *Paraplegia*, **7**, 179–92.

FRANKEL H.L. & Mathias C.J. (1976) The cardiovascular system in tetraplegia and paraplegia. *Handbook of Clinical Neurology*, **26**, 313–33.

GUTTMANN SIR L. & FRANKEL H.L. (1966) The value of intermittent catheterisation in the early management of traumatic paraplegia and tetraplegia. *Paraplegia*, **4**, 63.

Chapter 8

Rehabilitation and Management of the Neuropathic Bladder

The care of the neuropathic bladder is bedevilled by confused terminology, inexact assessment methods, empirical attitudes and a preoccupation with cases of spinal trauma. Management has often been described in relation to a particular disease, or depending on the site of the clinically demonstrable neurological lesion. This approach is changing, perhaps for two particular reasons. First, as a more functional view of the urinary tract has developed, it has become evident that it is difficult to predict from the neurological signs how the bladder will behave. Second, close observation has shown that bladder function changes considerably at different stages of disease, and also in response to environmental factors, especially infection. Because of these facts optimal management requires functional investigation.

In this chapter we have not attempted to repeat the details of management that would be appropriate, for example, in a spinal injuries unit. Indeed we are not qualified by experience to do so. Rather we have tried to describe the principles of treatment in relation to what is pathophysiologically *observed* rather than expected. The first section of the chapter therefore concentrates on the structure and innervation of the bladder and urethra, and on the principles of functional investigation. The second section of the chapter discusses practical management in relation to physiological principles. Such management may perhaps be encompassed by two questions:

1   Has everything appropriate been done to preserve renal and ureteric function?
2   Can continence be restored or incontinence palliated without compromising renal function?

THEORETICAL CONSIDERATIONS

An understanding of how the system works is always a necessary prerequisite for putting right a fault. Because of the recent and continuing research into this area, much of it stimulated by the activities of the International Continence Society, understanding is improving. The following accounts must be regarded not as definitive statements of fact, but as a physiological stimulus to more rational treatment. Perhaps the greatest single contribution urodynamics has made has been to provoke thought about therapeutic dogma.

Vesico-urethral Structure and Innervation

The structure and innervation of the bladder and urethra in humans has been studied extensively by Gosling and his co-workers (Gosling *et al.*, 1977; Gosling, 1979), and the following account is based largely on their work.

DETRUSOR

The main bulk of the detrusor, including the condensation around the bladder neck, is a meshwork of smooth muscle. This is not layered as is the intestine. It is relatively rich in acetylcholine esterase, evidence for a dominant cholinergic innervation. There is little noradrenergic activity.

Excitatory motor nerves to the detrusor arise from the parasympathetic (cholinergic) ganglion cells in the pelvic plexus. The preganglionic fibres run in the sacral roots 2–4. Nerve-mediated detrusor inhibition has been described, occurring after stimulation of the perianal area, and it is suggested that such relaxation may be induced by β-sympathetic action (Sundin & Dahlstrom, 1973). Bladder relaxation evoked by bladder wall stretch (accommodation) may be similarly mediated. As little significant sympathetic innervation reaches the bladder dome in humans, it is suggested by Gosling that such inhibition may occur at the neurons in the pelvic ganglia where noradrenergic axosomatic terminals have been observed. These sympathetic nerves arise in the T10—L2 level and run in the pre-sacral nerves and hypogastric plexus.

Around the bladder neck the detrusor muscle is arranged in various loops and slings. No doubt these are involved in the mechanisms of closure and opening of the bladder neck. Several mechanical theories of function have been elaborated, but these are presumptive and should be interpreted with caution.

URETHRAL SMOOTH MUSCLE

At and below the vesico-urethral junction the smooth muscle of the proximal or preprostatic urethra is histochemically distinct from that of the detrusor. In the male (Fig. 8.1) this muscle also forms the prostatic capsule and is richly provided with noradrenergic terminals, but relatively little acetylcholine esterase is found. In the female (Fig. 8.2) the fibres are longitudinally arranged along the urethra, and in contrast to the male the dominant innervation is cholinergic. In both sexes experimental studies using α blockers (Donker *et al.*, 1972) suggest that up to 80% of the resting urethral pressure depends on α adrenergic

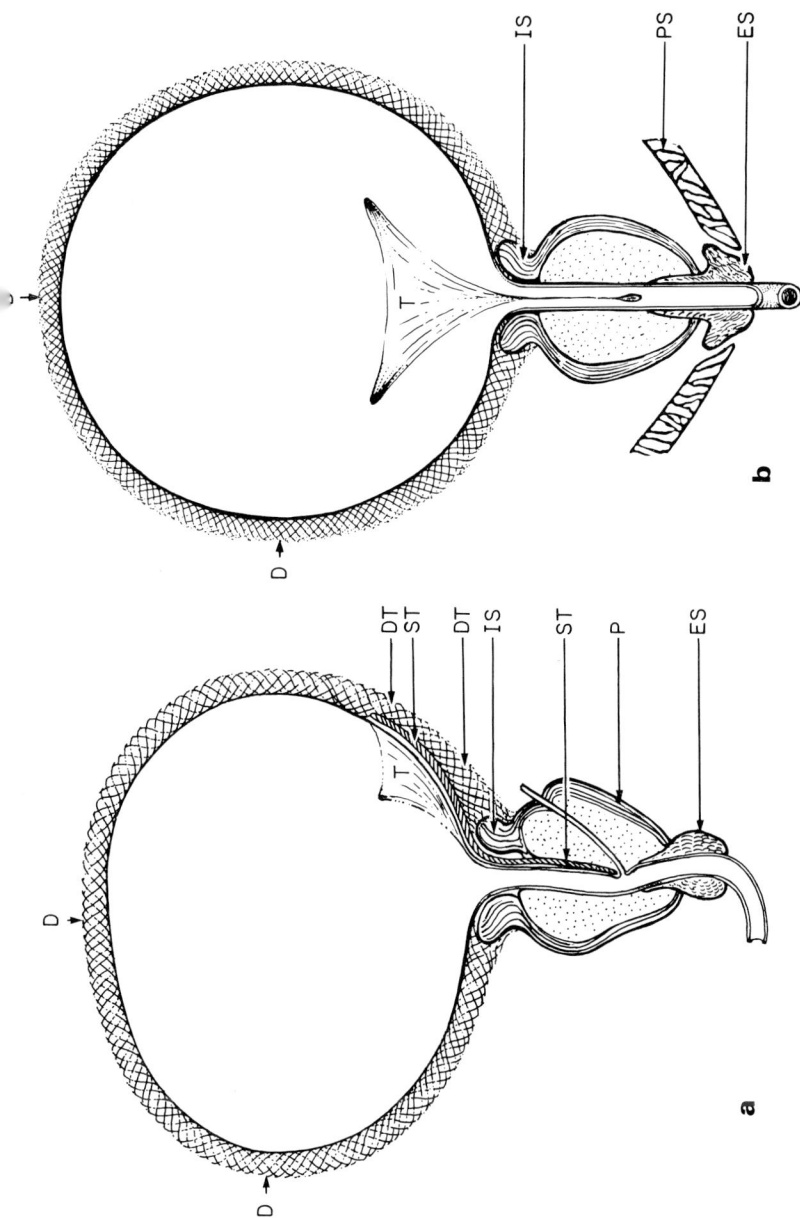

Fig. 8.1 (a) The male lower urinary tract in midline sagittal section. The detrusor (D) is condensed behind the bladder neck as the deep trigone (DT). This is distinct from the superficial trigone (ST). The smooth muscle at the bladder neck (IS) forms the proximal part of the urethral sphincter mechanism and is continuous with the prostatic capsule (P). The intramural striated muscle (ES) is condensed around the postprostatic urethra and forms the striated part of the distal urethral sphincter mechanism, or 'external sphincter'. (b) Viewed from the front the intramural (ES) and periurethral (PS) striated muscles are separated by a connective tissue septum. (From Gosling, 1979, with permission)

activity. As with the detrusor it is likely that the sympathetic influence on the
urethra occurs in part at the pelvic ganglia, especially in the female. In the male
the role of the sympathetic system in seminal emission is particularly significant
and the preprostatic urethra has been called a 'genital sphincter' preventing

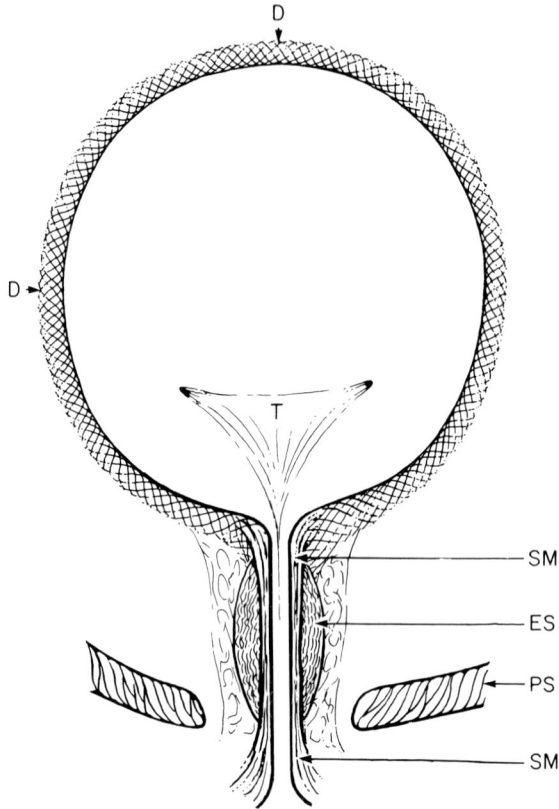

Fig. 8.2 The female lower urinary tract in coronal section. A thin layer of smooth
muscle (SM) extends the full length of the urethra. The intramural striated muscle
(ES) is thickest in the middle one-third of the urethra, and is anatomically separate
from the periurethral striated muscle (PS). (From Gosling, 1979, with permission)

reflux into the bladder. Stimulation of sacral nerves, perhaps involving preganglionic parasympathetic fibres, has been shown to cause urethral relaxation
(Torrens, 1978). These and other studies suggest that the autonomic innervation
promotes reciprocal activity between the bladder and urethra.

URETHRAL STRIATED MUSCLE

There are two groups of striated muscles in relation to the urethra, called by Gosling intramural and periurethral. Intramural fibre bundles are found close to the urethral lumen, sometimes inter-digitating with smooth muscle. In the male (Fig. 8.1) these fibres are orientated circularly around the postprostatic 'membranous' urethra. The muscle cells are smaller than usual and almost all of a 'slow twitch' type, rich in myosin ATPase. No muscle spindles have been seen. Evidently these fibres are adapted to maintain tone over a relatively long period of time. In the female (Fig. 8.2) the fibres are similar in type but form no such sphincter. Their density is greatest anteriorly and laterally in the middle third of the urethra. The intramural striated muscle is supplied by myelinated fibres from S_{2-4} passing through the pelvic plexus *not* running in the pudendal nerve. This explains why pudendal neurectomy does not abolish sphincter spasm.

The periurethral striated muscle of the pelvic floor is relatively remote from the urethra, separated from the intramural muscle by a connective tissue septum. This muscle is a mixture of slow and fast twitch fibres and is supplied by the pudendal nerve (S_{2-4}). This muscle is part of the levator ani complex or pelvic diaphragm. It can contract quickly, as on coughing or voluntary interruption of the urinary stream, but cannot maintain a long sustained contraction.

The urethra should not be regarded as a collection of sphincters, but as an integrated closure system relying not only on the active neuromuscular components described above but also on passive factors such as urethral elasticity and mural tension.

RECEPTOR SITES

Much recent effort has been directed towards the analysis of sympathetic receptors in the urinary tract. The distinction between experimentally demonstrable α and β adrenergic receptor sites and innervation is not always made clear. α adrenergic receptors, causing smooth muscle contraction when stimulated, are located mainly in the region of the bladder neck and proximal 4 cm of the urethra in both sexes. β receptors are very few in this area, being present mainly over the bladder dome. β stimulation encourages bladder relaxation. Appreciation of these functions aids the understanding of the action of drugs on the urinary tract.

The complex inter-relationship of nerves, transmitter substances and receptor sites may be beginning to be understood, after years of controversy about the relative roles of sympathetic and parasympathetic systems. Nergardh (1975) has shown that while acetylcholine always leads to a contraction of the detrusor fibres, resistance at the bladder neck may either increase or decrease. By selective blocking of receptor sites he has demonstrated that the actions of acetylcholine may be mediated by adrenergic receptors. It appears that a single transmitter substance can act on two adrenergic receptors producing opposite muscular responses. His hypothesis is that acetylcholine acts on sympathetic ganglion cells peripherally with the release of noradrenaline. The response to noradrenaline depends on its concentration. In low concentration receptors are stimulated allowing bladder neck relaxation whereas in high concentration α receptors are stimulated and contraction occurs. As Harrison (1976) notes, many other explanations are possible, and the next decade will show great advances in understanding, hopefully accompanied by corresponding improvements in treatment.

Central Nervous Influences

The central nervous connections of the lower urinary tract have been well reviewed recently by Nathan (1976) and by Fletcher and Bradley (1978).

SENSATION

In general there are no specialized sensory endings peripherally. Endings from the muscle (presumed mechanoreceptors) enter through the sacral roots (S2–4). Afferents in the hypogastric nerve and thoraco-lumbar roots (T12–L2) are most likely to originate in the submucosal layer. Clinical studies confirm that discriminatory sensation, both proprioceptive and enteroceptive, is mediated by sacral roots. Afferents with the sympathetic component of the thoraco-lumbar nerves produce a poorly localized feeling of distension or pain.

There is some dispute as to the pathways of sensation centripetally in the spinal cord. Most observations have been made on patients who have undergone anterolateral cordotomy. Nathan (1976) believes that all intrinsic sensations from the bladder and urethra pass up in the spinothalamic tracts. If these are sectioned the patient may retain the feeling that micturition is imminent and other sensation from the pelvic floor mediated by the posterior columns. Others (Hitchcock *et al.*, 1974) have shown preservation of bladder sensation after spinothalamic tractotomy producing bilateral sacral anaesthesia. Certainly experiments in animals suggest that some bladder afferents pass in the medial part of the posterior columns (Kuru, 1965), but the spinothalamic tract is the more significant conduit.

BRAIN CENTRES

Stimulation studies in animals, and analysis of the effects of ablation and tumours in man, have revealed a number of areas in the brain with an influence on micturition.

Since micturition is subject to social constraint the cortical control of lower autonomous centres is highly developed in social animals. The areas involved in man are the superior frontal gyrus and the adjacent anterior cingulate gyrus. Lesions here diminish the awareness of vesical events, allowing the lower centres to act autonomously. This is the territory supplied by the anterior cerebral/pericallosal artery, spasm or occlusion of which promotes incontinence. Otherwise local tumours may have the same effect, and similar manifestations occur in more generalized cerebral disorders such as cerebral atrophy and hydrocephalus. Lesions more posteriorly in the frontal region (paracentral lobule) may result in spasticity of the striated sphincters and levatores ani producing urinary retention.

In the subcortical brain are various areas that between them produce the balanced facilitation and inhibition necessary for coordinated bladder function. The organization is summarized diagrammatically in Fig. 8.3. The principal areas involved are the septal region and anterior hypothalamus, the pontine reticular formation and the cerebellum. This descending system is controlled not only by the frontal cortex but also by the limbic system, the reason why bladder function is so influenced by emotion.

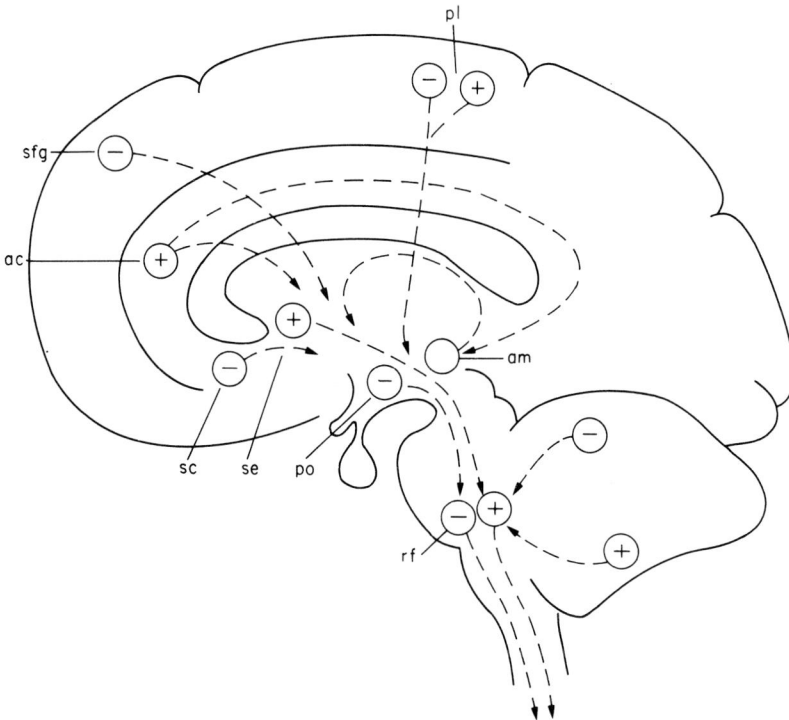

Fig. 8.3 Higher nervous influences on bladder function. ⊕ =facilitation, ⊖ = inhibition. ac—anterior cingulate gyrus, am—amygdala, pl—paracentral lobule, po—preoptic nucleus, rf—reticular formation, sc—subcallosal cingulate gyrus, se—septal area, sfg—superior frontal gyrus.

Efferent fibres from the reticular formation of the brain stem, concerned with bladder control, pass caudally in relation to the lateral corticospinal tract. Several authors place them laterally, and Kuru (1965) suggests that the vesico-constrictor and vesico-relaxor fibres are separate in the lateral and ventral reticulospinal tracts respectively. In man the position may be laterally close to the insertion of the dentate ligaments (Hitchcock *et al.*, 1974) or medially between the lateral corticospinal tract and the intermedio-lateral grey matter of the cord (Nathan, 1976). The fact that tract localization in the cord is difficult may suggest individual variability, or perhaps that the tracts are not localized to the expected extent.

SACRAL MICTURITION CENTRE

The so-called 'micturition centre' in the conus medullaris can also act autonomously. Unlike the centres in the brain, however, it cannot fully coordinate parasympathetic, sympathetic and somatic activity. This incoordination, or 'dyssynergia', is the basis of many of the complications to be described in more detail below. Under normal circumstances the reciprocal and integrated action of the autonomic and somatic systems, suggested by the observed peripheral innervation described above, is mediated by the conus. This activity is summarized below in Fig. 8.4, which must be regarded as an over-simplication.

Functional considerations

Normal urinary continence and voiding may be regarded as the balanced reciprocal interaction of the forces of expulsion and the forces of retention. These have been discussed by many authors (Bates, 1971; Yeates, 1972) and for simplicity they are tabulated below (Table 8.1).

These various forces do not depend solely on normal nervous control. Physical

Table 8.1.

Forces of expulsion	Forces of retention
Detrusor contraction	Detrusor relaxation
Abdominal muscle contraction	
Diaphragmatic contraction	
Bladder neck funnelling	Bladder neck closure
	Intra-abdominal urethra
	Urethral tension and elasticity
Urethral relaxation	Distal urethral closure
	1. involuntary
	2. voluntary

and hormonal factors are of great importance, influencing how the muscle and supporting tissue can respond. For example, detrusor relaxation (accommodation) depends on distensibility (compliance). Contractility depends on undamaged muscle. Sensation, and urethral contraction vary with the hormonal state, especially in females. Muscle hypertrophy can influence physically the way that muscle behaves.

Bearing in mind the complexity of the situation it is facile to attempt a classification of neuropathic bladder dysfunction based only on the type or level

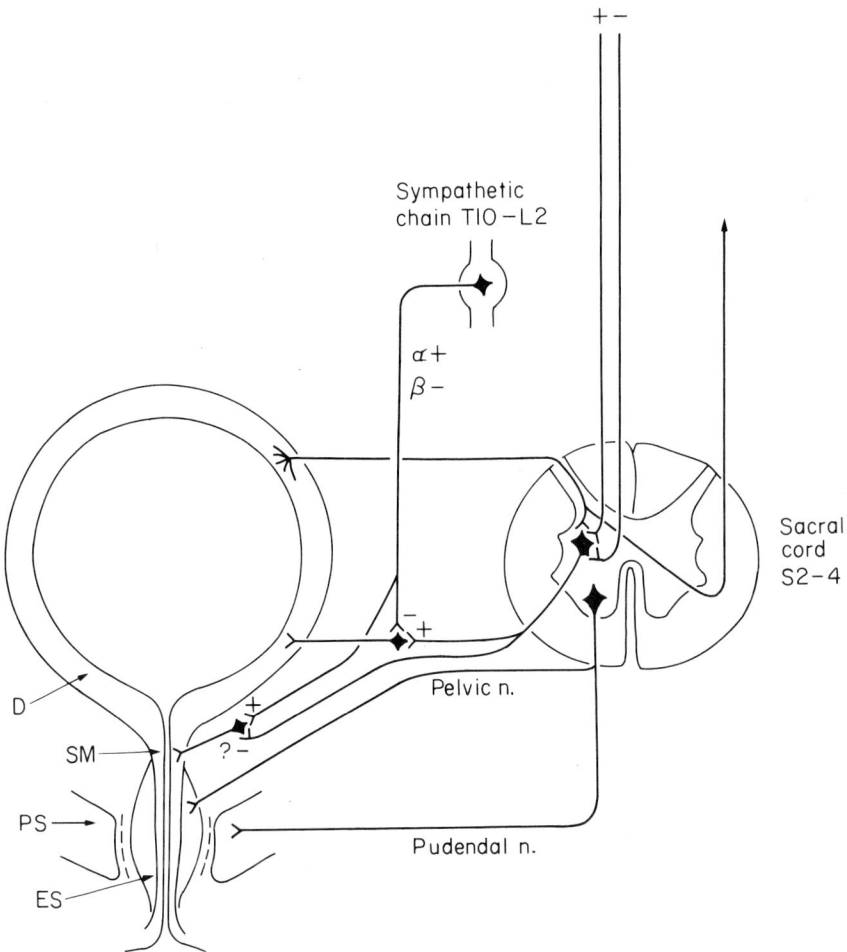

Fig. 8.4 The peripheral innervation of the bladder and urethra. Abbreviations as in Fig 8.1.

of the neurological lesion. It is necessary to measure the various factors and to build up an objective picture of bladder function, for each case is different. For this appropriate investigation is needed.

Urodynamic Technique

The micturition cycle, storage and voiding, can very well be regarded as a pressure volume loop (Fig. 8.5). The filling part of the curve is equivalent to the

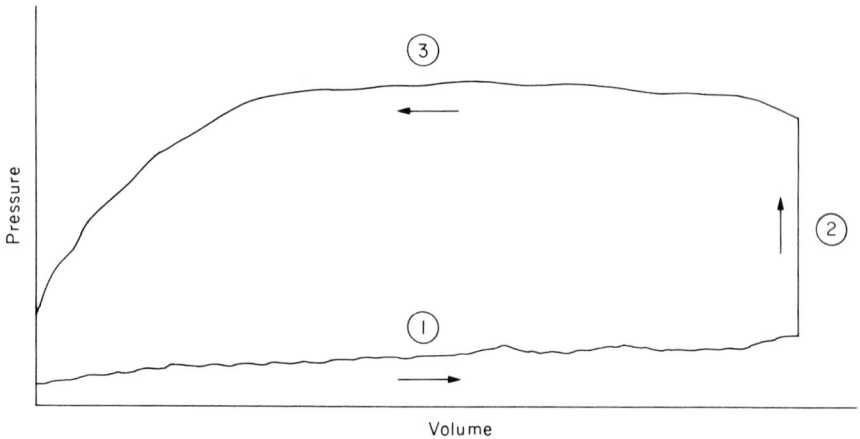

Fig. 8.5 Bladder function expressed as a pressure/volume loop. (1) Filling cystometrogram. (2) Micturition contraction (isometric phase) termination at the opening pressure of the bladder neck. (3) Micturition contraction (isotonic phase), the bladder pressure is usually fairly constant during micturition.

inflow cystometrogram. Logically the cycle must continue after bladder contraction as the micturating cystometrogram. The bladder contraction is isometric until flow starts and is relatively isotonic thereafter. Variations in bladder behaviour can be represented by loops of different shapes. The curve can, be plotted automatically during investigation on an XY plotter.

Investigation must consider outflow tract function as well as bladder function. The value of such urodynamics has been reviewed by Thomas (1979). The important tests in neuropathic bladder disorders include:

Filling cystometrogram $\pm$ Synchronous video or
Micturition cystometrogram   cinecystourethrography
Urinary flow
Urethral pressure
Sphincter electromyography

In addition to these standard investigations, electrophysiological studies of bladder function may be undertaken. These tests are still in the stage of development, but include measurement of the sensory threshold to stimulation, nerve conduction times across the sacral reflex arc, and the analysis of electroencephalographic changes following bladder distension, contraction or other stimulation.

CYSTOMETROGRAM AND FLOW STUDIES

The filling and micturition cystometrograms are often regarded separately but, in our opinion, should always be considered together. To test the storage phase (the ability of the bladder to accommodate) an infusion of saline is usually employed via an urethral or suprapubic catheter. Recently bladder distension by Co_2 has become popular. The intravesical pressure is monitored continuously, and if there is concurrent measurement and subtraction of the intrarectal pressure (representing intra-abdominal pressure). This allows an estimate of

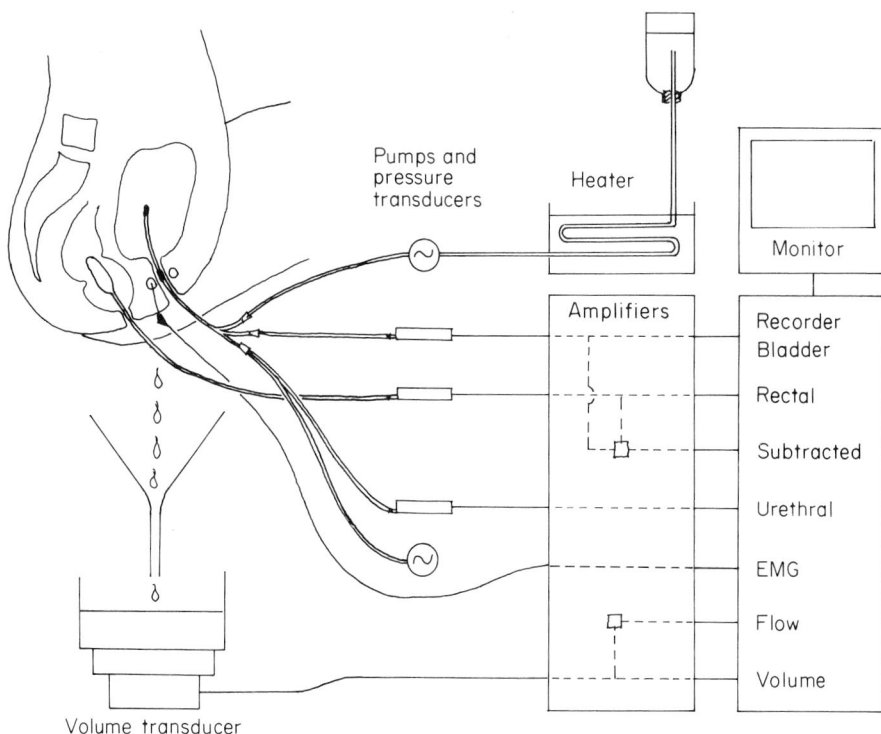

Fig. 8.6   The arrangement of apparatus for urodynamic testing of the neuropathic bladder. In this case a triple lumen Portex 'Rossier' catheter is in place recording both bladder and urethral pressure. X-ray equipment is not included in this diagram.

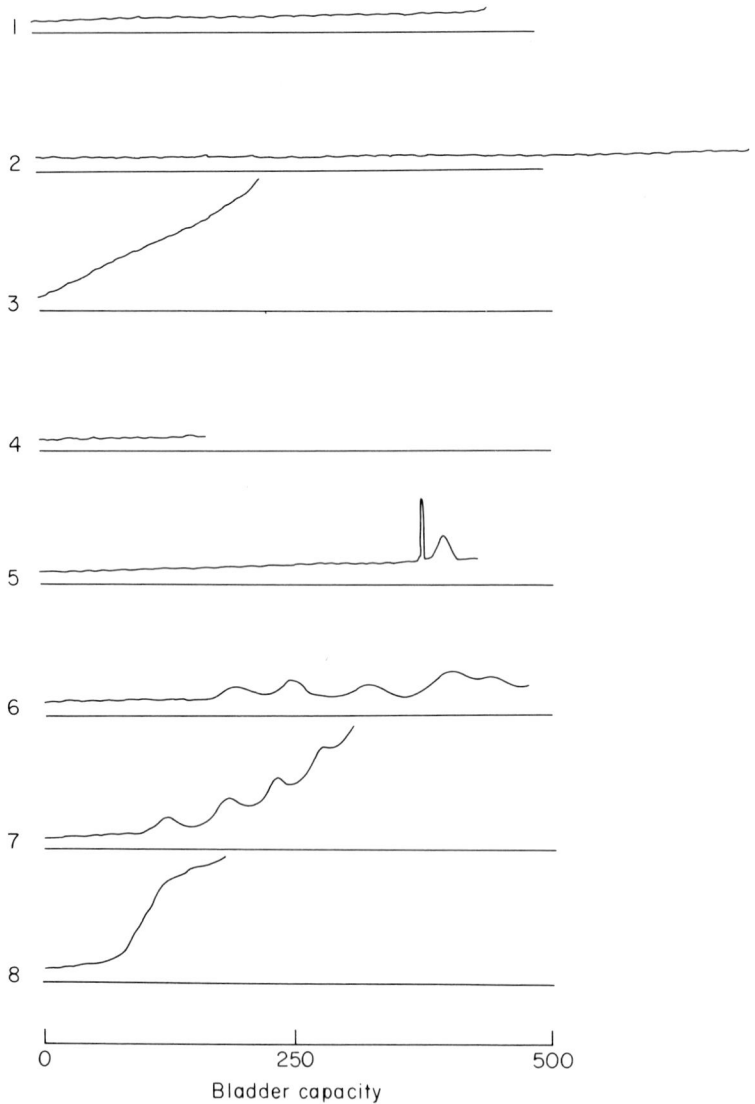

Fig. 8.7 Pattern of filling cystometrograms. Types 5–8 show various stages in the development of hypercontractility. (After Torrens & Abrams, 1979)

  1. The normal situation. compliant and with no contractions until the patient voids voluntarily.

  2. Capacity large, highly compliant, with no contraction on voluntary effort and reduced sensation: the denervated or overstretched bladder.

  3. Capacity small, low but constant compliance: the physically indistensible bladder.

  4. Capacity small because of increased sensitivity, compliant, no involuntary contraction: the inflamed or idiopathically hypersensitive bladder.

  5. Capacity normal or a little reduced, compliance normal, abnormal contractions provoked by coughing and physical activity.

  6. Capacity normal or a little reduced, compliance normal, contractions appear spontaneously.

the intrinsic bladder pressure (detrusor pressure). When the patient feels that his bladder is normally full voluntary initiation of voiding is encouraged and the intravesical pressure and urinary flow monitored during evacuation. The arrangement of apparatus is represented in Fig. 8.6.

The results of investigation (Figs. 8.7, 8.8) should be described in terms of

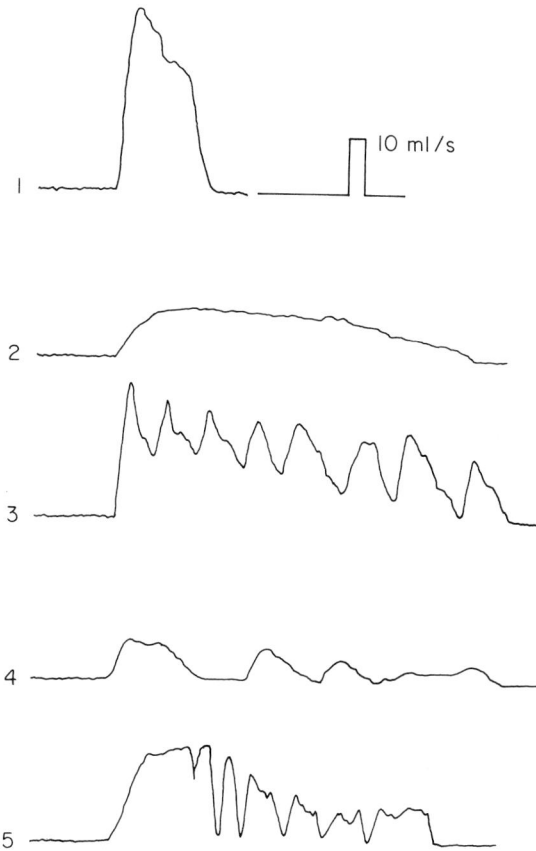

Fig. 8.8   Urinary flow rate tracings to demonstrate both quantitative and qualitative variations.
1.   Normal
2.   Obstructed, prostatic hyperplasia
3.   Abdominal straining
4.   Intermittent weak detrusor contractions
5.   Obstructed detrusor–sphincter dyssynergia.

7.   Capacity reduced, compliance reduced progressively as capacity increases, contractions appear spontaneously but relaxation occurs. This usually indicates a hypertrophic bladder.

8.   Capacity very reduced, compliance difficult to assess as the bladder con tracts spontaneously at low volume and only relaxes slightly, maintaining a high pressure.

sensation, capacity, compliance, contractility and flow, all of which may be increased, normal or decreased (Torrens & Abrams, 1979). Sensation is tradi- tionally described as the capacity at the first desire to void, and the capacity at an urgent desire to void. Since sensation is such a subjective phenomenon, it is important to describe it clearly in subjective terms and to obtain a good rapport with the patient beforehand so that they can describe their feelings accurately. Without this rapport and without some understanding of the variability of sensation, the assessment can be of little value.

Provided that sensation is normal, the maximum cystometric capacity is that at which the patient feels a normal strong desire to void. The bladder should not be over-filled during cystometry because this will influence its contractility. Compliance is the volume increment for a given change of pressure. This is a defined parameter and does not have any of the physiological connotations of the word 'tone'. Since the word 'tone' cannot be defined absolutely its use leads to semantic confusion and therefore should be avoided. Compliance therefore describes the slope of the cystometrogram, which in the normal bladder should be virtually flat at a low filling rate and over the normal volume range.

The normal bladder should not contract under any provocation until the patient wishes to void. Spontaneous bladder contractions during the filling phase have been given many names. Currently popular are unstable, uninhibited, and detrusor hyper-reflexia. These contractions may lead to involuntary inconti- nence and whether or not the patient is aware of this will depend on the sensation. Decreased contractility must be judged from the response occurring at the initiation of voiding. An acontractile bladder is easy to identify. Deficient con- traction may be less easy to quantify unless one considers the relation between the pressure generated and the flow produced (Griffiths, 1974). Inadequate contraction will usually lead to a residual urine, and this must also be measured.

Flow studies (Abrams & Torrens, 1979) are informative not only for the maximum flow produced but also for the characteristics of the flow curve. Interrupted flow patterns are common in neuropathic bladder disturbances, and a consideration of pressure and flow together allows one to distinguish between interruption due to inadequately sustained pressure and that due to intermittent sphincter occlusion (detrusor–sphincter dyssynergia).

URETHROMETRY

In addition to the inferences regarding urethral activity made from the tests described above, the action of the sphincters can be investigated directly by the electrical activity and pressure they may produce. Electromyography of the pelvic floor tests only the voluntary striated muscle. EMG activity may be subject more often to misinterpretation than other urodynamic parameters. The value of the investigation is proportional to the skill of the investigator (Blaivas *et al.*, 1977). It should be remembered that the exact location of the end of the EMG needle is not known, and this is significant in cases where the various sphincter components may not be active together. Combination of electromyography with cystometry allows more accurate interpretation of detrusor–sphincter imbalance. A better idea of the total activity of the urethra, including the autonomic components, can be gained by measuring the urethral pressure by the urethral pressure profile technique (Brown & Wickham, 1969), or by means of a catheter tip transducer in the urethra. This method continuously registers

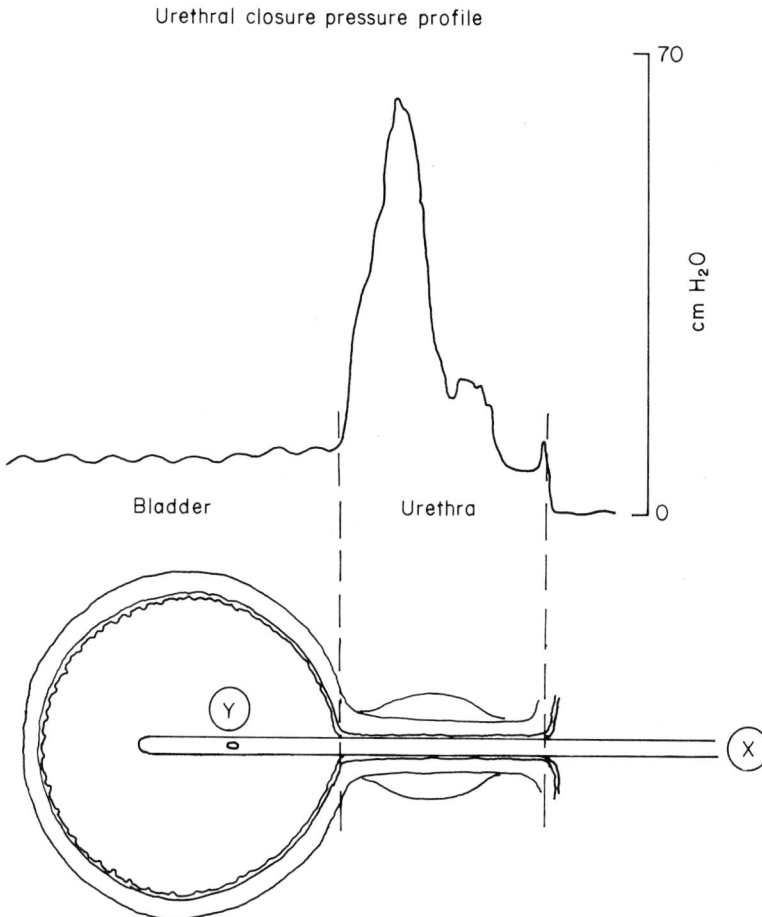

Fig. 8.9 Urethral closure pressure profile and a diagram of the recording catheter. At Ⓧ is situated the pressure transducer and the constant perfusion pump. Perfusion may be with water (2 ml/min) or carbon dioxide (130 ml/min). The perfusate escapes through small holes at Ⓨ, which is the point from which the pressure is recorded as the catheter is slowly withdrawn down the urethra.

the pressure as the measuring catheter is slowly (0.7 cm/s) withdrawn down the urethra (Fig. 8.9). Synchronous assessment of bladder and urethral pressure has been used by Rossier and Ott (1976) in spinal cord injuries.

VIDEO-CYSTOURETHROGRAPHY

Radiological studies taken during micturition are perhaps the single most valuable way of assessing function. When these are combined with studies of bladder pressure and urinary flow they produce the most comprehensive investigation presently possible (Thomas, 1976). The configuration and activity particularly in the region of the bladder neck and the distal urethral sphincter will usually complete diagnosis initiated by examination and other investigation.

PRACTICAL CONSIDERATIONS

As Thomas (1976) states, the neuropathic bladder is often in a finely balanced state which can easily be upset by infection, rapid filling or a change in the volume of the residual urine normally present. When investigating such patients the bladder should not be emptied first, serious consideration should be given to using the suprapubic route for monitoring pressure, and the filling rate should be low, 15 ml/min or even less. If the videocystourethrogram and urodynamic information can be recorded on the same tape, later reappraisal of the information is easier. It will be found necessary to repeat the assessment of storage and voiding at least three times to ensure that the results are representative. This assessment is not something which can be delegated to a technician, or indeed to a junior clinician. It is of its greatest value only when performed by the clinician with ultimate responsibility for management decisions.

Classification of Neuropathic Bladders

In dealing with this apparently complex subject it is important to bear in mind two fundamental considerations. First, use only terms capable of absolute definition. Secondly, do not confuse the classification of the patients' neurological condition with the classification of bladder function, they may not be the same.

CLASSIFICATION OF THE NEUROLOGICAL CONDITION

It is best if this is done in the simplest possible way. The alternatives are outlined in Table 8.2 below. In all cases it is necessary to quote the neurological level of anatomical positions of the lesion. This may influence the interaction of sympathetic, parasympathetic and somatic systems.

Table 8.2 Classification of the neurological condition

		Complete	Incomplete
Lower motoneuron lesion	Sensory		
	Motor		
Upper motoneuron lesion	Sensory		
	Motor		
Mixed lesions	Sensory		
	Motor		

Table 8.3 Measured urodynamic variables.

		Increased	Normal	Decreased
Bladder	Sensation			
	Capacity			
	Contractility			
	Compliance			
Urethra	Sensation			
	Contractility			
	Relaxation			
	Urinary flow			

Table 8.4

Complete lower motoneuron lesion

Senseless
High capacity ⎫
Acontractile ⎬ Low pressure
Hypercompliant ⎭
Inactive sphincter
Voiding by strain

Complete upper motoneuron lesion

Senseless
Low capacity ⎫
Hypercontractile ⎬ High pressure
Hypocompliant ⎭
Hyperactive sphincter
Voiding reflexly

CLASSIFICATION OF VESICO-URETHRAL DYSFUNCTION

This should be expressed in terms of the measured urodynamic variables (Table 8.3). If these two classifications are combined in the case of complete neurological lesions, a description such as that in Table 8.4 is obtained. It can be seen that the functional classification is far more informative.

In general neurological practice complete lesions such as these are the minority, many cases being incomplete. In spinal injuries the findings may be more predictable. Even if predictable, however, the situation may not be static, the condition varying especially with infection. In any patient the function may or may not be 'balanced' as discussed below, and this, too, requires objective assessment. Rather than attempt a more comprehensive classification the average clinician would be well advised to evaluate each case separately.

CLASSIFICATION BY SYMPTOMS

This is the least accurate way of representing function, but is very important if the patient's problem is to be viewed in perspective. The relevant symptoms are noted in the section on clinical assessment below.

Finally we submit a short list of adjectives which, in our opinion, should never be used to describe the bladder. These are hypertonic, atonic, systolic, cord, automatic, autonomous and autonomic. Other terms such as reflex uninhibited, paretic and spastic should be used with care. They describe *not* what is observed but what the observations are thought to mean. Such a subjective element may not be acceptable.

PRACTICAL MANAGEMENT

There are two main problems in management, and they may conflict one with the other. Urinary continence may be the most important goal for the patient, while the clinician is concerned with protecting the system from infection and from deterioration of renal function. Perhaps in his preoccupation with the long-term prophylaxis the clinician can fail to manage incontinence adequately, relegating the patient to yearly out-patient review. Certainly the aim for the future should be both continence and long-term renal preservation.

Much of the management of neuropathic bladder disorders has been evolved in relationship to spinal cord injury patients. Such cases do have rather specific problems, but at least a system for coordinated care has been worked out. The time is appropriate for a similar service to be provided for other neurologically disabled patients.

Pathology and prognosis

As any neurologist knows, the incidence of neuropathic bladder disorders in neurological disease is high. The exact incidence, however, seems very variably reported and has been summarized in Table 8.5. If the high incidence of bladder dysfunction is inconsistently reported, it is even more difficult to be sure of the ultimate pathological significance of the condition. The complications have been studied in relation to injuries of the spinal cord. Thomson-Walker (1937) reported on the outcome of spinal injuries in World War I and, of the 339 cases, 160 (47.2%) died from urinary infection within the first three months. He believed that septic catheterization was responsible. The situation had improved vastly by World War II, though the longer-term mortality remained. Donnelly *et al.* (1972) reported on the follow-up study of 170 spinal cord injury patients.

Table 8.5 Incidence of neuropathic bladder disorders.

Abdomino-perineal resection	10–44%
Radical hysterectomy	7–80%
Polio (almost always recovers)	4–42%
Diabetic neuropathy	2–83%
Lumbar disc disease	6–18%
Multiple sclerosis—presenting symptom	2–12%
—overall incidence	33–78%
Parkinsonism	37–70%
Stroke	34–53%
Meningomyelocele	97%

Twenty-five years following the injury 97 or 60% had died and renal disease accounted for approximately 40% of deaths. Pyelonephritis was, however, demonstrable in more than 90% of all the autopsy material available, whatever the primary cause of death. On analysing the mortality figures, it was shown that the prognosis was related to the type of neuropathic bladder and this was classified as either 'good' or 'poor'. A good neuropathic bladder showed no vesico-ureteric reflux, a residual urine less than one-third of the bladder capacity, and did not require an indwelling catheter.

Tribe (1963) reported post-mortem findings on 220 patients with chronic paraplegia and, after excluding those related to metastatic malignant disease of the spine, he found little difference whether the paralysis was related to trauma or to other diseases causing similar manifestations. Loss of sensation rendered the patient liable to develop pressure sores, and the bladder paralysis led to ascending infection in the kidneys. He concluded that death in 75% of chronic paraplegics was related to these two factors, producing a combination of pyelonephritis, calculosis, amyloidosis and secondary hypertension. In 174 necropsies 65 cases of amyloidosis were found.

The incidence of renal death in other neurological disease is less well documented. It is common experience that the majority of cases of meningomyelocele that escape death from the complications of hydrocephalus die from renal failure. Estimates of the incidence of renal death in multiple sclerosis range from 21% to 55% (Bors & Comarr, 1971).

The progression of the complications seems similar in most cases. If neurological damage prevents satisfactory bladder emptying, residual urine collects in the bladder and infection is liable to follow sooner or later. This infected residual urine, if associated with impaired ureteric emptying or with ureteric reflux, leads to renal infection. Ureteric stasis may be related to obstruction of the intramural ureter by hypertrophy of the detrusor muscle in high pressure bladders. Lee and co-workers (1978) found dilatation of the upper urinary tract in 19 out of 377 patients. Vesico-ureteric reflux is more common; 5% of patients with spinal cord injuries develop reflux within the first three years of the injury, this figure rising to 17% at the end of seven years (Pennisi *et al.*, 1959). The incidence of reflux in meningomyelocele is very much higher. This may partly be due to the fact that at least 20% of children with maldevelopment of the nervous system also have congenital anomalies of development of the urinary tract. The coincidence of hydronephrosis and infection leads to formation of renal calculi in 8.2% of patients (Comarr *et al.*, 1962). Other complications of infection are bladder neoplasia (0.6%), and in males periurethral abscesses (15%) and epididymo-orchitis (25%). It is perhaps worth commenting here that at least 5% of deaths are found to be iatrogenic (Tribe, 1963) and that the rate of suicide is at least twice that in the normal population.

Clinical Assessment

The objectives of management must be to minimize the social and medical consequences of disordered bladder function. With these aims in mind the urological management may best be conducted in a unit coordinating this aspect of care with that of the patient as a whole. A suggested scheme of management is outlined below in Fig. 8.10.

It is not our intention to separate management of the neuropathic bladder from that of the patient as a whole, but this chapter concentrates only on bladder function.

GENERAL AND SOCIAL FACTORS

The mental state, mobility and dexterity of the patient have a profound influence on management. Are they well motivated? Can the patient manage appliances? Would they be continent if more mobile and able to reach the toilet? Will they cooperate with follow-up or take drugs reliably? Such factors modify one's approach to the patient to such a great extent that it is appropriate they should be considered first.

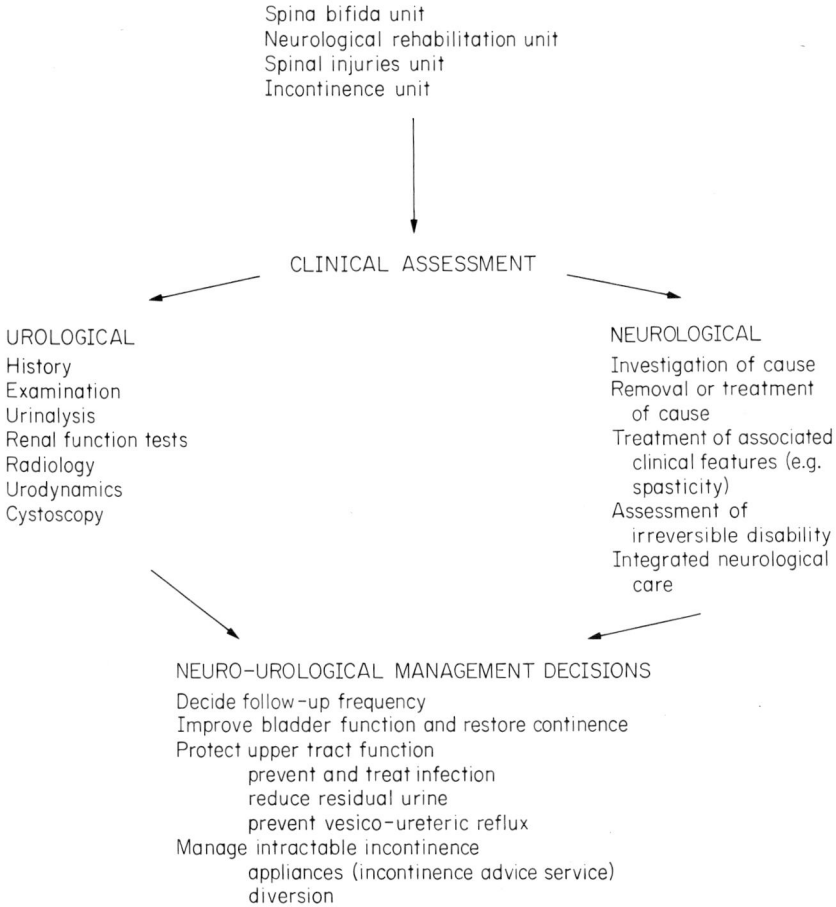

Spina bifida unit
Neurological rehabilitation unit
Spinal injuries unit
Incontinence unit

CLINICAL ASSESSMENT

UROLOGICAL
History
Examination
Urinalysis
Renal function tests
Radiology
Urodynamics
Cystoscopy

NEUROLOGICAL
Investigation of cause
Removal or treatment
    of cause
Treatment of associated
    clinical features (e.g.
    spasticity)
Assessment of
    irreversible disability
Integrated neurological
    care

NEURO-UROLOGICAL MANAGEMENT DECISIONS
Decide follow-up frequency
Improve bladder function and restore continence
Protect upper tract function
        prevent and treat infection
        reduce residual urine
        prevent vesico-ureteric reflux
Manage intractable incontinence
        appliances (incontinence advice service)
        diversion

Fig. 8.10   Management of neuropathic bladder dysfunction.

NEUROLOGICAL ASSESSMENT

In addition to classifying the type, level and extent of the lesion two particular questions need to be kept in mind. Will treatment of the primary neurological condition be the best treatment for the bladder? Is the course of the condition static or progressive, does it fluctuate, and what is its prognosis? Certain aspects of neurological examination are particularly relevant to the bladder and they are noted below.

This may help in the neurological diagnosis but should not be relied upon to do so. The pre-morbid history of bladder function may influence greatly the response to disease, and should include previous relevant surgery or other treatment. The onset and progress of the current complaints are recorded, bearing in mind the most significant problem for the patient.

Sensation requires evaluation separately from that made on the occasion of the cystometrogram. Sensory deficiency frequently contributes to incontinence. The sensation of bladder filling is separate from that of imminence of micturition, the latter occurring after the bladder neck has opened.

Voiding may take place on volition, spontaneously with or without sensation, reflexly to stimulation, or on voluntary straining only. Can the urinary stream be interrupted briskly by voluntary sphincter contraction? Is the stream interrupted involuntarily? On all occasions what force of stream is possible? Under what circumstances does incontinence occur? What is its degree and what social disruption does it cause? What steps are being taken to manage it? Not only are the answers to these questions important in themselves, but they guide the interpretation of urodynamic results. It is essential to be sure whether urodynamic results do reflect what happens under more normal circumstances.

Complications such as infection, pain, autonomic dysreflexia, and developing obstruction must be excluded. Infection must be taken very seriously, especially if accompanied by stones, debris or blood. As the patient may be unable to sense dysuria a subjective history of freedom from infection cannot be accepted.

Bowel dysfunction may parallel bladder dysfunction, and a similar sort of history should be obtained. Particular emphasis may be paid to sensory discrimination, questioning whether the patient is able to tell the difference between solid, liquid and gaseous material in the anal canal.

The sexual history can be of diagnostic value. It should be determined whether erection is absent, reflex or psychogenic. If ejaculation is present is it forceful and clonic or weak (emission)? Is there evidence of retrograde ejaculation? What is the character and acuity of orgasm if present? The significance of all these and other urological symptoms are summarized in Table 8.6.

Reflex erection is mediated by sacral roots and pelvic nerves whereas psychogenic erection may occur through the cholinergic fibres of hypogastric nerves. Ejaculation depends on the coordinated action of the somatic musculature of the pelvic floor and therefore the pudendal nerves. Orgasmic sensation is a combined afferent bombardment through the hypogastric (sympathetic) input and through the pudendal nerves.

Table 8.6 The significance of urological symptoms.

Lesion	Storage	Voiding	Sexual history
Complete UMN* lesion	Reflex incontinence, autonomic dysreflexia	Reflex voiding, intermittent spurting stream	Reflex erection (80%), no ejaculation, no orgasm
Incomplete UMN* lesion	Urgency, urge incontinence, storage decreased	Precipitate voiding	Variable
Complete LMN* lesion	Retention, overflow/stress incontinence, may feel abdominal sensation of fullness	Voiding by strain, unable to stop stream except by relaxing	Psychogenic erection (30%), no ejaculation, weak emission, no orgasm
Incomplete LMN* lesion	Storage increased, often continent	Infrequent slow stream, may feel bladder never empties	Variable, often impotent
Peripheral autonomic lesion (e.g. abdomino-perineal resection)	Stress incontinence, storage increased	Infrequent slow stream, may strain, feel urine passing	No erection, ejaculation possible, diminished orgasm

* UMN—Upper motoneuron, LMN—lower motoneuron.

EXAMINATION

The full neurological examination should include particular attention to the sacral segments. Certain other points on examination are particularly relevant to the status of the urinary tract. On abdominal examination the presence of bladder or renal swellings should be determined, and the existence of visceral sensation on deep palpation. Pelvic examination should consider particularly the anal tone and voluntary anal sphincter contraction, and in addition, as in any other case of incontinence, the prostatic size and the disposition of cervix and uterus. During anal examination the superficial anal reflex to stimulation with a pin should be tested. While examining the anal sphincter and the bulbo-cavernosus muscle the bulbocavernosus reflex can be elicited by squeezing the glans penis or clitoris. This reflex is present in 70% of normal subjects. The reflexes noted above can be quantified by using electrophysiological techniques for their demonstration. In addition to the bulbocavernous reflex the presence of urethro-anal and vesico-anal reflexes have been demonstrated by Rockswold and Bradley (1977). An elegant method for differentiation between the afferent and efferent parts of the reflex arc in relationship to human anal reflexes has been provided by Pedersen *et al.* (1978).

INVESTIGATIONS

Investigation is concentrated in relation to three main fields, urinary infection, renal function and vesico-urethral function.

Infection. As noted above, it is necessary to rely on regular urine culture for the absolute diagnosis of infection because disorders of sensation may prevent the appreciation of dysuria. Routine urine culture specimens frequently become contaminated and interpretation may be difficult. For this reason increased use of a dip inoculum in mid-stream is suggested. Suprapubic needle aspiration of urine provides a very accurate and relatively easy method of assessment, and is particularly applicable to patients who carry a residual urine.

Renal function. In addition to measuring the haemoglobin, blood urea and serum creatinine it is appropriate to perform excretion urography (IVP). This allows the identification of upper tract dilatation and of renal or ureteric calculi. Isotope renography and scintigraphy may give additional information on upper tract function. Urinalysis for protein is necessary, a loss of over 0.5 g a day being suggestive of renal amyloidosis. Thus amyloidosis may occur with a relatively small renal protein loss and a rectal biopsy is a more accurate method for diagnosis.

Vesico-urethral function. The IVP may give some idea of the capacity of the bladder, the thickness of its wall, and the residual present after micturition. Micturating video-cystourethrography is preferable. This also will demonstrate the presence of vesico-ureteric reflux. It may be undertaken in combination with urodynamic studies, and in this context provides the most complete assessment of lower urinary tract function.

Tests involving the modification of urodynamic parameters by drugs may give useful information. This is particularly true of the denervation hypersensitivity test (Glahn, 1970) and the phentolamine test (Olsson *et al.*, 1977). In the former an elevation of bladder pressure in response to carbachol suggests bladder denervation. In the latter, an increase in urinary flow rate in response to phenoxybenzamine gives a rationale for treatment with this drug when sphincter hyperactivity due to sympathetic imbalance is suspected.

The indications for urodynamic investigation are controversial at present. Some will state that the investigations are advantageous in all cases of neuropathic bladder. Others consider that useful information is seldom obtained. It is quite clear to us, however, that the use of urodynamic tests improves the accuracy of functional diagnosis. In many cases, particularly, for example, meningomyelocele, it may be impossible to predict bladder status from other clinical investigation. We are, therefore, of the opinion that these investigations should be performed as freely as radiology. As the facility for performing urodynamics becomes more widespread, it would seem that treating the neuropathic bladder without them is similar to treating anaemia by assessing the pallor of the skin.

Cystoscopy may not always be a particularly productive investigation. It should not be neglected, however, and should certainly be performed as part of the initial assessment, and later whenever there is persistent infection or haematuria that could be related, for example, to bladder calculi or to secondary urothelial changes.

FOLLOW-UP

Bearing in mind the importance of preventing deterioration in function, a regular and well-organized follow-up is essential. Specialized reassessment should occur every 3–12 months with investigation as appropriate after clinical examination. It is difficult to be dogmatic about the frequency at which particular investigation should be performed as every case of neuropathic bladder dysfunction is different. However, we would stress that it is better to over-investigate the patients rather than to neglect them, and in this context regular urinalysis is important despite the difficulties in obtaining good specimens. Renal function should be tested formally at least every year by some or all of the investigations noted above. In particular, the IVP gives much information relatively simply and the test can be modified to avoid excessive radiation exposure.

Dynamic Functional Diagnosis

The aim of diagnosis must be to bring together the clinical features and the results of investigation to provide a rational basis for management. The classification of neuropathic bladder dysfunction described earlier is one stage of this diagnosis. In this classification there are four particular areas of abnormality which may or may not coexist:

Bladder hyperactivity   (high pressure)
Bladder hypoactivity   (low pressure)
Urethral hyperactivity   (increased outflow resistance)
Urethral incompetence   (decreased outflow resistance)

Treatment will be discussed later in relation to these four groups of dysfunction, and aspects of this are summarized in Fig. 8.11.

To exemplify the contribution of urodynamics to this functional diagnosis we present this case report.

MULTIPLE SCLEROSIS

The coexistence of abnormalities occurs particularly in multiple sclerosis, and indeed all of the four groups noted above have been found together in this case.

A woman of 40 presented with a three year history of incontinence, transient dysarthria and ataxia. Examination revealed generalized hyperreflexia, extensor plantar responses, mild truncal ataxia and

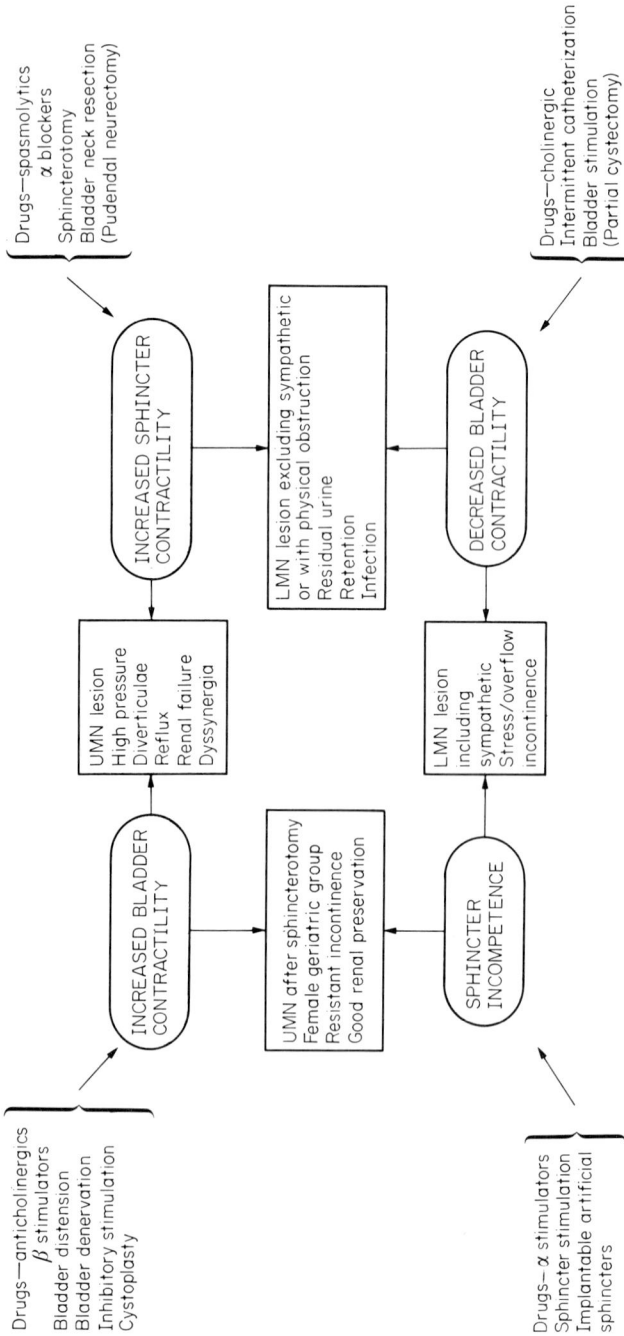

Fig. 8.11   The functional basis for treatment.

nystagmus. No sensory deficit was observed. There were increased latencies of visual evoked responses. The urine was not infected though there was a history of dysuria. The kidneys and ureters were normal on IVP. The resting maximum urethral pressure was 94 cm H_2O. She was unable to increase this by voluntary effort but it contracted strongly by reflex on moving the catheter in the urethra. Bladder filling (50 ml/min) produced no sensation, there was no rise in pressure, and at an average volume (300 ml) she was unable to initiate a voiding contraction. Further filling (440 ml) produced spontaneous bladder contractions which she was unable to feel until the bladder neck opened and the urine filled the posterior urethra. Then a sensation of urgency occurred and the external sphincter contracted firmly (Fig. 8.12). While attempting to remain continent the bladder pressure elevated, the posterior urethra distended, the bladder diverticulum appeared (Fig. 8.13) and there was reflux up the left ureter. Very soon an involuntary relaxation of the sphincter occurred and she was incontinent. She then continued voiding and achieved a normal flow rate (25 ml/s, 72 cm H_2O), but this was soon stopped by involuntary sphincter contraction, and an intermittent obstructed flow ensued (7.5 ml/s, 60 cm H_2O). A residual volume of 50 ml remained.

Summary

Deficient bladder sensation
Normal capacity
Decreased voluntary bladder contractility
Increased involuntary bladder contractility (unstable bladder)
Normal compliance
Involuntary sphincter relaxation (unstable urethra)
Involuntary sphincter contraction
Intermittent outflow obstruction (detrusor–sphincter dyssynergia)

This case exemplifies how different functional abnormalities can occur at different parts of the filling and voiding cycle. This, of course, complicates treatment considerably, but shows how important it is to have an appreciation of the dynamic situation. It was also evident on repeated investigation that the pattern of activity varied from one void to another. This is typical of neuropathic states, but occurs much less commonly in non-neuropathic bladder disorders.

REHABILITATION

We have considered management in relation to three areas, that designed to improve bladder and urethral function, that designed to prevent complications and especially to protect renal function, and that to palliate incontinence if it is inevitable.

Substantial disturbance of function, including incontinence, can exist before

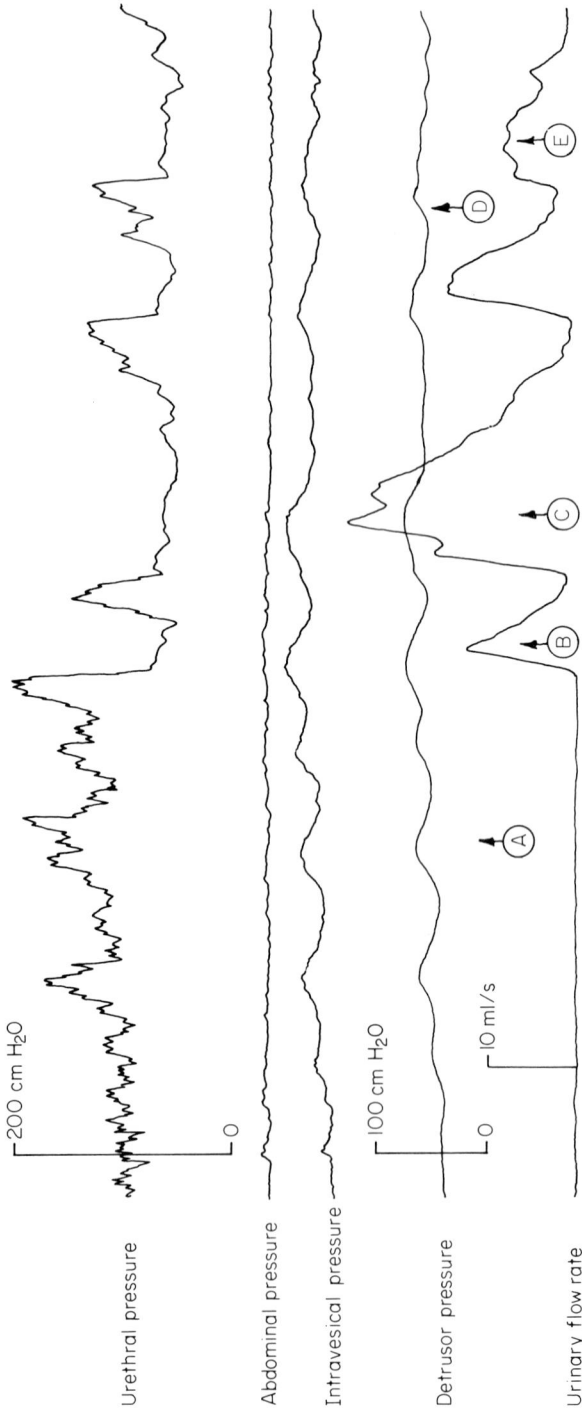

Fig. 8.12 Urethral pressure, bladder pressure and flow rate in a case of multiple sclerosis. Detrusor pressure is intravesical pressure minus abdominal pressure. Nearing capacity the bladder contracts spontaneously (A) and urine enters the posterior urethra producing urgency. At (B) the urethral pressure drops involuntarily and incontinence occurs (Fig. 8.13a), followed by a normal void at (C). This void is soon interrupted by involuntary sphincter contraction as at (D) (Fig. 8.13b) and this detrusor–sphincter dyssynergia produces an obstructed flow pattern (E).

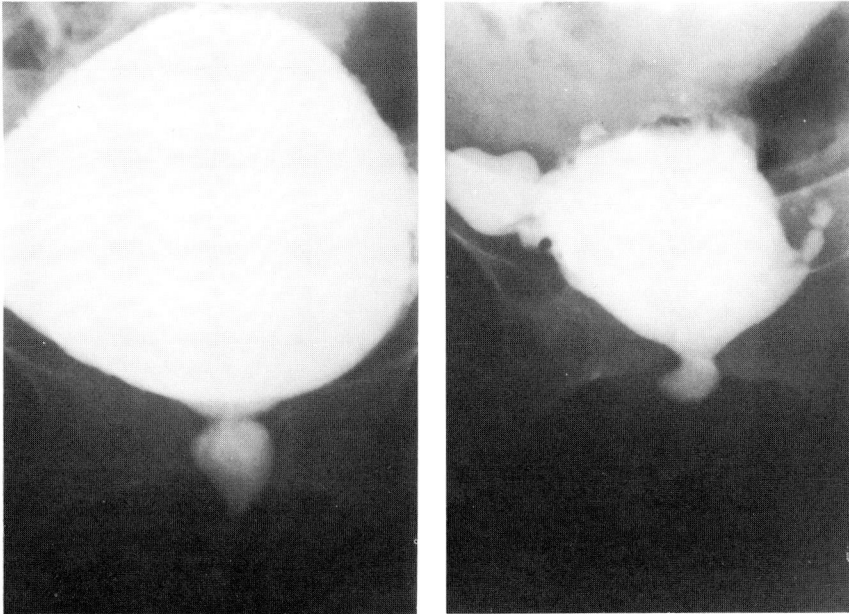

Fig. 8.13   Micturition cystourethrography in the case recorded in Fig. 8.12. **(a)** shows the 'spinning top' distension of the posterior urethra with continence not quite maintained by the external sphincter. **(b)** at lower capacity, shows the trabeculation and diverticulum formation, with a little reflux into the left ureter. The urethra is occluded by an involuntary sphincter contraction.

the bladder fails in its purpose of storage and voiding. Investigation must indicate, therefore, whether the bladder still functions acceptably in this respect. This state is often referred to as a 'balanced' bladder and as such is the principle aim of rehabilitation. It has been defined most often in relation to spinal cord injured patients:

'Bladder emptying without an in-dwelling catheter, a radiographically normal urinary tract and a sterile urine' (Morrow & Bogaard, 1977).

'Normal voiding pressure, a small pressure gradient across the sphincters and a residual urine of 50 ml or less' (Fam *et al.*, 1978).

Though the definition varies the concept remains valid, that optimal function should be maintained, or achieved by a physiological re-balancing process.

Both incontinence and the complications, principally urinary infection leading to renal failure, will be treated in part by improving bladder balance. If sensation is present there is a chance that continence may be restored, though not at the expense of worsening upper tract function. If incontinence is inevitable or untreatable then effective palliation by appliance or by diversion must be considered.

Improvement of Bladder Function

BLADDER HYPERACTIVITY

The failure of the normal storage function of the bladder usually occurs because of increased phasic or tonic contractility. This reduces bladder capacity and produces either a high intra-vesical pressure or urinary leakage, or both depending on the function of the outflow tract. When the bladder hypercontractility is associated with a hyperactive obstructive sphincter (Fig. 8.11) the bladder wall will hypertrophy and become trabeculated due to the extra work being performed. This hypertrophy affects particularly the bladder neck, sometimes to the extent of producing a secondary obstructive element. As the bladder pressure increases and the bladder fails, diverticulae and ureteric reflux develop and the residual urine increases. Muscle hypertrophy makes the bladder wall physically less distensible. Indistensibility also occurs in chronic infection due to fibrosis.

If the bladder is potentially distensible (compliant) as assessed under anaesthetic, the storage may be improved by counteracting the contractility. Inhibitory drug treatment (Table 8.7) consists mainly of anti-cholinergic agents and perhaps

Table 8.7.   Drug treatment of bladder and urethra.

	Bladder	Urethra
Inhibition	Propantheline	Phenoxybenzamine
	Oxybutine	Diazepam
	Dicyclomine	Baclofen
	Empromium	Dantrolene
	Imipramine	
	Isoprenaline	
Stimulation	Carbachol	Ephedrine
	Bethanechol	Phenylpropanolamine
	Distigmine	Imipramine

β sympathetic stimulators. Many drugs can be shown to produce an objective improvement when given parenterally. The few double blind controlled trials with oral administration show less, and frequently no effect. The side effects of anti-cholinergic agents, thirst and constipation, often lead to cessation of treatment. Nevertheless, such drugs are always worth trying, and anticholinergics may work better in combination with sympathomimetics. In our experience empromium (Cetiprin) and propantheline (Probanthine) are drugs of first choice. They may need to be given in larger than recommended dosage, and combined when appropriate with orciprenaline, ephedrine or phenylpropanolamine. Imipramine (Tofranil), effective especially in enuresis, has two peripheral actions. In addition to an anticholinergic effect it blocks the re-uptake of noradrenaline in the region of the bladder neck, thus enhancing the effect of noradrenaline and promoting bladder neck closure. Hyperbaric bladder distension, to near systolic blood pressure for up to two hours, has been effective in reducing contractility in some patients with non-neuropathic hyperactivity. Other series have found no benefit. One group of neuropathic bladders has been treated with encouraging results initially.

Since the bladder hyperactivity is mediated by nerves, bladder denervation as a treatment has been used for many years, especially in spastic paraplegics where intrathecal phenol or rhizotomy can convert the spastic bladder into a lower pressure, more flaccid one. Bladder denervation has been the subject of a recent comprehensive review (Torrens & Hald, 1979). Long-term follow-up of denervated bladders shows a recovery of tone, perhaps related to proliferation of α sympathetic terminals (Sundin & Dahlstrom, 1973). Despite this a small proportion of patients are much improved (Diokno *et al.*, 1977) and selective denervation, usually of the third sacral nerve, carries little morbidity. The technique is inferior to sphincterotomy in complete upper motoneuron lesions, but where sensation is preserved and incontinence is troublesome, especially in females, denervation may be considered. The bladder must be potentially distensible and outflow tract obstruction must be absent or treatable. The effects can be judged pre-operatively by selective block of the sacral nerves with local anaesthetic. It is particularly applicable to those with a cystometrogram showing hyperactivity only in the initial stages of filling, a not uncommon finding in multiple sclerosis. It may also prevent the expulsion of catheters in females with bladder spasticity.

Less destructive and physiologically much more attractive is the use of inhibitory perineal stimulation. Inhibition of bladder contraction has been noted following anal distension and electrical stimulation of the anal canal (Kock & Pompeius, 1963) and the vagina (Fall, 1977). Fall has worked out the optimal parameters for electrical stimulation and these are intermittent ramped trains of biphasic pulses (10 Hz, 1.5 ms duration) occurring every 30 seconds and each train lasting 10 seconds. The position of the vaginal electrodes is critical. Fall (1979) reports that the majority of his patients were cured or greatly improved by this technique, though the benefit sometimes appeared only after several weeks. Others have confirmed this work (Godec *et al.*, 1976) and it deserves wider application.

The hypercontractile and physically indistensible bladder may be enlarged by some form of enterocystoplasty using a segment of bowel from the caecum, ileum or sigmoid colon. This forms an iatrogenic diverticulum to the bladder (George *et al.*, 1978), but micturition is inefficient (Gleason *et al.*, 1972), so that an increase in residual urine occurs. The segment of bowel used does not seem to influence the results (Smith *et al.*, 1977). Cystoplasty is of value in selected cases of hypercontractile neuropathic bladder with incontinence, as long as outflow obstruction, secondary to a dysfunctional bladder neck or a spastic pelvic floor, does not exist or can be modified by pharmacological or surgical means. However, it should only be used after all other methods of controlling the unstable contractions have been exhausted. Cystoplasty decreases the magnitude but not the frequency of involuntary pressure spikes, as well as increasing the functional capacity of the bladder. A creatinine clearance of at least 40 ml/min is mandatory for any procedure in which the bowel is interposed within the intact urinary tract. A patch cystoplasty, using ilium or sigmoid colon, is superior to a tubular form. The overall failure rate of 35% may be expected to improve with more accurate preoperative screening using urodynamic techniques.

BLADDER HYPOACTIVITY

Decreased contractility may be consequent upon denervation or over-distension, or more often both. Because the parasympathetic motoneurons are located peripherally near the bladder, true denervation almost never occurs. The interruption of preganglionic parasympathetic fibres could more properly be termed decentralization. This explains why the bladder retains autonomous neurogenic tone after lesions of the cauda equina or pelvic nerves, though this tone and feeble contractions are seldom enough to empty the bladder. However, such peripheral preservation does mean that drugs have a better chance of working, particularly in view of the phenomenon of denervation hypersensitivity (Lapides *et al.*, 1962; Glahn, 1970).

Over-distension of the bladder acts in two ways. When the capacity exceeds about 700 ml the organ is at a physiological disadvantage and even under normal circumstances the pressure and flow generated are reduced. In addition more severe over-stretching disrupts muscular and neural elements in the bladder wall leading to permanent changes, in particular interstitial collagen deposition (Mayo *et al.*, 1973). This all exaggerates and perpetuates the problem of chronic neuropathic retention.

Patients with residual urine can be considered in this section also. The problem may be due to bladder hypoactivity, but also may occur with high outflow tract resistance. In each case the dominant causative factor needs most attention.

The neurotransmitter causing bladder contraction is acetylcholine. Drug treatment depends therefore on cholinergic agents (carbachol, urecholine) or drugs inhibiting anti-cholinesterase (distigmine). Carbachol and urecholine are most effective when given subcutaneously; intramuscular injection may lead to unpleasant gastrointestinal side effects. Oral administration, even high dosage, is less effective. Distigmine bromide is supposed to be long acting, requiring only a once daily dosage, but this may be increased with benefit. From comments earlier it is evident that acetylcholine acts on sympathetic ganglion cells to release noradrenaline, which in turn acts on α and β receptors. It is logical that α and β blockers should improve the pharmacological response to acetylcholine, though no controlled clinical trials have been performed which prove this.

A radical change in the management of the underactive bladder has occurred recently. This is the introduction of 'clean' intermittent self-catheterization. Sterile intermittent catheterization was advocated by Guttmann and Frankel (1966) in spinal injuries, and Herr (1975) summarized its use in establishing a bladder balance and a catheter-free patient following traumatic cord lesions. It was used in patients with temporary post-operative bladder atony following neurosurgical or other procedures, and in the long-term treatment of patients with large-capacity atonic bladders as an alternative to permanent indwelling catheters. The technique, which is most effective, puts an appreciable strain on medical and nursing services. Since Lapides *et al.* (1962; 1976) described the use of clean non-sterile intermittent self-catheterization an increasing number of reports have appeared. Both male and female patients may be taught to pass a fine catheter (FGB-14). Light and von Blerk (1977) describe its use in the congenital neuropathic bladder, using a catheter which is rinsed in tap water after use and kept in a dry container. The incidence of patients with sterile urine was 52.5% compared with 48% in Lapides' (1976) series. Complications such as traumatic urethritis and epididymo-orchitis are surprisingly infrequent. The technique is relatively easy to teach, even to children, and is becoming more popular in myelodysplasia (Schoenberg *et al.*, 1977; Withycombe, 1978). It certainly provides an acceptable alternative to diversion. Indeed it has been found appropriate to convert the hyperactive bladder to hypoactivity using drugs, and then use intermittent self-catheterization (Raezer *et al.*, 1977).

Electrical stimulation to improve bladder function may be directed either at the bladder nerve supply or the bladder muscle itself. Electronic devices may be, as in other fields, implanted or used transcutaneously. Nerve stimulation is probably the more effective method. It has been applied on the sacral nerves (Habib, 1967), or to the spinal cord in the region of the sacral micturition centre (Nashold *et al.*, 1972). Despite adjustment of position, and electrical parameters, stimulation in these regions causes both bladder contraction and sphincter contraction. This means that a high bladder pressure may occur and this is detrimental. Brindley (1973) has attempted to improve bladder emptying by intermittent trains of stimulation allowing continued bladder contraction but intermittent sphincter relaxation. Detailed urodynamic assessment of implanted stimulators is notably absent. In addition nerve stimulation requires an intact nervous system as far as the conus and sacral nerves are concerned. In these circumstances it is probably true to say that bladder rehabilitation can achieve reflex voiding in virtually every case. There is therefore little theoretical indication for electrical stimulation, except to trigger micturition and thereby assist maintaining continence.

Direct bladder stimulation has been technically less successful. It was developed in dogs where there is a definite trigger zone from which impulses spread through the bladder. No such trigger zone appears to exist in man. Even with multiple electrodes (Merrill & Conway, 1974) the intensity of stimulation is such that it causes pain and there is spread of the current to the pelvic floor with muscular contraction and obstruction. The impedance of the electrodes often increases progressively with fibrosis, requiring still larger currents. Alexander (1976), reviewing the situation, concluded results were best in incomplete upper motoneuron lesions and not unfortunately in the flaccid lower motoneuron bladder. He thought that improvement was due to 'modification of the reflex activity of the bladder' and this brings to mind the work of Fall (1977) quoted above. Indeed, it has been shown recently that external transvaginal or transrectal stimulation can produce both bladder contraction and bladder relaxation under different circumstances (Godec *et al.*, 1977). Therefore it would seem that the use of implants is contra-indicated, especially if it is only to trigger micturition. External stimulation deserves much greater investigation, but it does also depend on an intact sacral nervous arc. Spinal cord stimulation for the neuropathic bladder is discussed in Chapter 14.

Partial resection of the bladder should be mentioned if only to be dismissed. For some time large atonic bladders have been electively reduced in size by excision or infolding of part of the bladder wall. The object, in theory, is to make the remaining muscle more efficient in its action. Though the muscle may work more effectively for a short time, sooner or later further bladder distension occurs and the situation reverts to its previous state.

Despite all that has been written above, many patients with inadequate detrusor contraction require no intervention. Voiding may be facilitated by raising abdominal pressure, with or without added manual compression. In any case the presence of an uninfected residual urine does not make treatment obligatory, provided observation can be closely maintained.

HYPERACTIVE URETHRA (HIGH OUTFLOW RESISTANCE)

Static obstruction, caused for example by prostatic hypertrophy or stricture, may occur in patients with neuropathic bladders as in any others. It should respond to conventional treatment and will not be considered further. Dynamic obstruction, implying phasic or tonic hypercontractility of the sphincters, may be sympathetic or somatic in origin. Relative sympathetic overactivity occurs typically with a cord lesion below L2, especially when it includes the sacral segments. It is common in myelodysphasia. Somatic overactivity may occur with any upper motoneuron lesion. The two may therefore appear together.

Treatment depends on identifying the level of obstruction, perhaps best performed by micturating cystourethrography. Urethral pressure profiles and electromyography also help (McGuire, 1978), particularly if repeated after the therapeutic trial of drugs and perhaps differential anaesthesia. Thereafter the chief modes of treatment are drugs and endoscopic urethral surgery.

Sympathetic hyperactivity tends to be confined to the proximal urethra, and is due to α adrenergic agents. Modest success has been claimed recently by several workers using α blocking drugs (Awad & Downie, 1977; Olsson *et al.*, 1977). This treatment may be most relevant in myeolodysplasia. In spinal injuries Yalla *et al.* (1977) finds such 'internal sphincter dyssynergia' mainly in cases with autonomic dysreflexia. Certainly α blockers are very useful in the treatment of autonomic dysreflexia (McGuire *et al.*, 1976), but Yalla had disappointing results when treating bladder neck obstruction.

Somatic (striated) sphincter spasm is almost universal in upper motoneuron lesion, provoking what is popularly termed detrusor–sphincter dyssynergia (Yalla *et al.*, 1977). The appearance in micturating cystourethrography is typical with pre-sphincteric ballooning of the posterior urethra, sometimes likened to a spinning top especially in children. Drugs which relax striated muscle such as Dantrolene and Baclofen have been used, but without conspicuous success. Perkash (1978) states that non-surgical management with drugs succeeds in only 9.5% of patients.

Much has been written about sphincterotomy since it was introduced by Ross (1956). Following the observation that striated muscle fibres were found at the bladder neck in 19 out of 21 resections and that the striated fibres were found only at the 12 o'clock position, Ross concluded that 'it would therefore appear logical to perform a myotomy of the striated muscle at 12 o'clock, in a patient in whom bladder neck resection and pudendal neurectomy had been unsuccessful' and he reported having performed such a myotomy. Although pudendal neurectomy at one time was considered a logical approach to the problem of the spastic 'external' sphincter, impotence occurred in 50–60% of cases. From the observations of Gosling noted above it is evident that the pudendal nerve does not supply the intramural striated sphincter.

In 1967 Ross and co-workers published the results of division of the external sphincter over a 10 year period. Of 764 neurological patients admitted to Liverpool, 177 (23%) required sphincterotomy, producing elimination or considerable reduction of residual urine in 157 patients (89%). In a further 51 patients hydronephrosis disappeared following sphincterotomy in 14 and in another 14 it was improved. Many variations to the technique of sphincterotomy have now been reported. Ross *et al.* (1976) described posterolateral myotomy from an upper limit at the level of the verumontanum extending downwards for about 3 cm and 6 mm deep. Minimal coagulation current is used for the electrode knife and a few muscular fibres are divided at a time. The cutting current is avoided at any stage. In this way, the major problem of arterial haemorrhage is rarely troublesome and any venous bleeding is controlled by the introduction of a 22 Ch catheter. They conclude that it is safer to do too little rather than too much. The usual proportion of spinal injury patients needing sphincterotomy is 30% (O'Flynn, 1976; Fellows *et al.*, 1977). Fam *et al.* (1978) reported that 18% of incomplete lesions and 61% of complete ones required surgical intervention, but they used more rigid criteria for bladder balance, in particular normal voiding bladder pressure. Operation rates as high as 90.5% (Perkash, 1978) perhaps deserve reappraisal. The indications for sphincterotomy include:

1. high residual urine volume.
2. high voiding pressure due to detrusor sphincter dyssynergia.
3. autonomic hyperreflexia.
4. vesicoureteric reflux.
5. upper tract dilatation.

Division of the sphincter at several points, for example at 2, 4, 8 and 10 o'clock, has been reported (O'Flynn, 1976) but is probably unnecessary. Thomas (1976) reported a 56% incidence of impotence after division at 3 and 9 o'clock, and this was confirmed by Madersbacher (1976) whose incidence was 21%. The majority of workers now advocate anterior/median sphincterotomy. The use of sphincterotomy in other conditions such as myelodysplasia (Koontz & Smith, 1977) has been less popular, but in appropriate and fully investigated cases it deserves further analysis.

Bladder neck resection may need to be added to sphincterotomy, but is the operation of choice in lower motoneuron lesions. Early distal sphincterotomy may help to avoid later bladder neck resection (and therefore retrograde ejaculation) by preventing reactive hypertrophy (Fam *et al.*, 1978). When surgery is necessary, no agreed criteria for resecting the bladder neck, incising the distal sphincter, or combining the two operations as advocated by Smith and co-workers (1971), are available. Rossier and Ott (1974) add bladder neck resection to sphincterotomy if detrusor pressure is low. Fellows *et al.* (1977) suggested that the appearance of bladder neck on cystogram was of no help in the choice of operation. He concluded that the combined operation of bladder neck resection and internal membranous urethrotomy (sphincterotomy) has the greatest chance of initial success and should be performed in all cases if no attempt was to be made to preserve sexual function.

URETHRAL INCOMPETENCE

A totally inadequate urethra is relatively less common in neurological disease. Combined somatic and sympathetic inactivity necessitates a lesion extending between T10 and S3, for example spinal cord infarction. Somatic hypoactivity is more common. Otherwise decreased sphincter function may be related to urethral inhibition, or to non-neuropathic inadequacy as is common in elderly females.

Since neuropathic urethral incompetence is usually associated with bladder hypoactivity, procedures to increase *permanently* urethral resistance are inappropriate and will lead to urinary retention. It is thus necessary to perfect a technique that provides controlled *intermittent* urethral closure. Drug treatment is not adjustable in this way, but may help in minor degrees of disorder, as an adjunct to drugs acting on the bladder. α sympathetic stimulators work occasionally (ephedrine, orciprenaline, phenylpropanolamine), and imipramine has a similar action. β blockers may enhance this effect.

Sphincter stimulation was introduced by Caldwell *et al.* (1965). It involves implantation of a radio receiver subcutaneously, connected to electrodes attached to the pelvic floor muscles. About half the cases show some improvement, and a cure occurs in a few patients which may persist when stimulation is discontinued (Alexander, 1976). Neuropathic problems probably respond less well than non-neuropathic ones, and very few successes have been achieved in lower motor lesions where they are most needed.

Most interest at present is centring on implantable artificial sphincters. Operations and devices designed to produce passive continuous urethral compression (Kaufman, 1978) are not really appropriate in neuropathic states as noted above. This had led to the development of variable resistance devices (Rosen, 1978; Scott, 1978). These involve an inflatable cuff or paraurethral balloon, which can be deflated at will to allow voiding. A pump is needed, usually located in the scrotum or labia, and the Scott device includes an intra-abdominal reservoir so that intra-abdominal pressure is transmitted to the urethra. Initial implants had problems with mechanical failure and infection. Even including these failures the incontinence was cured in 60–80% (Cook *et al.*, 1978). With improvement in technique and experience, 90% success rates are being achieved (Scott, 1978). Bladder hyperactivity is a contra-indication to implantation, for it may produce upper tract dilatation.

Management of Complications

URINARY TRACT INFECTION

The maintenance of a sterile urine is an important principle in patients with a neuropathic bladder, but it can be impossible to achieve in the presence of structural abnormalities. Furthermore it is preferable to ensure a well-drained urinary tract in the presence of infection rather than an obstructed system with sterile urine, so far as the prognosis of renal function is concerned (Freeman *et al.*, 1975).

Escherichia coli is the most frequent infecting organism, but proteus, pseudomonas and klebsiella organisms are relatively common. There are now a wide range of antimicrobial agents available and it is advisable to choose the one with the narrowest appropriate spectrum of activity for the initial treatment. Recurrent relapse of infection is a major problem and then the use of long-term therapy should be considered. Treatment for six weeks, six months or longer may be indicated. Trimethoprimsulfamethoxazole or nitrofurantoin are of particular use because the emergence of resistant bacteria is less likely (Stamey *et al.*, 1977) and these agents may be used effectively at a reduced dosage of one tablet at night (Bailey *et al.*, 1971). Trimethoprim is of particular value in men with prostatic infection as the drug appears to enter the prostatic fluid in effective concentration (Reeves & Ghilchik, 1976).

Guttmann and Frankel (1966) used a combination of hexamine-mandelate and methionine as an acidifying agent for long-term prophylaxis as the antibacterial activity of urine increases with pH values below 6.5. This principle attracted renewed interest with the introduction of the compound Hiprex, but such agents can only achieve a low urinary pH so long as the acidifying capacity of the kidney is retained. In a group of 24 patients with a well-documented history of recurrent urinary tract infection, Nilsson (1975) showed that Hiprex reduced the recurrence rate, but no patient was completely free from bacteruria throughout the period under study. Hiprex does not eliminate urease-producing organisms such as proteus, but it may reduce the precipitation of magnesium ammonium phosphate and calcium phosphate which form the associated calculi.

When urinary tract infection occurs in the presence of obstruction, the risk of bacteraemia and renal impairment is increased. Relief of obstruction, instrumentation and removal of associated calculi should always be undertaken with appropriate antibiotic cover.

VESICO-URETERIC REFLUX

In patients with neuropathic bladders, Bunts (1958) reported a 13% incidence of vesico-ureteric reflux and Damanski (1965) a 25% incidence. Successful operative correction of vesico-ureteric reflux requires careful selection of the patients. The first stage in management requires the elimination of infection and abolition of increased intravesical pressure, by appropriate procedures on the bladder neck and urethra. This alone may abolish or reduce the reflux. If it does not, and especially if upper tract drainage is impaired, reimplantation of the ureter should be considered. Reece and Hackler (1975) reported a success rate of 83% in patients with unilateral reflux and 70% in those with bilateral reflux, but Hirsch et al. (1978) claimed an overall success rate in 15 patients of only 30% with failures on at least one side of all bilateral reimplantations. Operation is technically more difficult in the thick-walled, contracted or infected bladder, and the coexistence of reflux with these features may mean that urinary diversion is necessary.

AUTONOMIC DYSREFLEXIA

This is seen mostly in patients with cervical and high dorsal spinal cord lesions, and consists of a hyperactive sympathetic response to stimuli below the lesion. Hypertension (sometimes fatal), sweating, piloerection and bradycardia occur, especially after bladder distension or contraction, during instrumentation, in detrusor–sphincter dyssynergia and after catheter blockage. Treatment involves avoiding or removing the cause if possible, or counteracting the sympathetic reaction with adrenergic blockade (McGuire et al., 1976). Sometimes the hypertension may be severe enough to require vasodilation with sodium nitroprusside (Kursh et al., 1977). Spinal cord stimulation (Chapter 14) may also be effective.

Palliation of Incontinence

Incontinence is a social disaster, and may be responsible for more misery than any other aspect of a particular neurological disorder. It still seems an unsavoury subject for discussion, sometimes even between patient and doctor, and perhaps doctors are not always aware of the options available. There has been little critical assessment of the various palliative methods and appliances, and still less effort expended on innovation. The number of advertisements in the national press suggests that many sufferers still seek advice through their pages.

In Bristol (UK) it has been possible to organize an 'incontinence advisory service' which depends on the expertise of nursing staff who have made this their special interest. This service complements the activities of the urodynamic investigation unit which serves all interested physicians in the area. The advantages of this arrangement are considerable, especially for the patient. The management of incontinence has been divided below into sections on catheterization, incontinence appliances and urinary diversion.

INDWELLING CATHETERS

A principle of management in non-progressive neurological disorders is to achieve a catheter-free status, and Jacobs and Kaufmann (1978) stress the high incidence of complications that follow long-term catheter drainage in this group of patients. The problems of bladder calculi, haemorrhagic cystitis and occasional bladder carcinoma, together with the incidence of epididymitis, periurethritis with peri-urethral abscess and penoscrotal fistulae, are well documented. O'Flynn (1974) states that every patient treated with continuous catheterization develops urinary infection. However, long-term catheter drainage to the bladder has an important place in the management of the chronic invalid with urinary incontinence when no other form of treatment is appropriate. Bruce *et al.* (1974) found that the silastic-coated catheters were associated with less encrustation compared to the latex catheters. Silastic-coated catheters have a latex balloon which will still become encrusted. Solid silicone catheters have an advantage in this respect. George *et al.* (1978) noted that 10% of patients persistently blocked their catheters, irrespective of the type of catheter, and this was also shown in other series (Wastling, 1974; Bruce *et al.*, 1974). The use of Hexamine-Hippurate, bladder washouts with Noxytiolin and a week's course of antibiotics were compared in a trial conducted by Brocklehurst and Brocklehurst (1978). They concluded that none of these methods is worth using to control infection and that the infection does not seem to be a serious matter in geriatric patients. The frequency of catheter change should be adapted to the individual patient.

The management of the patient on long-term catheter drainage is not a procedure than can be described on the basis of a standardized regime. It must be undertaken as a trial on an individual basis. It is often an advantage to admit the patient for two to three days, to acclimatize the patient and their relatives to the concept of catheter management. The stiff texture of silastic catheters was noted to cause trigono-urethral pain in 50% of men and 70% of women patients by George *et al.* (1978) and the initial use of a soft latex or silastic catheter is an advantage. The drainage bag should preferably not be visible when the patient is able to be ambulant or chairbound, and the use of a thigh bag or a sporran type of suspension from the waist is recommended under such circumstances. A high fluid intake is encouraged, to avoid urinary debris, and a diuretic administered at night can be of value during the hours when fluid intake is reduced. Urinary acidification with Hexamine mandelate or vitamin C may be an adequate prophylaxis against infection.

Leakage around the catheter is a major problem with patients who have small capacity or hyperactive bladders. This may be aggravated by constipation and can be helped by the judicious use of enemas to evacuate the distal colon and rectum. A familiar mistake in such cases is the use of a progressively larger catheter, so that the urethra becomes grossly dilated and patulous, and this should be avoided. Furthermore, the quantity of fluid used to fill the catheter balloon should initially be kept at a minimum volume (10–15 ml) sufficient to retain the catheter *in situ*. In some cases the catheter is repeatedly expelled by bladder contractions. Rather than proceed to diversion, this may be treated by bladder denervation. In this respect sacral neurectomy has less in the way of rectal and skin complications than intrathecal phenol. We have also found that catheter drainage through a suprapubic cystostomy, after operative urethral closure, provides a simple and effective alternative to diversion.

INCONTINENCE APPLIANCES

External appliances may be considered under the following headings: pants and pads, occlusive devices and drainage appliances.

Pants and pads. This is the commonest solution to the problem of incontinence used by upwards of 50% of sufferers. Indeed at present there is no other satisfactory appliance for the female patient. However, impervious plastic pants do not provide the best solution, and they lead to antisocial odour and skin problems. The development of the marsupial pants (Willington, 1976) has been an important contribution. They are made of a hydrophobic material with an exterior pouch into which an absorbent pad can be placed. The skin is kept dry and the pad can absorb up to 300 ml of urine before being changed. This is an area where a little advice to the patient can be of enormous benefit.

Occlusive devices. These are of more use in the male. However, Hall (1965) stressed the limited use of the penile clamp in the incontinent male patient. He suggested that it should only be used intermittently and should never be used in patients whose hygiene and intelligence are limited, because of the complications of penile swelling, urethral stricture and persistent urinary infection which may arise as a consequence. Vincent (1964) described an external perineal pressure apparatus which seemed to work both physically and physiologically, but it has not been widely accepted, perhaps because it is cumbersome. For the female the

Edwards pubovaginal spring device and the Bonnar intravaginal inflatable device have been described recently; again neither has had conspicuous success. Too much pressure may produce a urethro-vaginal fistula.

Drainage appliances. Collecting sheaths, using a principle of pubic pressure applied by means of a supporting apparatus with a belt and groin straps, have a limited place in the management of the ambulant incontinent patient. However, there is a risk of erosion of the skin at the penoscrotal junction and the development of urethrocutaneous fistulae. There are difficulties with the adjustment of the apparatus and, in the case of the tetraplegic patient, other persons are required to fit the collecting apparatus. The penis is inserted into the sheath and, to prevent leakage, adequate pubic pressure must be applied. Troublesome inflammation of the glans penis and prepuce can arise and the foreskin may require to be trimmed, but circumcision should be avoided.

The condom sheath is the most commonly used device in the male paraplegic. It is a thin latex condom, connected to a piece of rubber tubing by means of a plastic adapter and drained into a leg-bag. There is complete freedom from straps with this appliance, which is a considerable advantage. The condom may be held in place by means of a skin adhesive cement or by Elastoplast and it usually requires to be changed every one to three days. The problems that may arise with this type of drainage system include the occasional splitting of the condom, usually as a result of the patient manœuvring himself or exerting traction upon the drainage system on movement. Twisting of the condom causes a failure of urinary drainage, giving rise to a macerated penile skin, and in some cases circumcision may be an advantage. A new adapter was described by Pearman and Shah (1973) to overcome this problem and it provided an internal diameter which allows a high urine flow rate and holds open the end of the condom, thus avoiding obstruction. To prevent accidental detachment of the condom, Lawson advised the application of two pieces of adhesive tape, placed longitudinally on either side of the penis, and a circumferential tape applied lightly over that. In some patients it may be necessary to shave the pubic hair, to prevent its being included in the piece of material, and care needs to be exercised to avoid undue pressure from the circumferential tape.

URINARY DIVERSION

Bricker (1950) reported on the substitution for the urinary bladder by use of an isolated ileal segment, and Mogg (1967) reported on the use of the colon conduit in 75 cases of incontinence of neuropathic origin. The indications for such diversion are:

1.   otherwise uncontrolled incontinence
2.   to provide a low pressure drainage system, especially in cases of vesico-ureteric reflux, when this cannot be managed òtherwise than by using the lower urinary tract.

Of 78 patients with multiple sclerosis reported by Desmond and Shuttleworth (1977), 12 (15%) underwent urinary diversion with an ileal conduit. Prior to diversion, 5 of the 12 patients were being managed by indwelling catheters, the remainder with appliances—pants, pads and sanitary towels. The indication for diversion was severe urinary incontinence, which was not controlled by other means. The need for specialized and adequate nursing care of these patients, to prevent pressure sores and to assist in restoring the patient's mobility to its pre-operative level, was stressed. The results were very satisfactory, in spite of a high incidence of post-operative complications. Pyocystitis, a purulent infection in the remaining bladder, developed in 3 out of 12 cases and required secondary cystectomy. The surgical trauma did not result in neurological deterioration of the patient. They concluded that the only absolute contra-indication was bed sores, and it was suggested that urinary diversion should be considered much earlier rather than as a last resort.

Stark (1977) reported that some degree of urinary incontinence occurred in 90% of unselected patients with myelomeningocele. In a review of 90 children with ileal conduits, followed over a 10–16 year period, 75 were still alive and Shapiro *et al.* (1975) stressed the need for lifetime follow-up. Stomal ulceration occurred in 38% of cases, ureteroileal obstruction in 22.3%, pyocystitis in 17.8%, renal calculi in 15.6% and intestinal obstruction in 18.9%. The post-operative mortality was 4.5%, but all these patients were in chronic renal failure. After 10–16 years 76% of 144 renal units remained improved or unchanged.

Altwein *et al.* (1977) reported 64 children with colon conduits over a 4.6 year follow-up period. These authors maintained that the colon provided a safer anastomosis because of thicker musculature, the availability of a redundant colon and a large stoma, not prone to stomal stenosis, rare occurrence of conduit elongation and less electrolyte reabsorption as compared to ileal loops. Stomal stenosis was reported in only 4.2% of cases.

Whenever possible, urinary diversion should be undertaken before there is any radiological evidence of the deterioration of the upper urinary tract. At present there is a swing away from diversion to more conservative methods, especially intermittent 'clean' self-catheterization, combined if necessary with drugs. It may be some time before it can be proved that this is in the patient's best long-term interest.

REFERENCES

ABRAMS P.H. & TORRENS M.J. (1979) Urine flow studies. *Urologic Clinics of North America*, **6**, 71–9.

ALEXANDER S. (1976) Electronic stimulation of the urinary bladder and sphincter. *Scientific Foundations of Urology*, pp. 107–10. Heinemann, London.

ALTWEIN J.E., JONES U. & HOHENFELLNER R. (1977) Long term follow-up of children with colon conduit, urinary diversion and ureterosigmoidostomy. *British Journal of Urology*, **118**, 832–6.

AWAD S.A. & DOWNIE J.W. (1977) Sympathetic dyssynergia in the region of the external sphincter, a possible source of lower urinary tract obstruction. *Journal of Urology*, **18**, 636–40.

BAILEY R.R., ROBERTS A.P. & BOWER P.L. (1971) Prevention of urinary tract infection with low-dose nitrofurantoin. *Lancet*, **ii,** 1112–14.

BATES C.P. (1971) Continence and incontinence, clinical study of the dynamics of voiding and of the sphincter mechanism. *Annals of the Royal College of Surgeons of England*, **49,** 18–35.

BLAIVAS J.G., LABIB K.L., BAUER S.B. & RETIK A.B. (1977) A new approach to electromyography of the external urethral sphincter. *Journal of Urology*, **117,** 773–7.

BORS E. & COMARR A.E. (1971) *Neurological Urology*. S. Karger, Basel.

BRICKER E.M. (1950) Bladder substitution after pelvic evisceration. *Surgical Clinics of North America*, **30,** 1511–21.

BRINDLEY A.S. (November 1973) Emptying the bladder by stimulating ventral roots. Communication to the Physiological Society.

BROCKLEHURST J.C. & BROCKLEHURST S. (1978) The management of indwelling catheters. *British Journal of Urology*, **50,** 102–5.

BROWN M. & WICKHAM J.E.A. (1969) The urethral pressure profile. *British Journal of Urology*, **41,** 211–17.

BRUCE A.W., CLARK A.F. & AWAD J.A. (1974) The problem of catheter encrustation. *Canadian Medical Association Journal*, **111,** 238–41.

BUNTS R.C. (1958) Vesicoureteric reflux in paraplegic patients. *Journal of Urology*, **79,** 747–50.

CALDWELL K.P.S., FLACK F.C. & BROAD A.F. (1965) Urinary incontinence following spinal injury treated by electronic implant. *Lancet*, **i,** 846–7.

COMARR A.E., KAWACHI G. & BORS E. (1962) Renal calculosis in patients with traumatic cord lesions. *Journal of Urology*, **87,** 647–57.

COOK W.A., BABCOCK J.R., SWENSON O.S. & KING L.R. (1978) Incontinence in Children. *Urologic Clinics of North America*, **5,** 353–74.

DAMANSKI M. (1965) Vesico-ureteric reflux in paraplegia. *British Journal of Surgery*, **52,** 168–77.

DESMOND A.D. & SHUTTLEWORTH K.E.D. (1977) The results of urinary diversion in multiple sclerosis. *British Journal of Urology*, **49,** 495–502.

DIOKNO A.C., VINSON R.K. & McGILLICUDDY J. (1977) Treatment of the severe uninhibited neurogenic bladder by selective sacral rhizotomy. *Journal of Urology*, **118,** 299–301.

DONELLY J., HACKLER R.H. & BUNTS R.C. (1972) Present urologic status of the World War II paraplegic. Twenty-five year follow-up. Comparison with status of the twenty years. Korean War paraplegic and five year Vietnam paraplegic. *Journal of Urology*, **108,** 558–62.

DONKER P.J., IVANOVICI F. & NOACH E.L. (1972) Analyses of the urethral pressure profile by means of electromyography and the administration of drugs. *British Journal of Urology*, **44,** 180–93.

FALL M. (1977) Thesis: Intravaginal electrical stimulation. *Scandinavian Journal of Urology and Nephrology*, Supplement **44.**

FALL M. (1979) Personal communication.

FAM B.A., ROSSIER A.B., BLUNT K., GABILONDO F.B., SARKARATI M., SETHI J. & YALLA S.V. (1978) Experiences in the urologic management of 120 early spinal cord injury patients. *Journal of Urology*, **119,** 485–7.

FELLOWS G.J., NUSIEBEM I. & WALSH J.J. (1977) Choice of operation to promote micturition after spinal cord injury. *British Journal of Urology*, **49,** 721–4.

FLETCHER T.F. & BRADLEY W.B. (1978) Neuroanatomy of the bladder/urethra. *Journal of Urology*, **119,** 153–60.

FREEMAN R.B., SMITH W.M., RICHARDSON J.A., MENNELLY P.J., THURM R.M., URNER C., VAILLANCOURT J.A., GRIEP R.J. & BROMER L. (1975) Long-term therapy for chronic bacteriuria in men. *Annals of Internal Medicine*, **83,** 133–47.

GEORGE N.J.R., DUNN M., DOUNIS A., ABRAMS P.H. & SMITH P.J.B. (1978) The late symptomatic and functional results of enterocystoplasty. *British Journal of Urology*, **50,** 517–20.

GEORGE N.J.R., FENELEY R.C.L. & SLADE N. (1978) Trial of long-term catheterisation in the elderly—initial findings. *Proceedings of the International Continence Society*, pp. 19–20. Manchester.

GLAHN B.R. (1970) Neurogenic bladder diagnosed pharmacologically on the basis of denervation supersensitivity. *Scandinavian Journal of Urology and Nephrology*, **4**, 13–24.

GLEASON D.M., GITTES R.F., BOTTACCINI M.R. & BYRNE J.C. (1972) Energy balance of voiding after faecal cystoplasty. *Journal of Urology*, **108**, 259–64.

GRIFFITHS D.J. (1974) The mechanical functions of bladder and urethra in micturition. *International Urology and Nephrology*, **6**, 177–82.

GODEC C., AYALA G.F. & CASS A.S. (1977) Electrical stimulation of the ampulla causing reflex voiding. *Journal of Urology*, **117**, 770–2.

GODEC C., CASS A.S. & AYALA G.F. (1976) Electrical stimulation for incontinence technique selection and results. *Urology*, **7**, 388–97.

GOSLING J.A. (1979) The structure of the bladder and urethra in relation to function. *Urologic Clinics of North America*, **6**, 31–8.

GOSLING J.A., DIXON J.S. & LENDON R.G. (1977) The autonomic innervation of the human male and female bladder neck and proximal urethra. *Journal of Urology*, **118**, 302–5.

GUTTMAN L. & FRANKEL H. (1966) The value of intermittent catheterisation in the early management of traumatic paraplegia and tetraplegia. *Paraplegia*, **4**, 63–84.

HABIB H.N. (1967) Experience and recent contributions in sacral nerve stimulation for voiding in both human and animal. *British Journal of Urology*, **39**, 73–83.

HALD T. (1975) Problem of urinary incontinence. In *Urinary Incontinence* (Ed. Caldwell K.P.S.). Sector Publishing, London.

HALL M.H. (1965) Appliances for the incontinent patient. *British Journal of Urology*, **37**, 644–6.

HARRISON N. (1976) Mechanisms of micturition. *British Journal of Hospital Medicine*, **17**, 454–61.

HERR H.W. (1975) Intermittent catheterisation in neurogenic bladder dysfunction. *Journal of Urology*, **113**, 477–9.

HIRSCH S., CARRION H., GORDON J. & POLITANO V. (1978) Ureteroneocystostomy in the treatment of reflux in neurogenic bladders. *Journal of Urology*, **120**, 552–4.

HITCHCOCK E., NEWSOME D. & SALAMA M. (1974) The somatotrophic representation of the micturition pathways in the cervical cord of man. *British Journal of Surgery*, **61**, 395–401.

JACOBS S.C. & KAUFMAN J.M. (1978) Complications of permanent bladder catheter drainage in spinal cord injury patients. *Journal of Urology*, **119**, 740–1.

KAUFMAN J.J. (1978) The silicone-gel prosthesis for the treatment of male urinary incontinence. *Urologic Clinics of North America*, **5**, 393–404.

KOCK, N.G. & POMPEIUS R. (1963) Inhibition of vesical motor activity induced by anal stimulation. *Acta Chirurgica Scandinavica*, **126**, 244–50.

KOONTZ W.W. & VERNON SMITH M.J. (1977) Transurethral external sphincterotomy in boys with myelodysplasia. *Journal of Urology*, **117**, 500–000.

KURSH E.M., FREEHAFER A. & PERSKY L. (1977) Complications of autonomic dysreflexia. *Journal of Urology*, **118**, 70–2.

KURU M. (1965) Nervous control of micturition. *Physiological Reviews*, **45**, 425–94.

LAPIDES J., DIOKNO A.C. & SILBER S.J. (1962) Clean intermittent self-catheterisation in the treatment of urinary tract disease. *Journal of Urology*, **107**, 458–61.

LAPIDES J., FRIEND C.R., AJEMIAN E.P. & REUS W.S. (1962) Denervation supersensitivity as a test of neurogenic bladder. *Surgery, Gynaecology and Obstetrics*, **114**, 241–4.

LAPIDES J., DIOKNO A.C. & GOULD F.R. (1976) Further observations on self-catheterisation. *Journal of Urology*, **116**, 169–71.

LEE I.Y., RAGNARSSON K.T., SELL G.M., MORALES P. & WHELAN J. (1978) Transurethral bladder neck surgery in spinal cord injured patients. *Archives of Physical Medicine and Rehabilitation*, **59** (2), 80–3.

LIGHT K. & VON BLERK P.J.P. (1977) Intermittent catheterisation in congenital neurogenic bladder, a preliminary report. *British Journal of Urology*, **49**, 523–6.

MADERSBACHER H. (1976) The twelve o'clock sphincterotomy; technique, indications, results. *Paraplegia*, **13**, 261–7.

MAYO M.E., LLOYD-DAVIES R.W. & SHUTTLEWORTH K.E.D. (1973) The damaged human detrusor. Functional and electron microscopic changes in disease. *British Journal of Urology*, **45**, 116–25.

McGUIRE E.J. (1978) Neurogenic incontinence in males. *Urologic Clinics in North America*, **5**, 335–46.

McGUIRE E.J., WAGNER F.M. & WEISS R.M. (1976) Treatment of autonomic dysreflexia with phenoxybenzamine. *Journal of Urology*, **115**, 53–5.

MERRILL D.C. & CONWAY C.J. (1974) Clinical experience with the mentor stimulator of patients with upper motor neurone lesions. *Journal of Urology*, **112**, 52–6.

MOGG R.A. (1967) Urinary diversion using the colonic conduit. *British Journal of Urology*, **39**, 687–92.

MORROW J.W. & BOGAARD T.P. (1977) Bladder rehabilitation in patients with old spinal cord injuries by bladder neck incision and external sphincterotomy. *Journal of Urology*, **117**, 164–7.

NANNINGA J.B. & ROSEN J. (1975) Problems associated with the use of external urinary collectors in the male paraplegic. *Paraplegia*, **13**, 56–61.

NASHOLD B.S., FRIEDMAN H., GLENN J.F., GRIMES J.H., BARRY W.F. & AVERY R. (1972) Electromicturition in paraplegia. *Archives of Surgery*, **104**, 195–202.

NATHAN P.W. (1976) The central nervous connections of the bladder. In *The Scientific Foundation of Urology* (Eds Williams D.I. & Chisholm G.). Heinemann, London.

NERGARDH A. (1975) Autonomic receptor function in the lower urinary tract. A survey of recent experimental results. *Journal of Urology*, **113**, 180–5.

NILSSON S. (1975) Long term treatment with methenamine hippurate in recurrent urinary tract infection. *Acta Medica Scandinavica*. **198**, 81–5.

O'FLYNN, J.D. (1974) Neurogenic bladder in spinal cord injury. Management of patients in Dublin, Ireland. *Urologic Clinics of North America*, **1**, 155–62.

O'FLYNN J.D. (1976) An assessment of surgical treatment of vesical outlet obstruction in spinal cord injury: a review of 471 cases. *British Journal of Urology*, **48**, 657–62.

OLSSON C.A., SIROKY M.B. & KRANE R.J. (1977) The phentolamine test in neurogenic bladder dysfunction. *Journal of Urology*, **177**, 481–5.

PEARMAN J.W. & SHAH S.K. (1973) A new adaptor which obviates problems associated with condom external urinary drainage of male patients. *Paraplegia*, **11**, 25–9.

PEDERSEN E., HARVING H., KLEMAR B. & TØRRING J. (1978) Human anal reflexes. *Journal of Neurology, Neurosurgery and Psychiatry*, **41**, 813–18.

PENNISI S.A., MAGEE J.H., BUNTS R.C., UNGER A.M. & HOLLADAY L.W. (1959) Renal clearances in paraplegics with recent and old injuries. *Journal of Urology*, **82**, 442–8.

PERKASH I. (1978) Detrusor sphincter dyssynergia and dyssynergic responses. Recognition and rationale for early modified transurethral sphincterotomy in complete spinal cord injury lesions. *Journal of Urology*, **120**, 469–74.

RAEZER D.M., BENSON G.S., WEIN A.J. & DUCKETT J.W. (1977) The functional approach to the management of the paediatric neuropathic bladder. A clinical study. *Journal of Urology*, **117**, 649–54.

REECE R.W. & HACKLER R.M. (1975) Vesicoureteroplasty in the paraplegic. Long-term follow-up in 77 patients. *Journal of Urology*, **113**, 474–6.

REEVES D.S. & GHILCHIK M. (1970) Secretion of the antibacterial substance Trimethoprim in the prostatic fluid of dogs. *British Journal of Urology*, **42**, 66–72.

ROCKSWOLD G.L. & BRADLEY W.E. (1977) The use of evoked electromyographic responses in diagnosing lesions of the cauda equina. *Journal of Urology*, **118**, 629–31.

ROSEN M. (1978) The Rosen inflatable incontinence prosthesis. *Urologic Clinics of North America*, **5**, 405–14.

ROSS J.C. (1956) Treatment of the bladder in paraplegia. *British Journal of Urology*, **28**, 14–23.

ROSS J.C., GIBBON N.O.K. & DAMANSKI M. (1967) Division of the external sphincter in the treatment of the neurogenic bladder. A ten year review. *British Journal of Surgery*, **54**, 627–8.

Ross J.C., Gibbon N.O.K. & Sundar G.S. (1976) Division of the external urethral sphincter in the neuropathic bladder; a twenty years' review. *British Journal of Urology*, **48**, 649–56.

Rossier A.B. & Ott R. (1974) Urinary manometry in spinal cord injury: a follow-up study. Value of cysto-sphincterometrography as an indication for sphincterotomy. *British Journal of Urology*, **46**, 439–48.

Rossier A.B. & Ott R. (1976) Bladder and urethral recordings in acute and chronic spinal cord injury patients. *Urologia Internationalis*, **31**, 49–59.

Schoenberg H.W., Shah J.P., Kyker J. & Gregory J.G. (1977) Changing attitudes towards urinary dysfunction in myelodysplasia. *Journal of Urology*, **117**, 501–4.

Scott F.B. (1978) The artificial sphincter in the management of incontinence in the male. *Urologic Clinics of North America*, **5**, 375–91.

Shapiro S.R., Lewbowitz R. & Colodny A.H. (1975) Fate of 90 chilren with ileal conduit urinary diversion a decade later: analysis of complications, pyelography, renal function and bacteriology. *British Journal of Urology*, **114**, 289–95.

Smith P.M., Cook J.B. & Arrowsmith W.A. (1971) Transurethral resection of the bladder neck and external sphincter after spinal injury. *Proceedings V.A. Spinal Cord Injury Conference*, pp. 168–169. Boston, Mass.

Smith R.B., van Cangh P., Skinner D.G., Kaufman J.J. & Goodwin W.E. (1977) Augmentation cystoplasty, a critical review. *Journal of Urology*, **118**, 35–9.

Stamey T.A., Condy M. & Mihara G. (1977) Prophylactic efficacy of nitrofurantoin macrocrystals and trimethoprim-sulfamethoxazole in urinary infection. *New England Journal of Medicine*, **196**, 780–3.

Stark G.D. (1977) *Spina Bifida. Problems and Management*. Blackwell Scientific Publications, Oxford.

Sundin T. & Dahlstrom A. (1973) The sympathetic innervation of the urinary bladder and urethra in the normal stage and after parasympathetic denervation at the spinal root level. *Scandinavian Journal of Urology and Nephrology*, **7**, 131–49.

Thomas D.G. (1976) The effect of transurethral surgery on penile erections in spinal cord injury patients. *Paraplegia*, **13**, 286–9.

Thomas D.G. (1979) Clinical urodynamics in neurogenic bladder dysfunction. *Urologic Clinics of North America*, **6**, 237–53.

Thomson-Walker J. (1937) The treatment of the bladder in spinal injuries in war. *British Journal of Urology*, **9**, 217–30.

Torrens M.J. (1978) Urethral sphincteric responses to stimulation of the sacral nerves in the human female. *Urologia Internationalis*, **33**, 22–6.

Torrens M.J. & Abrams P.H. (1979) Cystometry. *Urologic Clinics of North America*. **6**, 79–85.

Torrens M.J. & Hald T. (1979) Bladder denervation procedures. *Urologic Clinics of North America*, **6**, 283–93.

Tribe C.R. (1963) Causes of death in the early and late types of paraplegia. *Paraplegia*, **1**, 19–47.

Vincent S.A. (1964) Treatment of enuresis with a perineal pressure apparatus. The irritable bladder syndrome. *Development Medicine and Child Neurology*, **6**, 23–31.

Wastling G. (1974) Long-term catheterisation. *Nursing Times*, 3rd January, 17–18.

Willington F.L. (1976) *Incontinence in the Elderly*, pp. 230–44. Academic Press, London.

Withycombe J.F.R. (1978) Intermittent catheterisation in the management of children with neuropathic bladder. *Lancet*, **ii**, 981–3.

Yalla S.V., Blunt K.J., Fam B.A., Constantinople N.L. & Gittes R.F. (1977) Detrusor-urethral sphincter dyssynergia. *Journal of Urology*, **118**, 1026–9.

Yeates W.K. (1972) Disorders of bladder function. *Annals of the Royal College of Surgeons*, **50**, 335–53.

Chapter 9

Rehabilitation of Peripheral Nerve Disorders

Peripheral nerves can be affected by a very wide variety of diseases—infective, metabolic, immunological, toxic, malignant and heredofamilial—and these are considered in Chapter 2.

This chapter deals with injuries to peripheral nerves. The classic work of Seddon (1972) described three major types of disorder—neurapraxia, axonotmesis and neurotmesis.

Neurapraxia

Neurapraxia is defined as a temporary block to conduction commonly due to pressure—voluntary impulses fail to traverse the block, but there is no Wallerian degeneration. Electrical excitability is retained below the site of block, but the nerve usually is inexcitable above the block. Although motor paralysis is complete, some sensation may be spared. There is no wasting and no trophic lesions develop. It used to be thought that neurapraxia always recovered within six weeks, but it is now recognized that such blocks can be very prolonged. We have seen patients with compression of the ulnar nerve at the elbow with virtually complete sensory and motor paralysis which lasts 18 months, but who have recovered almost full function within a few days of decompression.

Ochoa et al. (1972) have shown that compression blocks are associated with mechanical changes in the nerve such that a node of Ranvier is invaginated into the myelin sheath. Metabolic changes occur under the block and it is possible that ischaemia also plays a part.

Electromyographic studies will help to demonstrate the block—the amplitude to supramaximal stimulation recording over a muscle supplied by the nerve will be markedly reduced above the point of compression compared with that below, and the mixed nerve action potential will be similarly reduced.

Axonotmesis

In axonotmesis, damage is more severe. The nerve sheath is intact, but the axis cylinder distintegrates, Wallerian degeneration occurs and regeneration

251

takes place at the usual rate of 1mm a day in adults, 2mm in children. As the internal architecture is maintained intact, little or no misrouting of axons occurs and the functional result is nearly perfect.

However, in traction lesions of nerves, particularly the brachial plexus, there may be a considerable degree of torsion with disorganization of the architecture of the nerve; cross innervation and disordered function are then inevitable.

Axonotmesis usually follows a severe closed injury in which the nerve is crushed, e.g. paralysis of the radial nerve in a fracture of the mid-shaft of the humerus.

Neurotmesis

In neurotmesis the whole nerve is divided including the sheath, and recovery is impossible without surgical suture. Each peripheral nerve has a special vulnerability to particular types of damage. Some common situations are listed below.

Median nerve. At the wrist lacerations due to a fall on glass, putting the hand through a window, suicide attempts, compression in the carpal tunnel by malunited or badly reduced colles fracture, myxoedema, rheumatoid flexor tenosynovitis or idiopathic thickening of the ligament.

Ulnar nerve. Vulnerable at the wrist in falls on glass or putting the hand through a window. Prolonged pressure in the palm in carpentry, dispatch riders, lorry drivers crashing their gears can damage the deep branch. It is liable to damage in fractures and dislocations around the elbow joint either immediately or as the result of late deformity stretching the nerve in the cubital tunnel (tardy palsy), pressure by Osborne's band, occupational palsy due to prolonged leaning on the elbows, pressure of osteophytes in osteoarthrosis and joint effusions or destructive changes in rheumatoid disease.

Radial nerve. Temporary block is common when compressed over the arm of a chair—'Saturday night palsy'. Axonotmesis is seen in mid-shaft fractures of the humerus when the nerve is compressed as it travels around the spiral groove and in dislocations of the shoulder, and also after too vigorous attempts to reduce them.

Musculocutaneous nerve. A rare lesion, but occurring in humeral fractures and in some cases of shoulder dislocation. It may coexist with traction lesions of the upper trunks of the brachial plexus and is thus difficult to diagnose.

Axillary nerve. This nerve is commonly involved in dislocations of the shoulder and in neuralgic amyotrophy. Owing to inadequate clinical examination circumflex nerve palsies can be diagnosed when the true disorder is a traction lesion of the C5 root. It is surprising how often the wasting of the spinati is missed. Abduction and elevation are often possible in pure deltoid paralysis using trick movements (page 254), whereas it is never possible if the external rotators are paralysed.

Brachial plexus palsies are considered in a separate section (page 262).

Femoral nerve. This can be damaged in fractures of the femur or organizing haematomas after direct violence injuries.

Common peroneal nerve. This is commonly involved in direct violence injuries to the knee, in dislocations of the knee and of the hip, and in too tight plasters in the treatment of fractures of the lower limb. It is not uncommon after operations for total hip replacement.

Sciatic nerve. This is easily damaged in dislocations and fracture dislocations of the hip. Sometimes only the lateral popliteal branch is affected and the localization of level of damage can be difficult.

All peripheral nerves are liable to damage by gunshot wounds either by direct violence or by the cavitation effect of a high velocity missile passing close by. Regeneration always takes longer and is often incomplete owing to the considerable degree of intraneural fibrosis. Nerves are liable to pressure by intrinsic tumours (neurofibroma, schwanoma) or extrinsic factors (ganglia, lipoma) or tight bands. A whole group of entrapment neuropathies are now known, such as compression of the median nerve in the carpal tunnel, the ulnar nerve in Guyon's canal at the wrist and by Osborne's band in the elbow, the median nerve by the ligament of Struthers at the elbow or between the two heads of pronator teres and the medial plantar nerve in the tarsal tunnel. A comprehensive review is given in Staal (1970).

TREATMENT

If a nerve is divided, it must of course be repaired. In closed injuries it may not always be necessary—for example 70% of radial nerve palsies associated with fractures of the mid-shaft of the humerus recover spontaneously.

The decision to explore depends on a sound knowledge of the natural history of injuries associated with nerve lesions (Seddon, 1972). If a nerve is compressed it usually requires release. The decision will depend on the degree of clinical involvement—sensory loss or wasting is an absolute indication for surgery, but one is interested in preventing such a degree of damage by prophylactic surgery and here electromyography has proved of great value. If, for example, the distal motor latency stimulating the median nerve at the wrist and recording in abductor pollicis brevis is more than 7 ms, surgery is indicated as it is known that spontaneous recovery will not occur (Goodman & Gilliatt, 1961).

In many situations the EMG studies indicate a much more profound degree of nerve involvement than appears clinically. Serial studies will show if the lesion is progressive and if it will require urgent surgical treatment.

There is at the present time a spirited controversy over the correct techniques for surgical repair of peripheral nerves. The classical method is epineural suture using the disposition of the blood vessels to obtain correct axial alignment. Millesi and his co-workers (1976) have argued a case for the use of multiple nerve grafts to try and match proximal and distal bundles correctly—using the technique of interfascicular suture. There is no doubt that correct alignment of fascicles would lead to better results in adults, but none of the experimental work in animals or clinical results reported so far convincingly prove the superiority of the newer technique. As Sunderland (1968) has pointed out, the architecture of the nerve is very complex. Fascicles are changing course throughout the length of the nerve such that a cross-section of a nerve may be entirely different 2 cm further distally. There is also the argument that grafting involves the axons crossing two suture lines.

Only a carefully controlled prospective survey will establish the truth and, as will be discussed later, methods of assessing results will need to be more functional than in the past.

If there is marked loss of nerve tissue, then grafting may be inevitable, but considerable length can be achieved by mobilizing nerves and flexing adjacent joints, thus avoiding nerve grafting.

TRICK MOVEMENTS

In certain cases of muscle paralysis, other muscles can perform the movements normally carried out by those paralysed. They are worth careful study, for if one is ignorant of them one may be deceived into thinking the muscles are working when they are not. Moreover, absence of the typical trick movements in a presumed nerve lesion raises serious doubt as to the diagnosis and finally patients can often be taught to use trick movements for function.

SHOULDER

In paralysis of the deltoid, the external rotators, in particular the infraspinatus, will rotate the humerus allowing the clavicular head of pectoralis major to act as an abductor. The long heads of biceps and triceps, as they cross the joint, assist in the movement. It is very unusual not to be able to teach patients with deltoid paralysis in axillary nerve lesions to gain full elevation against considerable resistance. If the infraspinatus is paralysed also (C5 root lesion, combined suprascapular and axillary nerve lesions), this action is not possible.

ELBOW

Elbow flexion is still possible in paralysis of muscles innervated by the musculo-cutaneous nerve by using brachioradialis (radial nerve supply) and this can be a very strong movement.

In a C5, 6 palsy, all the usual elbow flexors are paralysed, but slight elbow flexion can sometimes be obtained by strong pronation, wrist extension and finger flexion. The long flexors and extensors and the pronator teres arise from the lower part of the humerus and by contracting from their insertion to their origin can flex the elbow joint. Just occasionally, this movement is strong enough to allow limited function. Its importance lies in realizing that the ability to bend the elbow does not mean that the biceps and brachialis (or brachioradialis) are necessarily working. The muscles must always be felt to see if there is a contraction.

HAND

In complete paralysis of radial or posterior interosseus nerves it is always possible to extend the interphalangeal joint of the thumb provided that the patient is allowed to abduct his thumb in the plane of the palm. This is because the abductor pollicis brevis and the flexor pollicis brevis both insert into the extensor expansion of the thumb. By applying a little resistance to the radial border of the thumb, the immediate attempt to abduct the thumb can be spotted.

Sometimes powerful wrist flexion followed by relaxation can result in wrist extension and fool the examiner into thinking that the wrist extensors are working when they are not. It is a sure sign of a trick movement when the patient produces the opposite movement to that desired in an effort to obtain a rebound. Again, attempted finger extension results in *flexion* of the metacarpo-phalangeal joints due to the action of the interossei pulling down on the extensor hood.

ULNAR

When the patient attempts to abduct the thumb, the flexor pollicis longus substitutes for the paralysed adductor and the interphalangeal (IP) joint of the thumb flexes (Froment's sign). The long extensors can imitate finger abduction and the long flexors imitate finger adduction. If the patient puts his hand on the table palm down, raises his middle or ring finger and tries to abduct it, he will be unable to do so as the extensor is now fully occupied by keeping the finger in the air. Instead the whole wrist and hand move on the immobile finger—a very characteristic sign.

MEDIAN

When the patient attempts opposition, the IP joint of the thumb is hyperflexed in an attempt to approximate the tip of the thumb to the finger tips by the action of flexor pollicis longus which is spared in a lesion at the wrist.

When the patient attempts abduction in the plane of the palm away from the index finger, the thumb goes into radial abduction by the action of abductor pollicis longus.

LEG

The knee can be extended in the presence of paralysis of the quadriceps (femoral nerve) by snap-back action of the gastrocnemius. We have seen a patient with poliomyelitis whose glutei and quadriceps were paralysed on one side yet was able to walk without sticks and only a slight limp by gastrocnemius action and strong contraction of quadratus lumborum raising up the pelvis.

In a complete lateral popliteal palsy it can look as if the toe extensors are working when the patient makes a strong flexion movement in the toes and relaxes them—rebound phenomenon.

SPLINTAGE

Paralysed muscles are liable to shorten due to overaction of the unopposed antagonists and splintage may be necessary if deformity threatens. Much the most important reason for splinting is to provide function and lively splints can harness some of the trick movements described to allow function.

MEDIAN NERVE

Here one must splint the thumb so it is held away from the index finger in palmar abduction. This can be either by a static opponens splint or by a lively splint in which a spring is placed at the metocarpo-phalangeal (MP) joint of the thumb, thus helping the flexor pollicis longus to oppose the thumb to the fingers. This also prevents the thumb from being held adducted against the index.

ULNAR NERVE

Not all patients need splinting, but if there is a marked hyperextension deformity of the little and ring fingers at the MP joints then some device to prevent this is required. We use a splint which both prevents this hyperextension and allows active movements at the MP joints by a spring coil. As only a small palmar bar is used in this splint, the fingers are free for function. We prefer this lively splint to the static knuckleduster which is too cumbersome and less effective.

In a combined median and ulnar nerve lesion, the two splints are combined (Fig. 9.1). These lively splints are easy to make and are made in some centres by occupational therapists. They are cheap, easy to clean, comfortable, light, unobtrusive and patients really do wear them for work or hobbies.

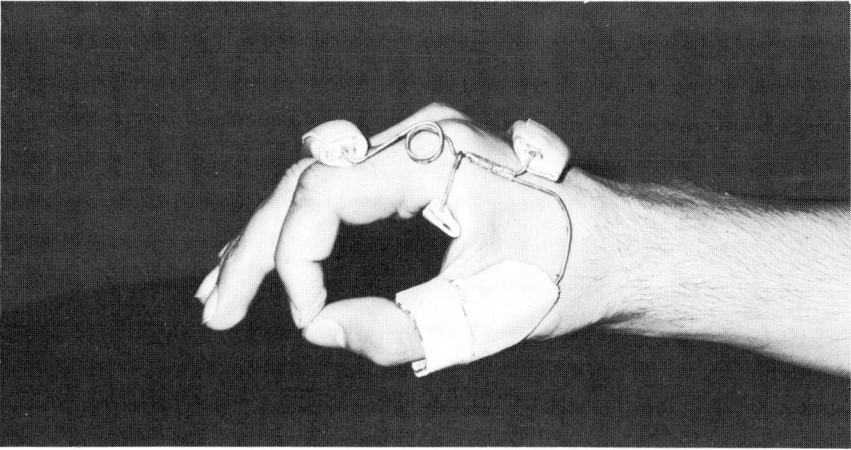

Fig. 9.1 Splint for combined median and ulnar nerve lesion.

RADIAL

The dropped wrist is a serious bar to hand function for the grip is weak in palmar flexion of the wrist. A lively cock-up splint is valuable, for this supports the wrist in dorsiflexion and by virtue of the spring at the wrist allows active movements. A spider attachment for the thumb and fingers is used by a few patients in an attempt to provide some release of finger flexion into extension. Some patients find their function is perfectly satisfactory wearing a simple wrist support like the Futura splint.

There is no indication to splint the shoulder in abduction in deltoid paralysis. There is no danger of deformity and no one has yet devised a lively splint to offer active abduction that does not prove a gross encumbrance.

In paralysis of elbow flexion (musculocutaneous nerve lesion, C6 root palsy) when there is no trick action to provide functional movements, such as brachioradialis or a strong Steindler effect, a splint can be provided to allow the patient to fix his elbow in one of the four desired positions of flexion. It comprises an upper arm and forearm trough joined by an elbow hinge with a ratchet which the patient locks himself. This splint thus puts the hand in the position of function. They can be provided in standard sizes which are altered to suit the individual patient and within a few hours of fitting the patient has mastered its use with the help of the occupational therapist or orthotist.

In C6 and 7 palsies where in addition there is paralysis of wrist extension a cock-up piece is attached to the forearm trough. In total paralysis of the upper limb a flail arm splint over the paralysed arm offers some function. It consists of the elbow splint already described to give variable fixed elbow flexion, which is attached to the upper limb by a shoulder support.

On the distal end of the volar surface of the forearm piece is a platform into which are slotted the standard devices for an artificial arm—split hook, pliers, dividers, driving attachment, etc. These are operated by a harness around the opposite shoulder. Thus the patient can put objects into the attachments and use the splint as a support, leaving the other arm free.

Whether the patient has had reconstructive surgery to the plexus—grafting or neurotization—or whether spontaneous recovery in time is expected it will be many months—even up to two years—before proximal muscle function can be expected. If the patient is not encouraged to keep the paralysed arm as part of his body image, he will become so one-armed that when recovery does occur he will not use it.

The use of the splint does just this and 70% of our 61 patients splinted used their splints regularly for work or hobbies or both. All of them found the support given to the shoulder valuable and found it cosmetically more acceptable than the dangling flail arm, (Wynn Parry, 1981).

Most patients whose arm has been amputated and a prosthesis supplied never use it. Few young men relish the loss of their arm and dislike being seen with a stump on the beach or by the pool. The flail arm splint we feel offers the best of both worlds—function and retention of the patient's own arm.

It may be that giant strides will be taken in the design of artificial arms in the future and this policy will need revision—at present we believe that amputation should only be offered if recurrent trophic lesions are a serious nuisance (and these are rare) or if the patient finds great difficulty in learning to use his non-dominant arm. Certainly only those with manual trades are likely to use the prosthesis.

LEG

In a few patients with permanent paralysis of the quadriceps, it may be necessary to prescribe a caliper. The Stanmore cosmetic caliper is light and easy to apply and well tolerated (Fig. 9.2).

In sciatic or common peroneal nerve palsies, the dropped foot needs support. The traditional iron and spring is heavy and requires a hole made in the heel of the shoe. It is always worth trying an ortholene (high density polypropylene) orthosis which fits into the shoe, stabilizes the ankle and by virtue of the inherent springiness of the thermoplastic provides a little movement at the ankle. Only if this proves too weak for the patient's demands is it necessary to provide a conventional caliper. Often well-fitting boots obviate the necessity for an orthosis at all. Sometimes fashions work in favour of patients.

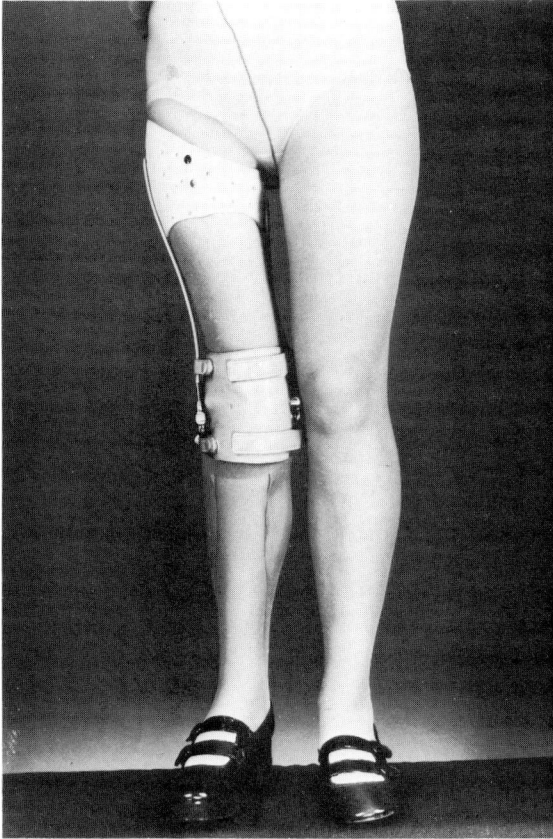

Fig. 9.2 Stanmore caliper for quadriceps paralysis.

RECONSTRUCTIVE SURGERY

When paralysis is permanent there are a number of surgical procedures which can offer excellent function. These are indicated, for example, when so much nerve tissue has been lost in an injury that nerve grafting is impossible, or when regeneration has not occurred because of intraneural fibrosis or the lesion is known to be irrecoverable as, for example, in avulsion of one or more roots of the brachial plexus.

The timing of these procedures is important. Clearly if it is known for certain that recovery is impossible, the sooner they are undertaken, the quicker the patient can return to normal life. But if recovery is possible then the statutory time is allowed to elapse for regeneration to occur, allowing 1 mm a day and a little over before an irrecoverable lesion is diagnosed.

During the period of waiting, use of functional splintage will allow the patient to return to work so that nothing is lost.

Surgical procedures can either offer stabilization of a flail joint-arthrodesis or tendon transfer to give movement. Obviously the transfer of a tendon implies loss of some of the transferred tendon's function and before embarking on such procedures a very careful assessment is made by the physiotherapist and occupational therapist. This is over a sufficient period of time and in a realistic environment to establish both that the planned procedure will improve function in the patient's everyday life and that the loss of the transferred tendon function will not obviate any benefit resulting. These decisions cannot and must not be made in the clinic. Usually we admit our patients to our rehabilitation ward and spend three days on a comprehensive assessment. Often a spell of intensive exercises and work in the workshops or occupational therapy department will build up more power in the muscles whose tendons are to be transferred, thus making the procedure more successful. No tendon whose power is less than 4+ on the Medical Research Council (MRC) scale should be transferred, as all muscles lose grade 1 on transfer.

The effect of an arthrodesis can be imitated by applying a plaster and observing the patient's function. Both he and the medical team can then be convinced of the value of the proposed operation.

SHOULDER

Arthrodesis of the shoulder is sometimes useful. It is always necessary if pectoralis is being transferred to biceps to restore elbow flexion.

To restore *elbow flexion* several procedures are available. If both the long flexors and long extensors are spared and strong, then the Steindler procedure is used. The origins of the long flexors and extensors are mobilized and reinserted higher up on the humerus.

If these muscles are unavailable, then the Clark-Brooks transfer is used in which the pectoralis major is inserted into the biceps. The drawback here is that elbow flexion is accompanied by adduction both because of the action of the pectorals as adductors and also because in brachial plexus lesions, which are the common indication for this operation, the external rotators are paralysed.

In this event if adduction is a bar to function, an external rotation osteotomy of the humerus allows a more natural arc of flexion.

Recently whole muscle transfer with its neurovascular pedicle has been used successfully—the latissimus dorsi being the most effective. The biceps is usually removed to allow room for the transfer.

Operations to restore shoulder abduction are disappointing, but occasionally the Zachery transfer can be valuable. The tendons of latissimus dorsi and teres major are inserted into the tendon of infraspinatus, thus converting internal rotators into external rotators. A full passive range of movement, an intelligent patient and an intensive rehabilitation programme are all essential if this operation is to succeed. Many patients feel that they can dispense with abduction, managing well with the normal arm, but just occasionally this procedure may make all the difference to a particular person with a particular problem.

PARALYSIS OF WRIST EXTENSION

In the pure radial nerve palsy with all other upper limb muscles spared, the standard procedure is flexor carpi ulnaris to extensors of fingers and thumb, pronator teres to extend wrist and palmaris longus to abductor pollicis longus.

If one or more tendons are unavailable for transfer, as happens in plexus lesions, then an arthrodesis of the wrist gives stability and releases a tendon for transfer to give active finger extension to release grasp.

PARALYSIS OF OPPOSITION

In pure median nerve lesions, this is usually only indicated if the patient has some functional sensation in the median distribution as otherwise he is unlikely to use the transfer.

The best transfer is flexor sublimis of the ring finger; the tendon is taken round the tendon of flexor carpi ulnaris as a pulley and inserted into the extensor expansion of the thumb. If flexor digitorum sublimis is unavailable, extensor pollicis brevis or extensor indicis can be used.

In a high median lesion when the flexors to the index and middle fingers are paralysed these tendons are connected to the flexor profundus of the ulnar two fingers (supplied by the ulnar nerve) and produce a mass flexor action.

CLAW HAND

Dynamic transfers to correct hyperextension at the metacarpo-phalangeal joints and to provide active flexion at those joints are disappointing—they usually act as a tenodesis. Zancolli's procedure is the simplest and in most cases the most effective. The volar plate is plicated, thus bringing the MP joints into slight flexion.

LEG

The most satisfactory reconstructive procedures are around the ankle. Arthrodesis of the hip or knee certainly offers stability in paralysis of these joints, but is a very major decision and may seriously impair the patient's comfort in daily life.

Transfer of tibialis posterior or peroneus longus to the insertion of tibialis anterior will correct the tendency to inversion or eversion and allow active dorsiflexion. A flail ankle can be made stable by arthrodesis.

BRACHIAL PLEXUS LESIONS

By far the commonest causes of lesions of the brachial plexus are road traffic accidents, with motor cycle accidents forming the majority. Most are traction lesions, the plexus being stretched between its two points of attachment at the transverse processes of the vertebrae proximally and the clavipectoral fascia distally. If the lesion is violent, there may be actual ruptures of one or more of the C5, 6 or 7 roots. Very violent injuries cause avulsion of the roots from the cord and this is commonest in C8 and T1 whose ligamentous attachment to the transverse process of the vertebrae is much looser or even non-existent.

In most cases the traction is caused by sudden distraction of the neck on the arm as the body is thrown off the machine while the arm tends for a fraction of a second to retain its hold on the handlebars. Pressure lesions can occur; drunk or comatose patients have been seen who have lain for many hours on their arm and suffered severe degenerative lesions, but almost always these recover nearly completely for there is no distracting force to cause intraneural fibrosis and the lesion is in continuity. Stab wounds and surgical errors cause clean division of the roots or trunks and should be repaired as a primary procedure and usually do well. It is traction lesions that cause the greatest problems in diagnosis and management.

The clinical patterns commonly seen in practice are:

Complete C5, 6 in continuity
Complete C5, 6, 7 in continuity
Rupture C5, 6/C7, 8, T1 in continuity
Rupture C5, 6/avulsion C7, 8, T1
Avulsion of all five roots.

However, all combinations are seen and two- or even three-level lesions occur; for example, rupture of C5, 6 avulsion C7, 8, T1, rupture of median and musculocutaneous nerves at the axilla.

The fact that the infraspinatus rarely recovers in plexus lesions may be due to damage to the suprascapular nerve round the suprascapular notch. In many instances there are two, three or even four separate accidents. The patient is thrown off his motor cycle on impact and stretches the plexus, then hits the oncoming car and may further damage nerves or roots, then is thrown on to the road suffering further injury and well-meaning bystanders may then inflict a fourth injury when moving the patient from the road.

CLINICAL PICTURE

C5 lesion	Inability to abduct, externally rotate or elevate the arm.
C5, 6 lesion	In addition, inability to flex the elbow or adduct the humerus.

C5, 6, 7 lesion	In addition, inability to extend the elbow, wrist, fingers or thumb.
C8 lesion	Paralysis of the finger flexors, some wrist flexors and sometimes the thenar muscles.
T1 lesion	Paralysis of the intrinsics.

Thirty years ago exploration of the plexus for possible repair of traction lesions was given up. So much fibrosis was found that it was impossible to recognize nerve tissue from fibrosis, ruptures were rarely found and yet, despite the gloomy operative findings, reasonable recovery in the upper roots did occur. The work of Narakas (1977) has shown that ruptures are now much more common— occurring in up to one-third of cases—possibly because now that crash helmets are obligatory many patients with injuries so severe that they would have been killed without wearing a helmet are now surviving and we are seeing much more damage to the plexus.

This is important, for ruptures are susceptible to nerve grafting and return of function to at least those muscles supplied by C5, 6 and 7 can be expected. Repairs of C8 and T1 are not undertaken as the time for regeneration is so long (three years) that muscle fibrosis occurs before reinnervation. It is significant that the author's series of 134 cases treated non-operatively (Wynn Parry, 1974) showed that one-third of upper trunk lesions did not recover and these may well have been ruptures.

The diagnosis of a rupture is therefore important in our service. We suspect a rupture of a root if the accident has been violent—high speed with multiple injuries—if the lesion of that root is complete and if there is a strongly positive neuroma sign at the root of the neck referred to that root's dermatome. By this we mean that tapping causes *painful* tinglings—much more violent than the standard Tinel and definitely unpleasant. If the roots are avulsed from the cord, then the prognosis is hopeless and it is important to establish this early on. The diagnosis depends on the fact that in such avulsion injuries the posterior root ganglion remains intact, and although the patient has complete sensory loss in the distribution of that root, the root and nerve will still conduct an impulse, therefore sensory conduction studies will show a response. If there is associated nerve damage more distally as is quite common, the amplitude of sensory action potentials will be lower than normal, but the detection of a measurable response in the presence of anaesthesia indicates a preganglionic component. These studies have replaced the histamine test which relied on the axon reflex producing a flare in a preganglionic lesion. If there is a complete lesion both proximal and distal to the ganglion, the electrical findings will be those of a postganglionic lesion and, taken on their own, underestimate the severity of injury.

A Horner's syndrome indicates involvement of the sympathetic supply at T1 and therefore a lesion proximal to the ganglion. Myelography shows filling of root pouches due to tearing of the dura away from the cord. It is not completely reliable. In some cases it underestimates the severity of damage and in other cases recovery has been seen despite a positive myelogram. If the patient suffers intense burning crushing pain this strongly suggests a preganglionic lesion.

If the lesion is a traction lesion in continuity, i.e. no rupture or avulsion, then spontaneous recovery is likely and surgical exploration not indicated, for it is generally agreed that neurolysis is likely to do more harm than good by risking damage to nerves and blood vessels.

In summary, the three types of lesion can often be distinguished as follows:

Avulsion: Very violent injuries, multiple injuries, severe burning crushing pain, Horner's syndrome (T1), complete lesion, retention of sensory conduction, positive myelogram.

Rupture: Violent injury. Complete lesion, negative myelogram, absent sensory conduction, no Horner's syndrome. No pain, positive neuroma sign.

Traction in continuity: Mild violence. May be complete lesion—if surviving units found on EMG or contraction detected clinically this indicates an incomplete lesion with an excellent prognosis (Wynn Parry, 1974). Absent sensory conduction, negative myelogram, no Horner's syndrome, no pain, progressive painless Tinel.

Treatment

It is important to establish an accurate diagnosis as surgery of the plexus is time-consuming and challenging—exploration and grafting can take 12 hours or more.

If the lesion is in continuity, it is left alone. If ruptures are found they are repaired with sural nerve grafts or using the ulnar nerve if C8 and T1 are known to be avulsed. If, however, there is extensive loss of nerve tissue or a two-level lesion (C5, 6 roots, and musculocutaneous nerve for example) then grafting may be impossible and neurotization indicated. This involves mobilizing the upper four or six intercostal nerves and implanting them into the distal stump of the upper primary trunk or the median and musculocutaneous nerves, whichever is surgically most appropriate. Alternatively the accessory nerve can be used provided it has not been damaged. In avulsion injuries of the whole plexus, neurotization is the only means of offering any return of function.

Objectives are perforce limited—all one can expect is reasonable elbow flexion and shoulder adduction and occasionally wrist and even finger flexion with some protective sensation in the hand. This may in carefully selected cases offer the patient worthwhile function, but preoperative assessment is vital. The patient must be absolutely clear in his mind that only limited function can be expected and be sure that he or she really needs that movement in daily life. Admission to the rehabilitation ward for close study and assessment in the physiotherapy and occupational therapy departments is essential.

During the many months while waiting for recovery to occur either sponta-neously or after surgical repair, the patient must retain full passive movements in all the paralysed joints and use any spared muscles (in partial lesions) to the full. All patients should be assessed by the physiotherapist and if joints are stiff treated with progressive passive mobilization. Once satisfactory movement has been restored, the patient continues them at home. It is the physiotherapist's task to teach the patient and a responsible relative or friend how to carry out these movements. She should check regularly that range has been maintained — monthly in the early stages, three-monthly later on.

Surgical exploration of the plexus requires a good range of external rotation of the shoulder and it is therefore necessary in most cases to undertake an intensive programme of passive movements before surgery is possible. This underlines the great importance of maintaining passive range from the earliest days after injury. This is often overlooked in the patient with multiple injuries whose life is threatened; understandable but not acceptable.

Functional splintage offers patients with plexus lesions a reasonable degree of function; even the patient with total paralysis of the arm can be given some help. Paralysis of elbow flexion in C5, 6 lesions can be helped by an elbow-locking splint allowing the patient to fix his elbow in one of four positions so as to facilitate function of the spared hand. An attachment to provide dorsiflexion of the wrist can be added if the C7 root is involved.

In complete upper limb paralysis, the flail arm splint offers supportive func-tion, being an artificial arm over the flail arm, and helps to keep the arm in the pattern of movement and the body image so that when recovery occurs the patient will use the arm (Fig. 9.3). These splints are ready made.

All patients are reviewed every three months to ensure that splints are satis-factory, passive movements are being maintained and no problems are arising at work.

As soon as recovery begins, physiotherapy is again prescribed. We favour short intensive periods of rehabilitation (10–14 days); half or full day's physio-therapy to relearn the use of recovering muscles and build up power and stamina, and occupational therapy to use the arm in realistic activities to relearn func-tional patterns. The patient can then carry on these activities at home. For patients unable to attend local physiotherapy departments we readmit them to our minicare five-day ward. This allows comprehensive reassessment, including follow-up EMG studies and prolonged functional assessments. These are com-plex specialized problems and cannot be sorted out in a busy out-patient de-partment.

Once it is clear that no further recovery will occur, and this implies at least three years since injury for proximal muscles and longer for more distal muscles, reconstructive surgery can be considered. This may be stabilization by arthro-desis or offering movement by tendon transfer. If surgery is not possible then a permanent splint may be the solution. If so, it is justified to make a special splint to measure and incorporate refinements that would be unjustifiable as a

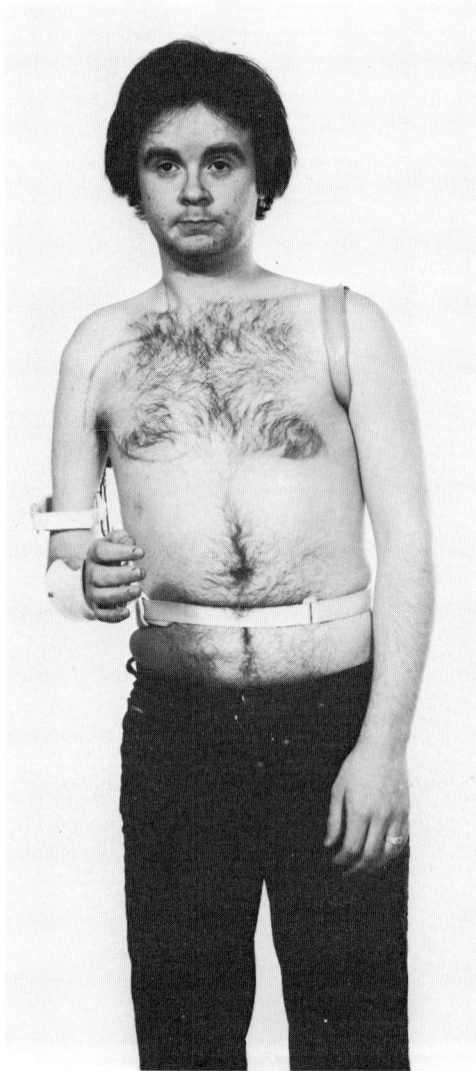

Fig. 9.3a   The flail arm splint.

temporary measure. A not uncommon pattern is a C5, 6, 7 palsy which shows only limited recovery—weak elbow flexion, no rotation or elevation of the shoulder, no recovery of wrist or finger extension and weakness of wrist flexion either due to C7 supply or partial involvement of C8. Neither a Steindler procedure nor tendon transfers for wrist or finger extension are feasible. A splint with a rotation element to allow positioning of the arm in variable rotation, elbow lock and wrist dorsiflexion piece can be worn as a permanent orthosis.

These splints are more expensive than the ready-made variety and require time and skill to produce, but are amply justified in such circumstances.

It used to be recommended that patients with flail arms due to avulsion of the plexus were best treated with amputation of the arm, arthrodesis of the shoulder and fitting of a prosthesis. Such a procedure was urged at an early stage before the patient becomes totally one-armed. This approach has been reversed of late; most patients with prostheses for brachial plexus palsy do not actually wear their arm (Randsford & Hughes, 1977) and almost all become fully one-armed within two months, and such early amputation is unjustifiable as it is impossible to assess the exact nature of the lesion and the prognosis so soon after injury.

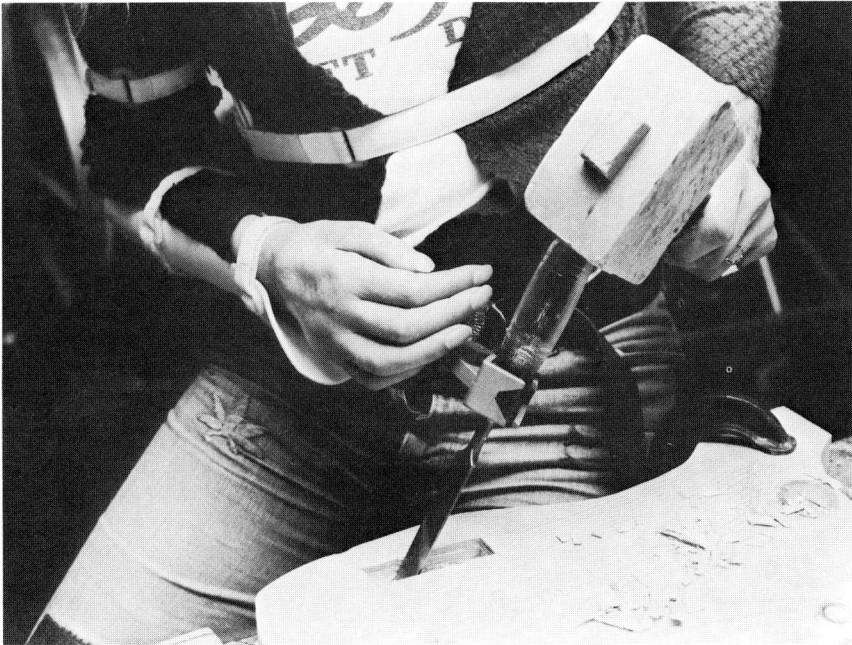

Fig. 9.3b Practical application of the flail arm splint.

Pain in Brachial Plexus Lesions

Avulsion of nerve roots is accompanied by one of the most distressing pains imaginable. Usually the pain starts two to three weeks after injury, though it can sometimes begin within a few hours of the accident. It is consistently described as burning, gnawing, gripping with often severe tinglings like unpleasant electric shocks. It is present continuously as a background and never remits by day or night. Many patients also experience periodic paroxysms of pain building up to a crescendo over several seconds until they feel as if they are about to burst. During these paroxysms they cannot continue conversations or activities. Some have paroxysms lasting minutes at a time and may have to retire to be alone. In some there is a regular pattern of crescendos, paroxysms, periods of increased pain, such that they can learn their particular pattern and adjust their activities to it.

Strangely enough, the pain does not usually prevent them from sleeping, although many like to take nitrazepam to help induction of sleep.

No outside stimulus has any effect on the pain—quite unlike causalgia. The pain appears to be *sui generis*—moreover few patients find any but mild relief from analgesics, however strong, and most give them up after a trial as they find the stupefying effect of drugs outweighs the minimal relief of pain. The few patients who have tried cannabis speak of its ability to modify the pain somewhat, but the effects on performance were quite unacceptable and all have given it up.

Distraction, in work, hobbies, conversation and sport, all damp down the pain and can even make it disappear during the period of strong involvement. This is why it is so important to encourage these patients to return to work or training as soon as possible as this may be the *only* way of helping pain. Some learn that total solitary relaxation in an armchair can take the brunt of the pain away, but meditation and hypnosis are surprisingly ineffective.

Presumably both relaxation and distraction bring in the patient's own central inhibitory tract from the thalamus via the raphe nucleus to the dorsal horn, and future research might do well to explore means of alerting and controlling this system (Chapter 4).

In 50% of 52 patients transcutaneous electrical stimulation relieved the pain, and in each case there was some afferent input to modulate.

> In one patient there was a total avulsion of C6–T1 with sparing of some of C5. Three months later, he was admitted to our rehabilitation ward where transcutaneous nerve stimulation was tried; stimulating over the back of the neck at C3–7 and the root of the neck. Pain was substantially relieved after two treatments and relief for most of the day followed regular use for two hours twice a day.

It is known that total deafferentation of a section of the cord causes the release of spontaneous discharges in the cells of lamina I and V in the dorsal horn some 10–30 days after section (Loeser *et al.*, 1968) and it is presumably this mechanism that is at work. This fits with the central nature of the pain, unrelieved by external events, and the timing after injury.

Patients are demoralized and disturbed by this pain—they cannot understand how a totally anaesthetic and flail arm can be painful. Some ask for amputation—but this, of course, never relieves the pain; the pain of phantom limbs should have warned surgeons off this field. They are helped by a careful explanation of the cause and at least the fact that the doctor does understand their problem and can give some reason for it. He can also, by listening to the experience of other patients' pain, recommend tricks and techniques that have been helpful.

Most patients either lose their pain after variable intervals or become so adapted to it that it no longer seriously affects their activities. It usually lasts at least a year—thereafter the proportion each year with severe pain lessens, leaving perhaps 10% with permanent intractable pain. It may be that in this group cerebral implants should be considered. In the past too many patients have been fobbed off by their doctor with the expression 'it is all in the mind' and regarded as 'functional' or depressed. We now know that the pain is indeed in the mind and it is here that relief must be found. Antidepressants have never helped these patients unless they do have a true depressive illness—which is very rare, the vast majority of these patients being extrovert cheerful young men.

Recently Nashold (1981) has reported excellent results from coagulation of the dorsal root entry zone. This procedure aims to destroy the abnormal firing cells.

RE-EDUCATION

Motor Re-education

During the stage of paralysis, while awaiting reinnervation, the patient is taught passive movements daily to keep a full range and appropriate lively splintage to encourage maximum function. Apart from periodic review to ensure that joints are supple, splints satisfactory and the patient at work, no formal physiotherapy is required. We are not impressed by the case for daily electrical stimulation of denervated muscle to prevent atrophy and it has never been shown to affect the work output of muscle in man. All experiments have been either on animals or have used plethysmography as a judge of muscle bulk and there are objections to this as a criterion of muscle function. One can have significant wasting with excellent power; bulk represents tissue fluid and fat among other ingredients. We have treated over 800 nerve lesions and have found that when reinnervation occurs muscle power and bulk return without the need for stimulation. When recovery is detected clinically, the patient should be encouraged to attend for a short period of intensive exercise to relearn the use of muscles that may have been paralysed for many months. He can continue these at home. Review should be frequent (two to three monthly) and periodic short spells of physiotherapy and occupational therapy instituted to capitalize on recovery. Splints can be discarded as soon as function allows and once muscle power has returned to MRC grade 3. The best form of treatment is realistic occupational therapy chosen with a mind to the patient's work or hobbies. Carpentry, metal work, gardening and printing with adapted handles are all popular with men and indeed with many women, but most women prefer household activities, typing, sewing and craft work. For lower limb injuries lathes and fretsaws can be adapted to provide progressive resistance. All types of games, both hand games such as blow football, weighted draughts, car race games (Wynn Parry, 1973) and gymnasium activities, can be encouraged. For nerve injuries in the leg, progressive cycle rides, walking, circuit training and later football are useful.

Regular muscle strength charting on the MRC scale and measurement of maximum strength and stamina using spring balances or strain gauges are valuable as a check on progress both for patient and doctor. The more objective measures that can be recorded the better.

Sensory Re-education

During the paralysed stage there will be anaesthesia in the distribution of the nerve. Quite soon after injury there is ingrowth of adjacent normal nerves into the denervated area and this can be quite extensive. The radial nerve has been seen to take over the pulp of the thumb and half the pulp of the index finger in median nerve lesions. Trophic lesions may occur in the anaesthetic area, particularly in median nerve and sciatic lesions. The patient must be carefully and repeatedly instructed by the therapist on avoiding these lesions: care in smoking, avoiding putting the hand on a radiator or hot stove, equal care in cold weather and when using the refrigerator. Gloves should always be worn in cold weather in nerve lesions involving the hand and thick woollen socks in sciatic or medial popliteal nerve lesions.

Functionally the most important sensory nerve is the median. It used to be thought that stereognosis never recovered after median nerve lesions, only protective sensation could be expected. It was believed that misrouting of axons was inevitable as they crossed the suture line and a high proportion would innervate the wrong receptors. Moreover it was believed that there was sensory specificity: special receptors and tracts with no overlap subserving the various modalities such as touch, pain, pressure, heat and cold.

The most widely used index of sensory recovery is two point discrimination (2 PD). As Onne pointed out in 1962, 2 PD is invariably poor, being over 20 mm in adults in the finger tips after median nerve sutures. In children, however, values of 2 PD can approach normal. There was thus an entrenched belief that the results of median nerve sutures might be satisfactory for motor recovery, but would always be poor for sensation.

Working in a military environment with highly skilled technicians, we found (Wynn Parry, 1966; 1973; Salter & Wynn Parry, 1977) that cooperative patients who needed their hands for skilled work could be re-educated to a level of stereognosis not far short of normal and that this was functionally most valuable.

As soon as some sensation returns to the finger tips, training is started. The patient is blindfolded and the unaffected part of the hand covered with gauze finger stalls. He is then presented with a number of wooden blocks of various shapes—square, rectangular, oval, etc.—and asked to feel around them and identify their shape. This is a good introduction to the patient in his first essay into learning again how to build up an image in the mind by tactile stimuli. If he fails to identify the object, he is asked to look at it and relate what he sees to what he feels. The process is then repeated with the blindfold on and continued until he has learned all the shapes. Next, different textures such as felt, wool, canvas, sheepskin and rubber are presented to the blindfolded patient and he tries to recognize these, describing out loud his impressions and building up a progressive image. He attempts recognition again and if he fails he looks at the texture and feels it, relating visual to tactile impressions. When successful with most textures he graduates to objects, thus summating texture, shape, temperature and density. Large objects are used first, then smaller ones. It is important to use objects with which the patient is familiar—it is no good giving most women a sparking plug. Table 9.1 shows our regime.

Table 9.1

Recognition times of objects 19 months after median and ulnar nerve suture at the wrist

	Seconds
String	17
Pencil	3
Small bottle	8
Nailbrush	4
Match	7
Shuttlecock	2

Two-point discrimination in mm 19 months after suture of the median nerve (figures in parentheses are 2 PD on equivalent site on normal hand)

	Index	Middle	Ring	Little	Thumb
Proximal	9 (2)	10 (3)	9 (3)	10 (3)	9 (1)
Middle	10	8	11	11	
Distal	8 (2)	9 (2)	15 (2)	13 (2)	12 (1)

Training sessions are short to avoid fatigue, 15 minutes twice a day, and a relative is taught the technique so the training can be continued at home. Quite quickly with training, patients become more aware of their hand and begin to use it for everyday activities which they had avoided previously. At regular intervals, usually three-weekly, tests are carried out using different textures and objects. The patient is not told the results so that there will not be a training effect from the tests. Most patients regain satisfactory stegnosis and some have been able to return to intricate skilled work requiring 'blind' finger activities and played keyboard instruments.

In 23 patients after median nerve sutures the average time for recognition of textures at the start of training was 34 seconds, most patients being able to recognize four textures.

After an average of 9 weeks' training seven textures could be recognized in an average time of 19 seconds.

Similarly, the average time for recognition of objects was 23 seconds and after 9 weeks' training this fell to 11 seconds—the patient being able to recognize seven more objects (Wynn Parry & Salter, 1976).

We have confirmed Onne's work that 2 PD is grossly abnormal in such patients and Table 9.1 shows that 2 PD can be poor yet sensory function excellent. 2 PD most probably measures nerve fibre density and as such is useful as an academic test to gauge proportion of fibres reaching the periphery, but it is no use as a test of *function*. We believe that clinical sensory testing should include the recognition of objects and textures. Finally it must be appreciated that when one attempts to feel an object to recognize it, one automatically moves it between fingers and thumb. Attempts to identify (correctly) something laid statically on the finger tip as in the 2 PD test always fail.

This gives the clue as to how retraining may work. Clearly the ability to regain stereognosis is incompatible with the specificity theory of sensation, for it is well recognized that there is considerable misrouting of axons. It is now believed that although there is certainly some degree of end organ specificity, many fibres respond to several different types of stimuli, and it is the pattern of activity both spatially and temporally that determines the nature of sensation. The pattern of impulses reaching the cord will depend on a large number of variables including the frequency, interval between discharges, and sequential firing of fibres.

In retraining one is attempting to train the patient to learn a new code, for the pattern of firing will be abnormal due to a smaller number of fibres firing with a slower conduction speed. Central remodelling certainly occurs and sensory re-education is eminently worth trying in all patients with median nerve lesions who need that sensation in daily life. Sometimes hyperaesthesia is a serious problem for stereognosis and we have found that transcutaneous electrical stimulation proximal to the nerve applied for periods of one hour or more regularly several times daily can inhibit the hyperaesthesia and allow much improved stereognosis.

Localization is an important parameter of sensation and is always disordered after nerve sutures in adults. This too can be easily trained. The patient is blindfolded, touched in various places and asked to locate the touch. If wrong, he opens his eyes and relates what he sees to where he feels it; re-education usually only takes three weeks of training.

PAIN

A number of peripheral nerve disorders are associated with pain. These include painful neuromata, causalgia, irritative neuritis, painful amputation stumps and plexus avulsion. Even the most skilled suture of nerve does not prevent a number of fibres escaping from the sheath and forming a neuroma—this is usually painless although many patients have a persistent strongly positive Tinel's sign at the suture line. In some cases this may be very painful and cause severe painful paraesthesiae when knocked or rubbed and permanent tinglings in the distribution of the affected nerve. This may be so distressing as to exclude all use of the hand. Often resuture and even two attempts at resuture are tried and we have seen patients in whom, even after the highest class of surgery with interfascicular grafting under microscope cover, the pain returns often more severely than before.

If the neuroma is only painful on pressure or touch then a wrist band with a hole around the neuroma and a cover on top of it may be enough. But if there is spontaneous pain and paraesthesiae then other measures must be sought. It is possible that there are two mechanisms to this pain—one peripheral and one central. Wall and Gutnik (1974) showed that the terminal neuroma after cutting the sciatic nerve in a rat produces spontaneous discharges which can be suppressed by proximal electrical stimulation of the nerve.

Some deafferentation occurs with nerve lesions and the balance between large and small diameter afferent activity in the dorsal horn is changed so that there is excessive activity in laminas I and V and pain is felt. As Cevero *et al.* (1976) showed, electrical stimulation of the large diameter afferent fibres can suppress this activity. We have found transcutaneous nerve stimulation (TNS) most helpful in these patients.

We apply our electrodes just proximal to (never over) the painful area and adjust the parameters of pulse width, amplitude and repetition rate according to the patient's reaction. We stimulate for many hours at a time and feel sure that the reports of disappointment with this technique are due to inadequate stimulation time. Most patients are stimulated twice a day and are encouraged both during and between stimulation to use their hand normally. There is thus a big advantage in admitting such patients to a rehabilitation ward so they may have a full programme of stimulation and activity in phsyiotherapy and occupational therapy departments. It is believed that this allows normal movement patterns to replace the abnormal ones set up by the neuroma. Many patients are provided with their own stimulator, which in England is now available on the National Health Service, and wear it all day if necessary. Our experience is similar to those who have worked with central stimulation—a short period of stimulation (one to two hours) gives many hours of relief. Moreover the effect is cumulative and longer and longer periods of relief with less and less stimulation are found. The process is one of trial and error—each patient has his own pattern of response and his own characteristic setting of parameters for stimulation. Some patients need to use the stimulator for many weeks or even indefinitely, a few gain immediate and permanent relief after two or three sessions. Some 'escape' from the effect and the treatment becomes gradually less useful, so prolonged follow-up is necessary.

We find that about 65% of patients with painful neuromas or irritative neuritis, e.g. ulnar neuritis at the elbow, respond satisfactorily. Vibration, massage, acupuncture are all believed to work in a similar way, but in our hands TNS is pre-eminent, and only if it fails do we attempt other peripheral modulating techniques.

Painful paraesthesiae in the sole of the foot are common and very distressing after sciatic nerve lesions. Some patients prefer total anaesthesia to this spontaneous sensation and ask for nerve section. TNS can be helpful and is best used permanently, for the firm pressure of walking on the sole modifies the pain presumably by increasing afferent input. Repeated nerve blocks with long-acting anaesthetics are sometimes dramatically successful and can be used in combination with TNS. A firm ortholene anklet pressing on neuromas of the sural nerve have been helpful also. But these painful peripheral nerve conditions in our hands have proved much more intransigent than in the upper limb.

Hand surgeons are all too familiar with the painful amputation stump—often of a tip of a finger—leading to successive amputations at higher levels, only for the pain to return and even to spread to other unaffected fingers. In the same way as in painful neuromas, multiple operations must be avoided. Once pain has been present for any length of time, it becomes central and peripheral destructive surgery only adds to the deafferentation and compounds the issue. TNS and vibration are often dramatic in these cases and should always be given an extended trial.

We have seen extraordinary results from TNS in patients with painful phantom limbs even when treated many years after amputation. One patient whose pain had been present for 18 years was treated thus. First she felt the fingers of the phantom unclench, then straighten, then the elbow straightened and she then lost her pain completely after a week's stimulation, two hours twice daily. She now uses the stimulator a few times a week to keep the pain at bay. Similar spectacular results in avulsion injuries are alas rare, possibly because the avulsion produces much more severe central damage and sets off more reverberating circuits than a traumatic amputation.

Causalgia

This extraordinary condition follows partial nerve lesions and is commonly seen after missile wounds near the median and sciatic nerves. The term should be reserved for such cases and *not* used for pain in plexus avulsion—the nature and reaction to treatment are entirely different.

The patient feels a constant burning in the hand or foot, which is slightly relieved by applying moisture—some patients go around with the part wrapped in moist towels. Weir Mitchell's patient kept his feet wet in his boots to avoid jarring his body on walking—even trivial external stimuli can elicit excruciating pain—a puff of air, banging of a door, a car starting up and emotional situations can be desperately painful. The part is cyanotic and cold, osteoporosis develops and the patient's whole life is taken up with his pain. This is in marked contrast to the pain in plexus avulsion, where external stimuli have no effect. Blocking the sympathetic by intravenous guanethedine or stellate ganglion block can dramatically relieve pain, but often only temporarily.

Success is usually taken as an indication to proceed to sympathectomy, but the sympathetic nervous system has an unrivalled penchant for regeneration and most pain specialists prefer repeated stellate or lumbar sympathetic blocks. It is essential to incorporate these techniques into a planned rehabilitation programme so that the patient uses the limb when pain-free and re-establishes normal patterns of neural activity.

What is the nature of causalgia? Clearly there must be a sympathetic disorder, for the symptoms and signs are those of sympathetic over-reaction, and there must also be the peripheral and central effects of deafferentation. The whole panoply of techniques for peripheral nerve pain relief may need to be deployed — sympathetic blocking, TNS, vibration, acupuncture and intensive rehabilitation.

ELECTRODIAGNOSTIC TECHNIQUES

Electrodiagnostic techniques are of great value in the diagnosis and prognosis of peripheral nerve injuries. In clinical practice, the commonest situations where they are used are:

1.   to assess if regeneration has begun at a time after suture when reinnervation could be expected, for electrical signs precede clinical signs of recovery by many weeks

2.   to decide if denervation is present when symptoms of nerve damage are present but there are no objective signs

3.   to assess the extent of damage in a partial lesion and by serial studies to determine if a lesion is remaining static, deteriorating or improving; this is of particular value in lesions suspected of being due to compression—e.g. entrapment neuropathies

4.   to establish if a brachial plexus lesion is preganglionic or postganglionic

5.   to assess the presence of anomalous innervation

6.   to decide if neurological deficit is due to root or nerve involvement, e.g. distinguish in a patient with paraesthesiae in the thumb and index finger, between cervical spondylosis and median nerve compression at the wrist or in a patient with paraesthesiae in the big toe between L5 root pressure and a lateral popliteal palsy.

Electrodiagnosis uses two fundamental techniques: the activity of muscle at rest and on effort by recording with a needle electrode and displaying its electrical activity on the oscilloscope, and the response of motor and sensory nerve to electrical stimulation.

At rest a normal muscle is silent on EMG, on minimal contraction a few motor units fire, each unit comprising the axon and a variable number of terminal nerve fibres. Units are small in facial muscles (100 μV, 2–3 ms duration) and large in the proximal limb muscles (up to 5 mV and 10 ms in duration). As effort increases, so more units fire and their frequency increases until the whole base line of the oscilloscope trace is obliterated to produce the so-called full interference pattern. If motor units have been damaged then the interference pattern is incomplete.

Some 18–21 days after denervation, the muscle fibres no longer controlled by their nerve revert to their embryonic pre-innervation behaviour and start to contract spontaneously. This activity is picked up on EMG as spontaneous fibrillation, potentials of amplitude 100 μV and duration of 1 ms which, of course, cannot be detected by the naked eye. Thus the detection of these fibrillation potentials in a resting muscle are indicative of denervation. As the motor unit breaks up in active degeneration, the units are seen to be complex and polyphasic because the myelin is disintegrating, conduction in the distal terminals is slowed and temporal dispersion occurs. Exactly the same type of unit is seen in early regeneration, for the nerve terminals in the newly formed unit also conduct slowly because the myelin is immature. The detection of a few polyphasic units of low amplitude and prolonged duration in a clinically paralysed muscle is a sure sign of recovery. In chronic partial denervation, denervated muscle fibres are incorporated into adjacent normal motor units by sprouts from normal nerve fibres, thus producing motor units of much greater amplitude than normal. These so-called giant units are another sign of denervation—units may be seen of amplitude 10 mV or even greater.

Motor nerves conduct at an average rate of 50 m/s and sensory nerves at a slightly faster rate. It is easy to measure conduction velocities by recording muscle activity with needle or from surface electrodes and stimulating the nerve at various accessible points. By using surface electrodes and stimulating beyond a point when no further current produces any increase in the size of response, one can gain an accurate idea of whether all the motor units are responding as values are known for most muscles. In a suspected ulnar nerve lesion, for example, one can record over the abductor digit minimi and stimulate the ulnar nerve at the wrist, just below and just above the elbow and in the axilla. Latencies are thus obtained at each level, and by measuring the distances from the sites of stimulation, velocities are calculated for each segment of nerve. In this way, local slowing can be detected and the site of an entrapment neuropathy revealed.

Sensory conduction is measured in a similar manner. In the hand, sensory action potentials can be recorded by stimulating the digits with ring electrodes and recordings made over the appropriate nerves at the wrist. The radial sensory potential is obtained by stimulating the nerve antidromically in the mid-forearm over the radius and recording over the first dorsal inter-osseous space. The musculocutaneous nerve sensory potential is found by stimulating at the elbow and recording over the lateral border of the forearm. In the leg the sural potential is obtained by stimulating just lateral to the midline 14 cm proximal to the Achilles tendon and the recording along the lateral malleolus. Two examples of the value of these techniques in assessing the site of entrapment may be given.

In a suspected compression lesion of the median nerve in the carpal tunnel, the sensory action potential may be smaller than normal and delayed in time (latency). The distal latency or time taken from stimulus at wrist to the abductor pollicis brevis (chosen for its virtually invariable median supply) may be prolonged whilst the velocity in the forearm is normal. The normal latency from wrist to APB is 4 ms. A delay of more than 5 ms is significant of compression and more than 7 ms represents a severe lesion and needs surgical decompression. One of the earliest signs is reduction or loss of the median sensory action potential, which may occur well before there is any change in the motor response. These changes in conduction can occur before fibrillation appears or a substantial reduction in amplitude of the motor response.

In a suspected compression lesion of the ulnar nerve at the elbow, the sensory action potential from little finger to wrist may be reduced or absent, the mixed nerve action potential from wrist to above elbow also abnormal, while the response from above elbow to axilla is normal.

With recording electrodes over the abductor digit minimi, the response to supramaximal stimulation at the wrist might be 5 mV, just below the elbow 4.5 mV, just above the elbow and in the axilla 2.5 mV, thus indicating a pressure lesion at the elbow. The conduction velocities would be normal in the forearm but slowed across the elbow segment. If the lesion were more severe and involved a significant degree of Wallerian degeneration, the amplitude at the wrist would be markedly reduced and velocities slowed. Measurement of amplitudes is a helpful guide to the amount of denervation, and serial amplitude measurements will show recovery if they increase or deteriorate or if they diminish with time. We thus like to study conduction both by needles which allow detection of denervation by showing fibrillation and giant units and with surface electrodes to allow quantification of the response.

The detection of local blocks to conduction due to local segmental demyelination can be demonstrated in all the accessible nerves. For example, in a suspected pressure lesion of the median nerve between the two heads of pronator teres, conduction velocities and amplitudes will be normal when stimulating at the wrist and recording over abductor pollicis brevis, while conduction will be prolonged and amplitudes reduced when stimulating in the axilla.

Block of the lateral popliteal nerve will be shown at the knee by recording over extensor digitorum brevis and stimulating at the ankle, at the neck of the fibula and in the popliteal fossa.

Brachial Plexus Lesions

As discussed above, the key to prognosis is to distinguish the preganglionic lesion from the lesion distal to the posterior root ganglion—for in the preganglionic lesion the prognosis is hopeless, while in the latter there may be a prospect for recovery.

In preganglionic lesions, although there is total anaesthesia, the cell body of the sensory nerve is still intact and thus the peripheral sensory nerve will conduct an electrical impulse. Consequently sensory action potentials will still be present although sensation is absent. There is often some damage to the nerve in its postganglionic course and so the action potentials may be reduced in amplitude, but it remains true that any evoked action potential in sensory nerve in an anaesthetic area implies preganglionic involvement. Hence, recording sensory action potentials in the C5–T1 roots is an essential part of the investigation of plexus lesions.

It must of course be realized that if there is also a distal lesion, e.g. rupture or complete axonotmesis of nerves distal to the ganglion, the electrical findings will be those of a postganglionic lesion, i.e. absence of a sensory response.

Root Lesions

Proximal nerve or root involvement by pressure such as in cervical ribs and thoracic outlet syndromes or spondylosis or other causes of root pressure result in local demyelination, but not changes in distal conduction. Thus in a cervical rib, denervation may be found in abductor pollicis brevis and also sometimes in an ulnar supplied muscle, yet sensory conduction as judged by median and ulnar sensory action potentials will be preserved and motor conduction will be normal. The same holds true in spondylosis—tinglings in the hand with preserved sensory and motor conduction with denervation in small hand muscles will suggest root involvement as will preservation of sural and lateral popliteal nerve sensory potentials with tinglings in the foot and denervation in L5, S1 supplied muscles.

A lesion can be assigned to a particular root by demonstrating denervation (spontaneous fibrillation) in muscles supplied by that root, but not in other muscles.

Facial Nerve

There are certain situations when elaborate techniques such as have been described of motor and sensory conduction are not necessary and when simple techniques provide the answer. This is particularly true of the neurapraxias. A good example is Bell's palsy. Here, there is complete paralysis of facial muscles on one side. Five to ten days after onset, EMG will be of no help—denervation in the form of spontaneous fibrillation does not appear for 18 days and because of the block no units appear on effort on the oscilloscope.

However, if the facial nerve is stimulated at the stylomastoid foramen, contraction will be seen in all the facial muscles. The threshold can be compared with that on the normal side and should in a non-degenerative case be less than twice that of the affected side. Amplitudes to supramaximal stimulation can also be compared on the two sides by recording with surface electrodes over a facial muscle.

Wynn Parry and King (1977) showed that the vast majority of complete palsies in whom nerve conduction was retained at five days recovered completely. However, a few cases showed late denervation—after ten days—and the only way to pick these up is by serial conduction studies, so it is wise to study the response to nerve conduction, both qualitatively and quantitatively, up to three weeks after onset so as to detect these few patients who show late denervation. The same authors showed that if such patients had their facial nerves decompressed within four weeks there was a better chance of recovery than if treated conservatively. They also showed that electrical stimulation of the muscles when denervated in a degenerative lesion had no effect on the functional result, nor had splintage by lifting the corner of the mouth any effect on the ultimate cosmetic or functional result.

Ideally all patients in whom surgery for relief of pressure on peripheral nerves is planned should have EMG studies first to confirm the diagnosis. Many are the patients with pins and needles along the inner side of the forearm and in the ulnar two fingers whose ulnar nerves have been transposed at the elbow with no relief because their symptoms were due to a cervical rib or band, and many patients have had their carpal tunnels sectioned without relief of paraesthesiae in the median supplied fingers because the cause was to be found in the neck. In many patients too, the clinically obvious local pressure lesion was associated with a generalized neuropathy, the first signs being seen in sites vulnerable to pressure. In all these examples careful EMG studies looking at motor and sensory conduction in both clinically affected and unaffected nerves would have given the answer.

However, there are vast numbers of such patients and few centres to provide EMG services, so selection is inevitable. In most patients the diagnosis of compression of the median nerve in the carpal tunnel is obvious and EMG studies are not essential, but if there is any doubt operation should be delayed until EMG can be arranged.

It is the author's view that no operation on the ulnar nerve should be undertaken without full EMG investigations—many patients have been made worse by unnecessary interference with the nerve.

FUTURE

Clearly the most desirable advance will be in the field of prevention; reducing the frequency of motor cycle accidents, preventing injuries in the home and banning glass from public doors. We urgently need more sophisticated techniques to distinguish traction lesions in continuity from ruptures and avulsion of the brachial plexus. Far superior artificial limbs must be developed before it is justifiable to recommend amputation in a total preganglionic plexus lesion.

It is unlikely that microsurgery with interfascicular suture will significantly improve the results as compared with epineural suture in the best hands, but more universal adoption of intensive rehabilitation programmes would certainly improve results.

REFERENCES

CEVERO F., IGGO A. & OGAWA H. (1976) Nociceptor-driven dorsal horn neurones in the lumbar spinal cord of the cat. *Pain*, **2**, 5–24.

GOODMAN H.V. & GILLIATT R.W. (1961) The effect of treatment on median nerve conduction in patients with the carpal tunnel syndrome. *Annals of Physical Medicine, London*, **6**, 137–55.

LOESER J.D., WARD A.A. JR & WHITE L.E. JR (1968) Chronic deafferentation of human spinal cord neurons. *Journal of Neurosurgery, Chicago*, **29**, 48–50.

MILLESI H., MEISSL G. & BERGER A. (1972) The interfascicular nerve-grafting of the median and ulnar nerves. *Journal of Bone and Joint Surgery: American volume, Boston*, **54A**, 727–50.

MILLESI H., MEISSL G. & BERGER A. (1976) Further experience with interfascicular grafting of the median, ulnar and radial nerves. *Journal of Bone and Joint Surgery: American volume, Boston*, **58A** (2), 209–18.

NASHOLD B.S.,WITAN B., ZOREB D.S. (1976). Phantom pain relief, by focal destruction of the substantia gelatinosa of Rolando. *Advances in Pain Research and Therapy*. Ch. 1, pp. 959–63. Eds. Bonica J.J. & Albe Pessard D. Raven Press, New York.

NARAKAS A. (1977) Indications et résultats du traîtement chirurgical direct dans les lésions par élongation du pleaus brachial. I—Les indications du traîtement chirurgical direct. *Revue de Chirurgie Orthopédique et Réparatrice de l'Appareil Moteur, Paris*, **63** (1), 88–106.

OCHOA J., FOWLER T.J. & GILLIATT R.W. (1972) Anatomical changes in peripheral nerves compressed by a pneumatic tourniquet. *Journal of Anatomy*, **113**, 433–55.

ÖNNE L. (1962) Recovery of sensibility and sudomotor activity in the hand after nerve suture. *Acta Chirurgica Scandinavica*, Supplementum **300**. Stockholm.

RANSFORD A.O. & HUGHES S.P. (1977) Complete brachial plexus lesions: a ten-year follow-up of twenty cases. *Journal of Bone and Joint Surgery: British volume, London*, **59B** (4), 417–20.

SEDDON H.J. (1972) *Surgical Disorders of the Peripheral Nerves*. Churchill Livingstone, Edinburgh.

STAAL A. (1970). The entrapment neuropathies. In *Handbook of Clinical Neurology* (Eds. Vinken P.T. & Bruyn G.W.), Vol. 7, pp. 285–325. North Holland Publ. Co., Amsterdam.

SUNDERLAND S. (1968) *Nerves and Nerve Injuries*. Livingstone, Edinburgh.

WALL P.D. & GUTNICK M. (1947) Properties of afferent nerve impulses originating from a neuroma. *Nature, London*, **248**, 740–3.

WYNN PARRY C.B. (1966) *Rehabilitation of the Hand*, 2e. Butterworths, London.

WYNN PARRY C.B. (1973) *Rehabilitation of the Hand*, 3e. Butterworths, London.

WYNN PARRY CB. (1974) The management of injuries to the brachial plexus. *Proceedings of the Royal Society of Medicine, London*, **67**, 488–90.

WYNN PARRY C.B. & KING P.F. (1977) Results of treatment in peripheral facial paralysis. A 25 year study. *Journal of Laryngology and Otology, London*, **91** (7), 551–64.

WYNN PARRY C.B. & Salter M. (1976) Sensory re-education after median nerve lesions. The hand. *Journal of the British Society for Surgery of the Hand, Brentwood*, **8** (3), 250–7.

WYNN PARRY C.B. (1981). *Rehabilitation of The Hand*. Butterworths, London.

Chapter 10

Rehabilitation of Patients Suffering from Chronic Pain

INTRODUCTION

Pain is obviously a ubiquitous human experience and has been one of the most important aspects of medical practice for many centuries. The introduction of opiates and the development of anaesthetic techniques have brought remarkable changes in both surgical and medical therapies. At one time, management of acute pain was one of the most difficult and frustrating of all medical tasks. That is no longer the case and the horrors of post-injury, operative and post-operative pain are now largely of historical interest only. Nevertheless, management of the patient in chronic pain is far less satisfactory (Bonica, 1953). The opiates have limited value and there are few alternatives, except in pain of cancer origin. Delineating proper treatment for chronic pain of benign origin is an unsolved problem and represents a major part of medical practice now in virtually every country in the world. To complicate matters further, the expression of pain is very different in different nations and among different socio-economic groups. It is definitely influenced by the working environment, disability and social programmes, and the possibility of legal compensation for injury. Furthermore, the patient in chronic pain is poorly managed by otherwise competent physicians in virtually every medical system yet devised (Hackett, 1971). These patients tend to be over-treated, misunderstood, and finally rejected from the medical system because of their failure to respond to therapy. The experience described in this chapter is based on the USA, but the basic principles probably hold throughout most other countries. The major differences between our patients and those seen in other countries are likely to be in the psychosocial expressions of pain and suffering rather than in the pain itself.

The magnitude of the problem can scarcely be over-estimated. Low back pain is one of the most common reasons for being admitted to hospital in the USA. Pain in cancer is a major occurrence, though no one is entirely sure how frequently it complicates the treatment of neoplastic disease. Vocational disability causes huge expenditures in many countries of the world. Hospitalizations for medical and surgical therapy of pain add immense amounts to the yearly expenditures for health care in most modern industrial nations. Ineffectual surgery is often performed and ineffectual medicines are often prescribed. Only recently has it been understood that the patient complaining of chronic pain is likely to present a complex mixture of somatic injury, psychosocial abnormality and psychiatric disability, usually complicated by iatrogenic factors. In order to plan sensible therapy for the patient in chronic pain, it is necessary to carry out a rational assessment of these factors. We believe that this assessment must begin with an accurate physical diagnosis, complete assessment of psychiatric and psycho-social factors, institution of physical rehabilitation measures, elimination of drug dependence and misuse, while motivating the individual patients to assume responsibility for their own health and for facing the realities of their own situation. The material in this chapter will summarize our current methods of attaining these goals. However, it should be stressed that none of these tech-niques are considered satisfactory at the present time. All must be modified and improved as our understanding of pain grows. They all represent practical methods of solving the problems these patients present. There are no completely satisfactory techniques available at the present time and great improvements in the management of chronic pain are to be expected as research delineates the problem further.

The Patient in Chronic Pain

In the USA back pain and neck pain are by far the most common symptoms with which patients present for pain therapy (Sternbach *et al.*, 1973). Other common problems include spinal cord injury and post-thalamic stroke pain, peripheral nerve injury pain, the pain of metabolic peripheral neuritis, abdomi-nal or pelvic pain secondary to benign visceral disease and unusual forms of headache. Headache itself is usually treated by individual practitioners or in specialized facilities and patients with typical headache syndromes such as migraine rarely come to a pain treatment rehabilitation centre. Other specific problems such as trigeminal neuralgia are usually managed by individual prac-titioners without the need for the complicated pain therapy programmes. Pain in cancer takes a variety of forms, but again, these patients rarely present to the comprehensive pain treatment programme. It is more likely that patients with pain secondary to complications of cancer therapy, either painful surgical areas or post-irradiation pain, will make their way to a comprehensive centre.

Irrespective of the diagnosis, the consequences to the patient are approxi-mately the same. Our average patient has undergone six operations in the treatment of the underlying disease and the treatment of pain. Eighty-five per cent are addicted to narcotics either physiologically or psychologically and an equal number misuse a variety of medications, usually sleeping medications and tranquillizers. An extremely high percentage are depressed and suffer chronic anxiety. Nearly all are seriously insomniac and most have allowed the pain to become the primary fixation of their existence. They talk of nothing else, think of nothing else and orient their entire lives about the pain process. A rational approach to therapy must investigate all of these problems and attempt to deal with them (Merskey & Spear, 1967).

The Diagnosis

It is our belief that the most common error in the management of chronic pain arises in the original diagnosis. The most common mistake is to overlook a significant psychiatric or psychosocial abnormality and to apply a therapy for a physical diagnosis without regard to a serious psychological concomitant (Blumer, 1975). This is particularly true for low back pain. Therefore, it is mandatory when beginning therapy in the patient disabled by chronic pain, to be absolutely certain of the physical diagnosis and to be equally certain of present and past psychological factors. We begin with a scrupulous review of the physical abnormalities and the establishment of a physical diagnosis whenever possible. This will include review of previous studies and therapies and review of the current situation as seems indicated in the judgement of the attending physician. Equally important is a complete psychosocial history and psychiatric evaluation. Our evaluation of these patients begins with an out-patient psychological examination by a clinical psychologist and a psychiatric interview when it appears to be indicated to either the original examining physician or the clinical psychologist. In addition, the patients will be tested with a battery of psychological tests. These include the Hendler–Long Ten Minute Screening Test for chronic pain patients, the California Personality Inventory, the SCL-90, the Adjective Check List, the Minnesota Multiphasic Personality Inventory, the Wechsler Adult Intelligence Scale, the Bender–Gestalt Test and the Wechsler Memory Scale. The complete psychosocial history includes previous work records, marital history, relationships with parents, previous use of drugs and alcohol, and a careful review of the current marital situation. Equally careful drug intake histories are obtained. At the end of these two examinations, it is usually possible to assess the physical status of the patient and to determine the underlying cause of the apparent pain. It is also possible to determine whether the patients have any specific therapy which may be utilized for them. The influence of psychiatric and psychosocial factors can be clearly understood and the importance of all of these factors can be ordered into a reasonable treatment plan. At this point, we would make the following sample treatment plan. It begins with a physical diagnosis and determines what corrective or symptomatic measures may be applied to that diagnosis. It adds psychiatric and social factors and directs behavioural therapy at these factors. The importance of drug abuse or misuse is assessed and a corrective regimen begun. The patient's physical disabilities are reviewed and corrective exercise procedures commence. The overall aim of the programme will be treatment of pain, but with major behavioural changes irrespective of the achievement of pain relief.

Psychological Factors in Chronic Pain

There are three major psychological effects of chronic pain which occur ubiqui-
tously throughout our patient population. These are chronic anxiety, depression
and insomnia (Sternbach, 1974). Before discussing these three factors in detail,
however, it is well to review the preliminary results of psychological testing in
our patients carried out over a three-year period. The results of these tests have
been used in a pragmatic patient classification devised by Hendler and Long
which helps guide therapy. This classification is not meant to be psychodynam-
ically complete, but is currently employed only for therapy planning in the
context of our programme. On the basis of the physical examination and psychological testing, we divide our patients into four groups. The first of these we term
the *objective pain response*. These patients have a demonstrable cause of the pain
and respond to it in a reasonable way without significant psychological aberra-
tion. The second category we term the *exaggerated pain response*. This does not
imply that the pain is exaggerated, but rather that the patient's disability is out
of keeping with the level of abnormality discovered. In the USA such patients
usually have had an industrial injury and are seeking industrial disability or they
have suffered an injury in which litigation in the courts for personal injury is
under way. Such patients may well have a physical abnormality, but it generally
is not severe and the degree of incapacitation appears to be greater than the
physical findings warrant. The third classification is the *affective or psychiatric*
group. These patients appear to have pain as an expression of primary psychiatric disease. This is always a difficult statement to substantiate, but in any event
the psychiatric factors here completely overshadow the physical abnormalities.
Our fourth group we simply call pain of *unexplained origin*. In this group of
patients, we cannot find a physical cause of pain, but the patient's response does
not appear to be psychologically abnormal. These patients are generally managed in a symptomatic way and followed while we look for the underlying cause
of pain. On the basis of these same studies we also see that patients in chronic
pain exhibit much the same symptom stages as described by Kubler-Ross in
fatal disease. After our initial evaluations, we also describe our patients according
to the following classifications. Stage I, which is the subacute phase, is characterized by *anxiety*. The patients are usually unwilling to accept the abnormality,
do not wish to hear treatment plans which do not include total cure and return
to premorbid stage, and often go from physician to physician accepting therapies
which give promise of a cure. The second phase, which usually begins after six
months or more, is characterized by *anger*, hostility and a litigious mood. These
patients are angry with themselves and angry with the medical profession over
their failure to be improved. The third phase is the one in which the average
patient presents at a comprehensive pain treatment centre. This is characterized
by profound *depression* and may last for years. These patients have given up and
have resorted to complete inactivity, hypochondriacal fixation upon the pain,
the hopeless, helpless feeling of depression, and the misuse of drugs. The fourth

phase is that of *rational acceptance*. These patients have come to grips with their abnormality, accepted their limitations, and are able to be treated in a reasonable fashion.

This kind of patient characterization has great value in a practical sense. Patients with objective pain problems are candidates for interventional procedures, but only after they have been brought to the fourth stage of their disease. Patients with exaggerated and psychiatric pain complaints are rarely, if ever, candidates for interventional procedures, and therapy must be directed at the underlying behavioural problems. Unfortunately, in our series there is little difference between these groups in terms of the numbers of operations the patients have undergone and the kinds of drugs with which they are treated. Therefore, we are often in the position of attempting to correct an iatrogenic problem in a patient whose problem began with an exaggerated pain response or an affective pain complaint. Nevertheless, careful assessment of the patient's underlying problem and the current stage of the development of the pain complaint will be very valuable in planning therapy.

Beginning Therapy

Psychotropic drug use, from a practical standpoint, is necessary first to eliminate those symptoms which can be easily treated (Reiser, 1972). One of these is depression. It is mandatory to treat the patient's depression if any success in the overall programme is to be obtained. We usually employ a tricyclic antidepressant such as amitryptiline 75–100 mg at bedtime, employed in this way to take advantage of its sedative effect and also provide relief from insomnia. The tricyclic antidepressants are particularly effective in chronic pain states. Chronic anxiety should also be treated. The specific anti-anxiety agent is probably not important. We favour fluphenazine 1 mg three times a day, which is potent and has little sedative effect, but there are many other effective drugs. The combination of tranquillizers and antidepressant drugs will usually give symptomatic relief of insomnia in two to four days and great improvement in the other symptoms in two to four weeks. We usually employ these drugs for three to six months and then make an attempt to discontinue them as other behavioural aspects of the rehabilitation programme begin to bear fruit.

Patients in chronic pain characteristically exhibit a wide variety of other psychiatric abnormalities, including lack of empathy, defects in cognitive thinking, hypochondriasis, dependency, a belief that the rules do not apply to them, and hysteria. We believe that the majority of these reflect personality traits and not the effects of chronic pain. Behavioural therapy is more appropriate and will be dealt with separately (Sternbach, 1978).

Management of Drug Misuse and Abuse

The next important factor to consider is the effect of drugs upon the patient: 56% of our patients have abnormal electroencephalograms—the records showing a profound drug effect; 25% have significant defects in cognitive thinking and this can be related to drug therapy. Almost all those dependent upon narcotics, even in small amounts, have significant withdrawal side effects from their drugs. In the USA, the most common drug to which patients are addicted in oxycodone. The second most common drug is codeine and the other narcotics follow. Dextropropoxyphene and Pentazocine are commonly misused. The most abused non-narcotic is diazepam. Barbiturates and amphetamines are abused less frequently. Our programme begins with withdrawal from all narcotics and ordering of all other medications so that their therapeutic effects are maximal and their side effects are minimal. We utilize a voluntary withdrawal from narcotics; patients know that they are being withdrawn, and if the patient is receiving an intramuscular preparation, we usually convert them to an oral drug such as Methadone. Narcotic withdrawal schedules depend upon the severity of addiction. Seriously addicted patients are usually switched to a long-acting preparation such as Methadone or Levorphanol to obtain satisfactory blood levels, stable over many hours. This eliminates the high–low syndrome seen with the short-acting drugs. Most patients can have the narcotics eliminated within one week. Diazepam is discontinued in all patients. The drug potentiates depression and certainly interferes significantly with cognitive thinking. This drug is withdrawn in graduated amounts over a seven to ten day period as well. It is usually possible to discontinue other drugs much more rapidly, but any drug which is taken in significantly greater than usual amounts is discontinued slowly over at least several days to one week. As soon as drug intakes are down to reasonable levels, the psychotropic drugs planned for the patient, if any, are added. The anxiety of drug withdrawal is frequently controlled by the administration of Hydroxyzine 50 mg four times a day, and autonomic side effects may be treated effectively by the use of antihistamines. The withdrawal programme usually requires seven to ten days and is mandatory for any patient who wishes treatment. Any patient who decides that he or she does not wish to give up drugs is free to leave the programme at any time. Frequently, the simple elimination of narcotics, and dependency upon them, is enough to totally relieve the pain. The combination of elimination of harmful drugs and treatment of symptoms is often sufficient to give pain relief and nothing further is indicated.

The Comprehensive Pain Treatment Programme

Up to this point, there is nothing in the patient's evaluation and treatment that cannot be carried out by any competent practitioner in any medical setting where the physician has the confidence and trust of the patient and the patient has a sincere desire for self-help. However, there are some aspects of comprehensive pain management that are better done in a group setting with many kinds of health professionals available for care. This is not the only way in which such a programme can be carried out, but in our experience the aggregation of a group committed to the therapy of pain is significantly more effective than the management of the pain process through traditional medical channels (Bonica, 1953). In our programme, the patient evaluation is carried out individually, but all therapy is done in the group setting. The aims of the comprehensive management programme are drug withdrawal, group and individual counselling and psychotherapy, elimination of the hypochondriacal fixation upon the pain, return of physical competence, relief of distress, and improvements in social and vocational function. Pain relief is not necessarily a goal of this programme, except as it relates to these factors. Pain relief is more likely to be supplied through specific procedures which will be delineated separately. A comprehensive programme of this type can be carried out in almost any environment. Our current mode is in-patient, but this is primarily because we face serious drug misuse problems and feel more secure in having these patients under control. Much of this behavioural programme can be implemented on an out-patient basis, but we have not been successful with out-patient drug withdrawal with our seriously addicted and habituated patients. The programme we employ is not strict behavioural modification. Rather, it could be termed behavioural suggestion in which the problems are identified for the patients and their aid is enlisted in solving them. The first aim is eliminating the hypochondriacal fixation upon the pain and the overwhelming dependence that these patients have on physicians and the medical system. Patients are not allowed to talk about their pain, except under specific circumstances. A great deal of their immediate supervision is taken over by trained nurses, nurse practitioners, social workers and psychologists. The physicians involved in the pain treatment centre function as a group and all are involved in the patient's care. One is responsible for the diagnostic evaluation, but the therapeutic programme is managed by all. The patients are encouraged to be as active as possible and rewarded by attention for non-pain behaviour. Pain behaviour is discussed frankly with them and the problems they create for themselves are pointed out in detail. A second very important aspect of the group process is the technique of physical therapy. Our patients undergo 30–60 minutes of group exercises each morning. In addition, they all have a complete physical assessment by a physical therapist, and individual activity and exercise programmes are planned. These are both short-term and long-term. The group exercises serve to focus the entire group of patients on activities and patients reinforce each other in accomplishing the goals set by our physical therapist. These goals will include physical conditioning and muscle strengthening, walking and running, and learning new ways to accomplish physical activities without exacerbations of pain. Our average patient has been inactive 20 hours a day and so we begin at a very low level to restore function (Fordyce, 1973). The psychodynamics of the group are also important and taken into consideration. All kinds of patients with chronic pain are managed in the same ward. Those with objective pain responses and those with exaggerated pain responses are managed together. After identification, those judged to have affective pain states are transferred to psychiatric care. However, the other two groups are managed together and it is of significant value for them to see each other's therapies and to hear the discussions. Patients are admitted at daily intervals and kept for approximately two weeks. This allows those patients who have made progress during their stay to be helpful in the indoctrination of patients recently admitted. The patients often become the best therapists and the pressure of the group on a recalcitrant newcomer is extremely important. Group psychotherapy sessions are managed by clinical psychologists and psychiatrists. They are extremely important, and for many of our patients are the best aspect of the programme following drug withdrawal and correction of psychiatric symptomatology. These patients benefit greatly from learning that others have the same problems and need the same therapies. They are able to discuss their angers and frustrations and often, for the first time, are forced to come to grips with their own participation in their pain syndrome. Individual psychotherapy and counselling are available for those patients who require it because of specific aberrations. Social service is available to assist with vocational problems and often the first step in re-education begins in this phase of the programme.

This comprehensive therapy approach allows a multi-faceted attack on all of the things that are wrong with these patients. Ordering of drugs and improved physical function are very important, but the behavioural aspects of this part of the programme are the most important therapy techniques employed. Without them, it is doubtful if any of these patients will ever become candidates for pain-relieving procedures and great emphasis is placed upon this part of the programme.

Relief of Pain

It is an unfortunate fact that no therapy exists for the pain experience for a large number of the patients presenting to a pain rehabilitation unit. It is unusual for there to be a specific problem to be treated. Interventional therapies for symptomatic relief are applicable only to a relatively small number of patients incapacitated by the complaint of chronic pain. Quite obviously, the patient falling into our affective or psychiatric pain group does not require an interventional procedure. Psychotherapy is the treatment of choice (Blumer, 1975). Very few patients who are classified as exhibiting the exaggerated pain response should have interventional procedures. Some of these patients have underlying problems which can be treated effectively, but interventional procedures for pain alone are highly unlikely to solve the psychosocial problems that accompany the painful process. Interventional procedures, such as discectomy, are contra-indicated without evaluation of the psychological aspects which these patients present. It is also virtually useless to use interventional procedures alone in patients who are in the angry or depressive phases of their illness. The patient who is severely depressed cannot determine if the therapy has been of value and the patient who is excessively angry is very likely to be severely disappointed and made worse by a less than optimal result. In our opinion, the first step in planning an interventional procedure is to be certain that all of the ancillary problems we have discussed have been solved or are at least under treatment. Only then will interventional procedures be optimized.

Diagnostic Nerve Blocks

Diagnostic blocks are extremely helpful in deciphering complicated pain problems. Therapeutic blocks are rarely indicated in severe chronic pain of benign origin. Neither are multiple repetitive temporary blocks of great use in the management of most serious chronic pain states. There is very little evidence in the literature that therapeutic blocks provide long-lasting relief for more than a very small number of patients.

Diagnostic blocks, on the other hand, are extremely useful in establishing the cause of the pain and in helping to plan interventional procedures (Bonica, 1964). Peripheral nerve blocks and root blocks are useful in identifying the paths by which the pain is travelling and determining sites of injury. Segmental, epidural or spinal anaesthesia can be useful in the same way. Sympathetic blocks may be useful in determining the importance of an autonomic component in the pain problem. However, the response of pain to sympathetic blockade is capricious and not reliably predictable for the success of sympathectomy. Many unusual pains will respond for a short period of time to sympathetic blockade, but recur promptly after sympathectomy. In true causalgia, sympathetic block is predictive of pain relief by sympathectomy, but in other less well defined states, the response to sympathetic blocks is not always reliable (White, 1976). Temporary blockade of fusion donor sites, pseudoarthroses and similar areas of abnormality may be very helpful in determining the origins of pain in a patient with a chronic back pain or neck pain syndrome. Blockade of the trigeminal nerve and its branches can be very useful in determining the type and level of head and face pain. However, it must be emphasized that the results of an individual block are difficult to interpret and not at all predictive that section of the nerve involved will relieve the pain. When interpreting the results of block, it is important to carry out a careful repeat examination to be certain that the expected result of the block has in fact occurred and that no other neurological structures other than those blocked have been involved. The results of the blocks can then be incorporated into the overall physical diagnosis in order to add information about the cause of pain. It is important not to over-interpret the results of these procedures and not to ascribe undue physiological significance to the results of a variable technique (Bonica, 1964).

INTERVENTIONAL SURGERY FOR THE RELIEF
OF PAIN

There are a number of destructive procedures which have been used over many years for the relief of pain. Some are very effective in cancer pain, but few have anything to offer in the treatment of chronic pain of benign origin.

NEUROLYTIC AGENTS

Peripheral nerves, the sympathetic system and the spinal roots may be destroyed by the injection of neurolytic agents. Alcohol and phenol are generally used. Alcohol blockade of peripheral nerves runs a significant risk of a post-injection neuritic syndrome and rarely is successful for pain relief for more than a short period of time. Neurolytic sympathectomy is a much more successful procedure, particularly for destruction of the coeliac axis. Neurolytic injections into the gasserian ganglion and the branches of the trigeminal nerve are very successful, but better techniques now exist (Harris, 1940). The primary use of neurolytic agents has been for the destruction of spinal roots in the pain of cancer. The success rate is fair and the complication rate high. Pain relief is generally for three months or less and the technique has very little place in the management of chronic pain of benign origin (Papo & Visca, 1976). Chemical sympathectomy is useful in true causalgia and reflex sympathetic dystrophy when temporary sympathetic blockade has relieved pain totally on several occasions. Chemical destruction of the coeliac axis may be useful for chronic abdominal pain, particularly of chronic pancreatitis, but the risks of the procedure make it more appropriate for cancer pain (Bonica, 1964). Alcohol block of the gasserian ganglion or the branches of the trigeminal nerve is sometimes still indicated, but radio-frequency lesions are so much easier to perform that chemical blocks are rarely used now.

PERIPHERAL NEUROTOMY

Section of peripheral nerves is rarely indicated in the treatment of chronic pain of benign origin. There are exceptions, however. Thoracic neurotomy to relieve post-incisional pain is a useful technique. Destruction of the nerves may be by surgical section or by radio-frequency destructive heat lesions through percutaneously placed needles (Siebens, 1974). Section of nerve for neuroma pain is sometimes useful, particularly if the neuroma is in a location where it is liable to be traumatized. However, the overall success rate of neurotomy, even for neuroma pain, is less than 50%. Neurotomy may be useful in Morton's neuroma, trigeminal neuralgia and post-incisional pain. There is virtually no other reliable indication for peripheral neurotomy (White, 1946).

SPINAL RHIZOTOMY

Spinal rhizotomy is not very useful in the management of chronic pain of benign origin either. It has been most commonly employed for relief of intractable sciatica secondary to root injury with disc herniation and/or multiple surgeries. The success rates of 25–35% are disturbingly low and the procedure cannot be recommended (Loesser, 1972). Upper cervical rhizotomy for relief of intractable greater occipital pain is sometimes utilized, but is a drastic procedure for this symptomatology and patients must be chosen extremely well. Such a procedure should be planned only after all other techniques have failed to relieve intractable occipital headache. Posterior rhizotomy is not useful for most kinds of incisional pains or for post-herpetic neuralgia (Onofrio & Campa, 1972).

CORDOTOMY

Percutaneous or open cordotomy remain excellent procedures for the relief of cancer pain. With unilateral cordotomy pain relief occurs 85–95% of the time and the complication rate is small (Kahn & Peet, 1948; Ogle *et al.*, 1956). With bilateral cordotomies, success is significantly less, and the complication rate is much greater (Lin *et al.*, 1966). However, when the patient is to survive for more than one year, the success rate begins to fall and the incidence of post-cordotomy dysaesthesia is increased. Cordotomy is rarely used for pain of benign origin (Mullan *et al.*, 1968). There are still indications for it, however. In completely intractable situations, the pain relief which may be obtained through cordotomy is sometimes very valuable. The risk of failure of post-cordotomy dysaesthesia and the possibility of early success with later failure must be carefully explained to the patient. When the patient understands the situation, then cordotomy still can be valuable for unilateral pain. There are better alternatives now, however, that carry significantly less risk and the procedure is rarely used.

Another spinal cord operation which may have value in the treatment of chronic pain is midline myelotomy. The crossing fibres of the anterior spinal thalamic tract are severed to denervate a specified area of the spinal cord. The technique is mostly used in pelvic pain secondary to cancer. It has been employed for benign pain with good reported results, but the risks of the procedure and the small number of patients treated make it impossible to state that this is a technique which should be extensively employed. There may be individual cases where careful selection will make the patient a candidate for the procedure (Sourek, 1977).

OPERATIONS ON THE CRANIAL NERVES

Section of cranial nerves for specific pain problems such as trigeminal neuralgia and glossopharyngeal neuralgia has long been practised and is satisfactory therapy (Peet & Schneider, 1952). However, radio-frequency destruction of the gasserian ganglion via a percutaneous technique is now used as the primary therapy for tic douloureux which requires intervention. Division of the nervus intermedius may occasionally be indicated for unusual vascular head pain syndromes, but otherwise section of the cranial nerves is of little value in the therapy of head and neck pain. One of the most exciting areas which is now being explored is the concept of microvascular decompression for the relief of head and face pain. Janetta (1975) has reintroduced Walter Dandy's belief that compression of the cranial nerves in the posterior fossa by vascular structures may produce a wide variety of symptoms, including the trigeminal neuralgias. Microvascular decompression, or removing these vascular structures from the nerves using the operating microscope, has been very successful in Janetta's hands. There have not been enough patients reported outside Janetta's own programme to be certain of its applicability. However, the original data for trigeminal neuralgia are quite satisfactory and Janetta's division of the face pain problems into tic douloureux, trigeminal neuralgia, both surgical diseases, and atypical facial pain, an unexplained problem at the present time, is used as the diagnostic guide for selection of patients. The effects of microvascular decompression in other painful syndromes of the head have not yet been evaluated in a large enough number of patients for assessment.

STEREOTACTIC INTRACRANIAL PROCEDURES

The use of stereotactic lesions in the thalamus, hypothalamus and other areas of the brain is very difficult to assess. Enthusiastic reports have appeared, but not all stereotactic surgeons are able to reproduce these data. It now appears that stereotactic lesions which do not affect personality are of little value in the treatment of chronic pain of benign origin (Siegfried, 1977). Cingulotomy and limited frontal lobotomy may be employed in carefully selected patients where anxiety or depression is the most important consideration. However, review of the literature indicates that these procedures are unlikely to have a persisting effect and are much more useful in the patient who has been psychiatrically destroyed by the knowledge of a malignancy than in patients with long life expectancy (White, 1962; Nashold *et al.*, 1969).

THE NEUROAUGMENTATION TECHNIQUES

Melzack and Wall (1967) introduced a new theory of pain perception in which they pointed out that the perception of pain could be modified by non-painful sensory input. Wall and Sweet then demonstrated that electrical stimulation of the human nervous system could significantly modify pain perception and chronic pain (Sweet, 1977). Shealy devised implantable devices for stimulation of the human nervous system and the first of these were manufactured in the late 1960s. The original devices were for stimulation of the human spinal cord and peripheral nerve stimulators followed shortly. Transcutaneous electrical stimulators utilized externally on the skin had been available for many years, but in the early 1970s modern engineering techniques were applied to make these useful devices. Techniques for stimulating the brain were then developed. All of these have now been in use for nearly ten years and considerable data have been gained from them. In spite of all their shortcomings, these techniques remain the best pain-relieving techniques available in chronic pain once it has been determined that specific corrective procedures are not available (Long & Hagfors, 1975).

TRANSCUTANEOUS STIMULATION

This is the most valuable neuroaugmentation form for most patients. Huge numbers of patients have been treated using these techniques. The original studies were simply surveys of the application of the techniques on large numbers of patients. The patients appeared to have satisfactory control of otherwise intractable pain in significantly greater than placebo numbers. More circumscribed studies have since been carried out that demonstrate that placebo or sham stimulation is not helpful; that the response to electrical stimulation is greater than placebo effect; and that certain categories of disease respond better than others. Pain of peripheral nerve injury responds very well to transcutaneous electrical stimulation. Post-herpetic neuralgia and phantom limb pain, which is not long established, also may respond. The less specific back and leg pains suffered by the victims of multiple surgical procedures may also be helped, but the number responding is significantly less. Nevertheless, transcutaneous stimulation remains one of the most valuable techniques for the majority of patients suffering from otherwise intractable chronic pain of benign origin. In our clinic, it is our usual practice to begin stimulation immediately when the patient is seen in the out-patient department or is admitted. The stimulation has two purposes. It may be effective in relieving the patient's pain, but it serves another important purpose, which is to demonstrate to the patient that new and different techniques will be utilized in their care and it gives them a significant morale boost to begin what will be a very difficult programme for them. Stimulation is carried out in the surround of the painful area, over major nerve trunks or major plexuses. Our usual trial on an in-patient basis is three days before any decision is made about efficacy. On an out-patient basis, the patient is instructed in the use of the device and allowed to use it for a minimum of one month before any decision about efficacy is made. Such patients are usually enthusiastic in the first few days and their responses about pain relief are unreliable. If pain relief persists after several days of use, then a one month trial is advocated. Before determining purchase, we demand that the following criteria have been met. First, the patient must be using the device and must be capable of its continued use. Then it is necessary that the pain relief be significant so that the patient is significantly better off with the device than without it. We must have not only the patient's report about this, but evidence of increase in function and decrease in medication use. Purchase is not recommended until these trials are complete and until it is apparent that the device will be an important part of the patient's pain therapy. Ideally, the device should obviate the need for other forms of therapy as well. Transcutaneous stimulation will be of greatest value in patients who are less seriously incapacitated. In our experience, even in the worst of chronic pain states, it will be useful in from 25% to 35% of all patients referred to us. There are some specific groups of patients who cannot be helped. In our experience, pain of central nervous system origin and pain of metabolic peripheral neuropathy are highly unlikely to respond. Furthermore, the psychoneurotic will not only not respond, but is frequently worsened by the procedure. Hyperaesthesia is the only organic pain syndrome which is routinely worsened by the application of a transcutaneous stimulator. When such worsening occurs it is strong evidence that there is a major underlying psychological problem which is not yet resolved (Long & Hagfors, 1975).

The only known significant contra-indication is the presence of a cardiac pacemaker. Skin irritation can occur, but there has been no major complication attributable to transcutaneous stimulation reported.

IMPLANTABLE ELECTRICAL STIMULATORS

All of the implants are approximately the same at the present time. They consist of a passive radio-receiver attached to an electrode which varies in form. This is the system that is implanted within the body. There is an external signalling device which activates the implanted stimulator by means of an antenna placed near the receiver. The activation takes place through the intact skin and the patient controls the strength and duration of stimulation. New devices are just appearing which are totally implantable and programmable through the intact skin.

STIMULATION OF PERIPHERAL NERVES

The implantable stimulators for peripheral nerve injury have been very successful in pain relief. These are the best of all the stimulating devices. However, their use is very limited. They have been effective only for pain of peripheral nerve injury, and only when they can be placed proximal to the level of injury. Other placements will relieve pain for varying periods of time, but after one to several years the pain problem almost always recurs. When the stimulator can be placed proximal to the injury, it is usually effective. Temporary percutaneous stimulation of the nerve, if effective in pain relief, is highly predicative of a successful implant. The original devices have now been in use for pain of peripheral nerve injury origin for ten years. Success rates of 70% or greater are obtained with pain of peripheral nerve injury origin and the effect of the device appears to be long lasting. In our series where the patient selection criteria are met, there have been no long-range failures with recurrence of pain (Long & Hagfors, 1975).

SPINAL CORD STIMULATION

The first stimulators devised by Shealy were for stimulation of the posterior columns. About 450 of these were implanted by a confederation of neurosurgeons in the USA over a three year period. The results of these patients were carefully documented and reviewed regularly. It appears that approximately 50% of the patients chosen for the procedure achieve satisfactory pain relief. However, after three years, it appeared that there was a tendency for decline in efficacy. The technical difficulties with these devices and this apparent decline in efficacy led most to abandon them, except as therapy for highly selected patients. However, a retrospective analysis of these cases indicates that this decision may have been premature. In the first place, patient selection techniques were much less adequate then than they are now. The effects of narcotic addiction were not well understood. The role of depression and anxiety was not appreciated, and no techniques for satisfactory preoperative screening were available. Even with advances in all these areas, the magnitude of the operative procedure and the number of complications which accompanied it made the procedure undesirable in view of the 50% success rate (Fox, 1974). Fortunately, the situation was changed by the development of wire electrodes which can be inserted percutaneously into the epidural space. These electrodes can be implanted and temporary extensions brought out through the skin to allow testing to be certain that pain relief will be obtained with optimum electrode placement. The device can then be internalized and made permanent. The actual stimulator is the same as has been used throughout the history of implantable stimulators. The only thing which differs is the percutaneously implantable electrode system. This converts a major procedure, done under general anaesthesia, requiring a full laminectomy, to a minor procedure performed under local anaesthetic and requiring only two skin and subcutaneous incisions. It does not appear that the overall success rate will be significantly greater, but the procedure is of significantly less magnitude and can be employed in well-chosen patients because it offers very little risk to them. We currently employ percutaneously implanted electrode systems primarily in the treatment of patients with arachnoiditis secondary to multiple low back operations. Stimulators are not implanted until the psychological and drug problems are under therapy and permanent implantation is carried out only when temporary stimulation has brought excellent pain relief. Using these stringent criteria, our overall success rate has increased to over 70%. However, there are still many technical problems with the implantable stimulators which limit their usefulness now. The stimulators are currently envisaged for a three to five year life and pain control in patients who are desperate for pain relief when other techniques are not apparently available. The stimulator systems are used in preference to major reoperations unless very specific indications for reoperative surgery exist.

BRAIN STIMULATION

Adams *et al* (1974), Hosobuchi *et al* (1973) and Richardson & Akil (1977) have separately pioneered the use of brain stimulation for pain relief. Stimulating electrodes using the same stimulator systems employed for spinal cord and nerve stimulation have been implanted in several areas of the brain. Stimulation was first carried out in the specific sensory nuclei of the thalamus (Mazars, 1975). Since then electrode systems in the posterior limb of the internal capsule and in the periaqueductal grey area have been used (Adams *et al.*, 1974). Only patients with pain of central nervous system origin and somatic pain which was otherwise intractable pain have been treated. The potential hazards of brain haemorrhage limit the usefulness of the technique. However, it is extremely successful when one considers the types of patients that have been treated. Success rates varying between 60% and 70% have been recorded in disease states for which no other therapy exists. The possibility that these stimulators function by means of activation of an endogenous opoid system is an intriguing one. If true, this hypothesis may lead to great improvements in nervous system stimulating techniques. At the present time, these implantable brain stimulators are almost the only thing that can be done for anaesthesia dolorosa, thalamic pain, pain from widespread metastatic disease and some patients with pain from arachnoiditis which has not responded to any other means of therapy (Hosobuchi *et al.*, 1973).

Success of Interventional Procedures for Chronic Pain of Benign Origin

None of the interventional procedures which have been described are applicable to large numbers of patients, except in specific disease states such as trigeminal neuralgia. Most of the patients referred to a comprehensive pain treatment programme have disease states for which little therapy is available. It is extremely unlikely that the patient with five operations on the back can be benefited by yet another. Very few patients have mistaken diagnoses and correctable problems. Destructive procedures have virtually no place in this kind of pain problem. Peripheral block techniques may be helpful in diagnosis but are rarely of any value in therapy. There are a few exceptions to this, but these are rare. The neuroaugmentation techniques are of value because they represent almost the only thing that can be done to alleviate pain in seriously injured patients. Long-term success rates with transcutaneous stimulation vary between 35% and 50%. Peripheral nerve stimulators are very successful but only for a specific group of patients. Spinal cord stimulators are useful but are employed in a small number of patients and brain stimulators must be applied even more selectively. In our programme, between 5% and 10% of patients are candidates for significant interventional procedures of these types. For the remainder, no specific pain-relieving techniques exist. For this reason it is very important to establish as early as possible that the patient understands that it is unlikely that a rapid and complete cure for pain will be obtained and that their own abilities to control chronic pain will become an important aspect of their future.

There are several principles which guide the selection of patients for interventional procedures in our clinic. The first of these is an accurate physical diagnosis. This means that whenever possible therapy is directed at correction of an underlying problem. This kind of specific therapy should always precede any other interventional procedure. In planning specific interventions, however, it is extremely important to be certain about the underlying diagnosis. Such blanket phrases as 'chronic low back syndrome' or 'low back cripple' serve only to obscure the actual problem. The use of reoperation simply because there are post-operative changes demonstrated in X-ray studies is not warranted and careful correlation between symptoms and the underlying diagnosis must be made. Patients undergoing non-specific therapies for pain must be even more carefully evaluated. The psychological factors are of extreme importance and it is very important to determine the classification. Our classification serves as a useful, though pragmatically derived tool. In our classification, patients falling in the objective pain category are considered to be candidates for interventional procedures. Even then, major interventions are used only when the ancillary problems of anxiety, depression, drug dependence and insomnia have been treated. Patients in the exaggerated pain category are rarely candidates for any interventional procedure, except for the correction of a definitive underlying problem or the use of minor percutaneous techniques. Two pieces of data from our initial series of interventional procedures support these conclusions. The so-called facet denervation or radio-frequency medial branch neurotomy has been used for the treatment of certain types of low back pain for the past six to seven years. In a recent study of 230 such patients, all chosen because of an apparent mechanical back syndrome, a retrospective review of success or failure of the technique with respect to psychological factors was undertaken. One hundred and fifty of the patients fell within the objective pain category. The success rate of the procedure in relieving pain for at least one year was almost 70%. Eighty patients fell into the exaggerated pain category. These patients were otherwise similar to the larger group in every way. Not one of the 80 patients was improved by the procedure. Similar data have been obtained for the use of implantable stimulators for the pain of documented arachnoiditis. In a review of 50 such patients who underwent percutaneous implantation of a spinal cord stimulator for pain relief, it was discovered that 40 of the patients retrospectively analysed fell in the objective pain category and 10 in the exaggerated or affective pain category. At the time the stimulators were implanted, the decision for therapy was made by the physician involved without knowledge of the classification in order to help validate the test. In the 40 patients falling in the objective category, the success of pain relief at 31 months was over 70%. None of the patients who were in the exaggerated pain group received benefit from the stimulator and virtually all required removal of the stimulator for psychiatric reasons. We believe strongly that patients should be carefully examined from a psychiatric standpoint, categorized in this general way, and have their ancillary problems treated before major procedures are contemplated.

SELECTION OF PATIENTS FOR TRANSCUTANEOUS ELECTRICAL STIMULATION

Most patients are candidates for this form of therapy. The technique has been most useful in pain of peripheral nerve injury origin, myofacial pain syndromes and chronic back and neck pain uncomplicated by multiple operative procedures. The method is also of value in a significant number of patients with arachnoiditis or post-operative back and neck problems. Patients with pain of central nervous system origin or metabolic peripheral neuropathy are unlikely to be benefited and patients with significant hyperaesthesia may have that sensation worsened temporarily. Patients in the exaggerated and affective groups, particularly hysterics, are very likely to believe their pain has been worsened by the stimulator. Beyond the psychological factors, there are no other selection criteria for a trial of this form of therapy in any patient with chronic pain. However, pacemakers are a contra-indication and patients with cardiac arrhythmias should certainly be treated carefully.

SELECTION OF PATIENTS FOR IMPLANTABLE PERIPHERAL NERVE STIMULATORS

We now utilize these devices almost exclusively for patients with pain of peripheral nerve injury origin. Preferably, it should be possible to implant the device proximal to the area of injury. Narcotic intake must be eliminated. The ancillary factors must be well controlled. Once these are accomplished, the patient is tested as a candidate for an implantable stimulator by a temporary percutaneous stimulation of the nerve. Those patients who achieved satisfactory pain relief are considered good candidates.

SELECTION CRITERIA FOR IMPLANTATION OF SPINAL CORD STIMULATORS

Stimulation of the spinal cord may be utilized for any kind of pain in which the stimulation can be applied above the highest level of injury. Control of medication and ancillary factors are equally important as for all of the other interventional procedures. Patients are selected for implantation by percutaneous temporary stimulation of the spinal cord. It is a simple matter to implant a temporary stimulating electrode over the dorsal surface of the cord via percutaneous midline epidural puncture. One to a few days of stimulation covering the painful area will allow patients to judge whether they like the sensation and whether pain relief is achieved during stimulation. This selection process greatly improves the success of the general technique.

SELECTION CRITERIA FOR IMPLANTATION OF A BRAIN STIMULATOR

The major decision here is made after it is proven that the patient is completely intractable to other reasonable forms of therapy. The majority of patients treated have had pain of nervous system injury origin or such serious somatic pain that they were completely incapacitated by it. It is extremely important that all ancillary therapies be exhausted before this procedure is undertaken. Not that the complication rate is high, but the potential complications are significant as contrasted with the other forms of electrical stimulator. Once other therapies are exhausted, it is again possible to test the patient before committing him or her to a full implantation. An electrode is placed into the target area in the brain and externalized by a temporary system. Stimulation can then be carried out over a long period of time even up to months if necessary to optimize the device before final implantation takes place.

Other Techniques

There are a myriad of other potential minor interventional procedures for pain. These include the so-called therapeutic nerve blocks, neurolytic blocks, injection of steroids, particularly in the epidural space, radio-frequency destruction of the innervation of lumbar or cervical facets, radio-frequency neurotomy usually of the greater occipital nerves or upper cervical roots, radio-frequency neurotomy for incisional pain and many other therapies even less proven. The indications for most of these techniques are not clear. The results are not well documented and most require significantly more information to be available before it is possible to state with certainty how effective they are and what selection criteria should be employed. There seems little question that the techniques are effective enough to merit use. This is particularly true of the therapeutic nerve blocks and epidural steroid injection. Both techniques have been in widespread use for many years. Nevertheless, it is virtually impossible to determine current efficacy rates, patient selection criteria, and predictors of success or failure. There is a great need for critical reassessment of the use of interventional procedures for the relief of pain, particularly with regard to pain relief lasting one year or more.

SOCIAL AND VOCATIONAL REHABILITATION

The initial aims of the pain treatment programme are directly related to the complaint of pain and its relief, the elimination of the influences of harmful drugs, and the treatment of specific psychiatric symptoms which may be either primary or a part of the pain neurosis. Once this is accomplished, the major goal is the improvement of social and vocational competence. In order to realize this goal, it is important for everyone involved to understand that there are two groups of patients and that success in these two groups is markedly different. As described above, the first group are normal individuals who have had an accident or illness which has resulted in chronic pain. They may have been subjected to useless operations and become addicted to medications in fruitless attempts to relieve their pain. They may develop chronic anxiety, depression and insomnia as symptoms of pain, and pass through the stages of pain development described earlier. However, since their premorbid personality has been good, they should respond well to the treatment programme outlined. It will be sufficient to provide as much relief as possible from the iatrogenic problems, and utilize group and individual psychotherapy to bring the patients to the rational phase of understanding their disease and its potential treatment. As soon as these symptoms are controlled, these patients should regain their original motivation and will function within their limitations. It is important that family members be involved in this process so that they understand what has happened to the patient and can provide help and support. These patients usually retain their vocational skills and do not need great help in dealing with their vocational problems. However, even when they are well motivated, they may not be able to return to their original employment. This is particularly true of the patient who has done heavy or strenuous work and who now can no longer perform physically arduous tasks. Most employers are anxious to have competent employees return and most will be helpful in seeking new jobs or in attempting to retrain such individuals for different vocations. In this group of patients, control of symptoms and a rational treatment plan are usually all that is necessary. Long-term support may be indicated for six months to one year, but it is rarely necessary over a longer period of time. The patients may need refreshers as in-patients or out-patients periodically to help with residual pain, but continuing intensive therapy is usually not necessary.

Vocational assistance begins with a completely honest review of their current physical status and what their capabilities are. The patients need assistance in determining whether they can return to their original employment and what their employment chances are. They may need direction into vocational rehabilitation programmes and assessment of these programmes according to their particular capabilities. In our experience, a great many industrial vocational rehabilitation programmes provide work education for patients, which do not consider the patient's innate physical ability. (A typical example is a young right-handed white male with a non-functioning right hand, markedly hyperaesthetic, secondary to median nerve injury, with one of the most severe reflex sympathetic dystrophy syndromes seen in our unit. The vocational rehabilitation centre involved in assisting him planned small appliance repair as a potential job for this man who was unable to use his markedly dominant right hand!) This group of patients can show marked improvement even after multiple operations and our success rate with them is reasonable. The best candidate for pain therapy is the individual who has continued to work in spite of difficulties. A significant number of these in whom we have implanted stimulators fall into that category.

The major problem in return of social and vocational competence comes when one considers the large number of patients presenting with chronic pain who had limited competence prior to their apparent injury or illness. Our demographic studies are not yet complete, but preliminary data indicate that in the USA, at least, a significant number of patients who present to a comprehensive pain treatment programme have a long history of social and vocational incompetence. The usual profile indicates normal or better than normal ability, but poor function. There is a long history of difficulty with authority. A significant number of these patients are victims of child abuse and a surprising number are involved in spouse or child abuse. There is usually a history of minor confrontations with neighbours, police, schools, military personnel and employers. Alcoholism is common. In the younger age group, the use of drugs, particularly marijuana, is also common. Sexual disturbances are also extremely common. The sexual dysfunction is usually impotence or frigidity and/or excessively rigid or excessively promiscuous behaviour. In short, preliminary data indicate that a large percentage of patients who present complaining of chronic pain are marginal individuals who may be diagnosed as having character disorders or, at least, sociopathic tendencies. We do not have definitive data to prove this point, but it appears from our preliminary studies that a significant proportion of patients who come to the pain treatment centre seeking industrial related disability or government supported retirement fall into this category. The data are less definite, but our first information indicates that patients seeking to recover through third-party litigation without obvious serious injury also often fall into this category. These patients characteristically score in our exaggerated pain response group. The typical patient suffers from industrial accident and, in spite of the absence of physical abnormalities, is unable to return to work because of pain (nearly always back or neck pain). Multiple examinations by physicians indicate no significant abnormality and conservative care for the problem is recommended. In desperation after a failure of therapy, such patients are studied by myelography or discography. It is not uncommon for a degenerated disc to be discovered. The unwarranted treatment in response to these findings and the patient's symptoms is as follows. The patient is subjected to an operation for removal of the degenerated disc. The failure to recognize the overwhelming psychosocial factors which reinforce the patient's pain complaint lead to a diagnostic error and a therapeutic error. The diagnostic error is the supposition that the patient's pain is related to the demonstrated degenerated disc. The therapeutic error is a surgical procedure rather than an investigation of psychological factors and appropriate psychiatric intervention. All too commonly the first procedure fails to relieve pain and then reinvestigation and reoperation follow, often with multiple repetitions. Finally, the individual surgeon or surgeons recognize that this patient has deteriorated from a psychiatric standpoint and now state, after multiple fruitless operations, that the problem is psychiatric in origin. Psychiatric consultation is then obtained. A second major error is frequently made here. By this time, the patient has completely adequate structural reasons to have pain. Many psychiatrists are not skilled in the evaluation of pain patients and most are not involved in industrial disability in any great way. The psychiatrist discusses the situation with the patient, sees the disabled physical state, recognizes the anxiety and depression, but assumes, probably correctly, that these are related to the multiple operations and the failure of pain relief, and tells the patient, 'There is nothing wrong with you psychiatrically. You have an organic pain problem and you need to go back and have it treated.' The patient has now been rejected from the usual medical system. No one now will attempt to treat the underlying pain directly and the usual forms of psychotherapeutic intervention are not warranted. In addition, the patient is left with multiple iatrogenic problems. The consequences of multiple operations on the back are very real from a structural standpoint, and it is likely that the patient has severe pain now. Many patients describe their post-operative pain as significantly worse than any they have ever suffered before. This is very telling for, of course, the patient with an acute disc herniation is so grateful to be rid of that serious pain that the post-operative pain is generally considered inconsequential. In addition to the sequelae of multiple operations, the patient is left depressed, anxious and unable to sleep, and usually is addicted to multiple drugs. Such a patient is a candidate for a multi-disciplinary comprehensive pain therapy programme, but the goals of therapy are significantly different than for the competent individual who has undergone this same kind of therapy. It is not a matter of restoration of social competence. What is actually needed is an improvement in the patient's premorbid state. This is a difficult order for any psychotherapeutic programme and generally beyond the scope of any of the behavioural programmes now available in chronic pain. The psychotherapeutic approaches recommended by Crue or Seres may be the best devices for these individuals. It is important for all dealing with chronic pain to recognize the situation. The criteria of success for these individuals are different from those for individuals who exhibited normal premorbid function. It is entirely possible that the iatrogenic problems can be solved, drug abuse can be eliminated and much pain behaviour can be changed. However, the simplistic approach of the pain treatment programme is unlikely to change a character disorder.

The vocational rehabilitation of these patients is an even greater problem. The same differentiation appears to occur. Many of our patients have continued working in spite of significant physical disabilities and severe pain. This is obviously a good prognostic sign and these individuals routinely fall into our objective pain category. Most patients who undergo major procedures are in this category. When the actual physical disability will allow it, these patients can be returned to work. The important factors here are elimination of disability related to excessive or improper drug ingestion, correction of the depression and anxiety, and repair of disrupted interpersonal relationships. The motivated individual is then usually able to return to work. It is important to give these individuals guidance about physical limitations and future work capacity, and assist them in realistic vocational planning. Again, it is most important that vocational rehabilitation programmes be guided so that these patients will be trained in appropriate employment when it is not possible for them to return to their original jobs. The problem occurs with the marginal employee who falls into our category of exaggerated pain response. The individual who has exhibited social incompetence is likely to have the same history in the vocational sphere. Usually, these patients have sustained a minor injury and no significant physical abnormalities can be found. Nevertheless, a complaint of pain continues. Competent individuals suffering the same apparent injury have returned to work in a short time with minimal therapy. However, for some reason these individuals do not. It is always possible that they have suffered an injury that is beyond our capacity to diagnose at the present time, but there is no evidence that this is the case (Shaw, 1964). This group of individuals represent a huge cost. Their medical care, lost wages, and future support when the disability is permanent, represent a vast sum in the USA. There are no data currently available to determine how many such patients exist and what percentage of the disabled work force they represent. However, in our programme, they outnumber the individual with a clear-cut injury and bona fide disability by a significant factor. Review of the situation will usually indicate poor vocational record, with low achievement and frequent job changes. A great deal of data are available characterizing sociological aspects of the problem (Tibbits, 1954). It appears that there are three major syndromes (Brodsky, 1971). The first is termed the worn-out worker. They are usually individuals of marginal ability who have been self-supporting for many years. They are frequently involved in manual labour which has become increasingly difficult as they have grown older. They are often called upon to compete with young, vigorous individuals, and are finding it more difficult to do so. The injury and its required absence from work demonstrate to them the advantages of not continuing their current employment. Usually, their skills are limited and job retraining is not feasible or they have no interest in retraining. The second group tend to be younger and have generally decided that they are quite content to be supported by disability payments and/or perhaps a working spouse. A third major category are patients who simply wish to retire in order to change jobs. This is common among individuals with employments that allow early retirement and reasonable income so that they may then take a second job and greatly augment their total income. Of course, there are other reasons ranging from simple job dissatisfaction through to deliberate attempts to obtain money by fraud. Whatever the underlying cause, it appears that something happens to these individuals so that they never become functional again. What this personal crisis may be is not yet understood (Modlin, 1967). Nevertheless, vocational rehabilitation in this group of individuals is extremely difficult. At the present time, it is possible to achieve basic goals with these individuals. It is usually possible to eliminate drug use, though these patients characteristically resent the planned withdrawal of narcotics. It is frequently possible to increase their activities and make them personally more functional, though this is usually done without any admission of physical improvement. The patients can frequently be protected from further interventional procedures, though this is the group that tend to look for simplistic answers and seek out surgical procedures. We are considerably less successful in improving personal competence, though even this is possible with long-term supportive psychotherapy aimed at the modification of pain behaviour. What is virtually impossible in our current social system is return to meaningful employment. Several factors influence this. The psychological motives that we have discussed are especially important, but it is also important to realize that many of these patients, most of whom work in manual labour, are incapacitated by musculo-skeletal problems that would not bother a professional person. It is extremely unlikely that an individual with three or four operations on the back can return to any vigorous activity. The combination of real physical disability, at least in the industrial sense, and the psychological factors which appear to be paramount in this group of people currently conspire to make meaningful job retraining virtually impossible. The current social system is very much against worthwhile therapy in these patients. If there has been a personal injury and there is litigation involved, then the success of litigation depends upon the maintenance of symptoms. If there is an industrial disability and the Industrial Commission is involved, then again the size of a lump-sum settlement or continued disability payments depends upon the maintenance of symptoms. Relief of symptoms may mean return to work. Therefore, the patient has a vested interest in maintaining the symptoms. This is even more true with job-related claims for government employees (Social Security Disability); disability is likely to be permanent. In many cases the Social Security payment is reasonably large compared to the worker's ability to generate an income. This money obtained without work is significantly better than a slightly larger amount of money obtained with work. Relief of symptoms again will mean loss of disability payments and the necessity to return to a distasteful job.

It is extremely important that these psychosocial factors be recognized early in the therapy of an individual patient. If it serves no other purpose than the prevention of unnecessary operations and inappropriate drugs, the recognition will be worth while. At the present, this syndrome of lack of vocational motivation is virtually untreatable. The patient is currently rewarded for sick behaviour, and until the rewards are given for well behaviour it is unlikely that this major social problem will be solved (Tibbitts, 1954).

THE ORGANIZATION OF THE PAIN TREATMENT
PROGRAMME

The organizational problems and their solutions in a pain treatment programme
are an often overlooked aspect of pain therapy. Central to a well-organized
programme is a thorough knowledge of group process, ward behaviour, communication networks, leadership, entry phenomena, and basic assumption
groups. Bion (1959) has clearly outlined the criteria for good group function: (1)
common purpose, (2) common recognition of boundaries of the group and the
position and function of subgroups, (3) the capacity to absorb or lose members
without losing group identity, (4) the absence of undesignated subgroups, (5)
adequate recognition of each individual for his contribution, (6) the capacity to
manage discontent. In addition, we believe that in the problem of pain a similar
language for diagnosis and common therapeutic techniques is important (Wilson
& Meyer, 1965).

Any pain treatment programme has a variety of organizational needs which
have to be defined before the programme is organized. One of the most important
is *patient selection*. It does not make a great deal of difference what group of
patients are selected according to the individual goals of a programme, but the
problems in pain are so varied that it is well to have a selection procedure which
fits patients to the skills and aims of the individual programme. The second
major aim is to *describe the goals and to organize therapy around these goals*.
Some centres currently deal with pain relief, some with altering pain behaviour,
others only with diagnosis, and some management of patients by selected techniques. In our opinion, the diagnostic-eclectic treatment approach is most ap-
pealing, but these goal decisions must be made according to the resources
available. In addition to pain relief, improvement of function and elimination of
harmful drugs are general common aims. These should be within the skill of any
pain treatment programme. The next important aim is in *staff selection*. One
member must be selected as leader and must function in this fashion. The
speciality of this leader is not important. Blumer (1975) has suggested that the
senior surgeon is most appropriate because of the propensity of patients with
chronic pain to ask for and expect surgical procedures. It is also possible for the
senior surgeon to serve as consultant and for the leader to be from another area.
However, it is very important that the leader accept full medical responsibility
for all patients. Non-physician personnel can certainly manage specialized areas
of therapy, such as behaviour modification programmes, but the diagnostic
aspect requires physician control. As a minimum, a multi-disciplinary centre
should have available a neurosurgeon and orthopaedic surgeon, an internist, an
anaesthesiologist, a neurologist and a psychiatrist. Not all of these individuals
have to be full-time members of the staff and can serve effectively as consultants.
Additionally, a physical therapist, clinical psychologist, dietitian, technicians for
biofeedback and transcutaneous electrical stimulation and a social workers are
useful in most programmes. Nurses should preferably have psychiatric experi-

ence or education, and a knowledge of neuropharmacology, group process and behaviour modification.

Obviously, any such unit should have complete diagnostic capabilities to allow the thorough evaluation of every patient referred. This should include complete psychiatric and psychological evaluation.

Comprehensive therapy techniques should also be available. It is our belief that if the programme is truly multi-disciplinary and chooses an eclectic approach, it should have available transcutaneous electrical stimulation, biofeedback, physical therapy and an exercise programme, narcotic withdrawal capabilities, the possibility for appropriate psychotropic drug use, facilities for diagnostic and therapeutic nerve block, facilities for appropriate bracing and home therapy techniques, group psychotherapy, individual psychotherapy, family and couples counselling including sexual counselling, weight loss control, a form of behaviour modification, and the possibility of referral for definitive therapy to any appropriate speciality.

A major aim also must be to maintain the gains made in the initial or in-patient programme. It is obvious that our in-patient programme is a limited facility which only begins a process which will require months to years to complete. Follow-up of patients becomes very important. This follow-up may take several forms. Some patients will be followed individually by the consultants of the programme as in the usual medical mode. Some patients will be maintained in a group psychotherapy activity. Some will be monitored by the nurse specialists working in the programme. Some may only require the support of a patient group organized to maintain gains, and alter behaviour and attitude. In our experience, abandonment at the end of hospitalization means almost certainly that the patients will resume their original behaviour.

One of the major things to be considered in organization is the reaction of health professionals to the patient with chronic pain. It is most important for physicians dealing with chronic pain patients to examine these reactions carefully and plan their therapies around them. It is rare that the physician dealing with the patient with chronic pain can provide an absolute or definitive therapy for the patient. There is a great tendency for the physician to dismiss complaints that cannot be visualized by a diagnostic technique (Hackett, 1971). There is an equally dangerous tendency to substitute a procedure, especially surgery, for a detailed personal analysis of the patient.

The frustration which the physician faces in dealing with these patients whom he neither understands nor helps takes several forms. One is the retreat to a procedure. Another is resorting to medications in order to get the patient out of the office. A third is merely to reassure the patient that all studies are normal without any explanation of why the patient suffers the pain.

Many physicians also are prejudiced against certain classes of patients. Attractive females may be viewed as hysterical (Chodoff, 1974). Patients with pending litigation, especially industrial injury cases, are not even seen by some physicians. The industrial injury prejudices the physician against any care in many instances. It is equally possible that the advantage which accrues to the physician through dealing with an industrial injury patient also influences therapy for some.

Early in their experience of chronic pain, most professional personnel take on the role of patient advocate. They vigorously look for something to do to the patient to eliminate the complaint of chronic pain. As each successive therapy fails, enthusiasm for treatment wanes. The physician becomes frustrated, begins to feel inadequate and becomes angry at the patient, basically for not getting better in spite of the multiple therapies utilized. The physician is disenchanted with particular patients and frequently abandons them, usually by referral to another specialist. This situation often leads to an adversarial role for one physician against others involved in the patient's care. The newest physician is still searching for the magic treatment and functioning as the patient advocate. The disenchanted physicians are viewed as adversaries, both by patient and physician. As long as this situation exists, no adequate therapy is possible. Adversarial interchange between physicians involved in the care of such a patient is often elicited by careful history.

Physicians can usually be categorized accurately in their management of chronic pain problems. One of the most common types is the *helper*. This physician sticks by the patient providing help *and* medication. The patient usually is assisted in litigation and disability. The physician testifies on the patient's behalf, confronts and argues with other physicians in support of the patient, and generally provides unlimited medication to relieve the pain. The medications which the physician prescribes, usually narcotics and hypnotics, create more problems than originally existed. The physician in this category is motivated by a sincere desire to help the patient, but usually creates unnecessary disability and significant drug problems through this desire. The second major category is the *busy physician*. This individual has no time to listen to pain complaints, especially those which do not suggest immediate diagnoses. He usually simply prescribes whatever is necessary to move the patient through the office as rapidly as possible. The third type of physician is the *judge*. This physician is prone to consider only totally objective data and is frequently offended by patients who do not share his own admirable work habits. He is quick to make a psychiatric referral, though the referral is frequently made upon the absence of physical findings, rather than for objective reasons. Such physicians have a difficult time comprehending the patient's response to pain and have little understanding of the ineffectual, hypochondriacal, depressed and anxious patient who presents with the complaint of pain. Exposure to this type of physician firmly entrenches the symptoms since the patient is determined to prove that this physician is wrong in what the patient perceives as accusations. There are others who function solely as *analysts*. Such a physician makes little effort to examine the possibility of an organic basis for the complaint of pain or to consider the organic causes once assurances from referring physicians have been obtained that there are no obvious organic causes for pain. The *behaviourist* is equally limited. The approach of this individual is to attempt to alter pain behaviour regardless of the aetiology and to make the individual more functional. Behavioural therapy is obviously valuable, but its application to all chronic pain patients is inappropriate. Following the analytical or behavioural modes strictly may actually prevent adequate pain therapy for some patients.

It is our belief that an eclectic approach should be adopted by the pain physician. We believe that this physician, regardless of speciality, should retain an impartial approach. An accurate diagnosis should be made and then treatment selected according to the diagnosis. The physician should not make judgements but should exhibit empathy without being over-sympathetic. Personal warmth, a genuine concern for their patients' well-being and the ability to avoid an adversary relationship are extremely important features in the personality of the physician dealing with patients with chronic pain. It requires self-discipline and training to maintain such an approach and physicians should spend a significant amount of time examining their own attitudes and reactions if they are to be effective. A hostile or judgemental attitude is never productive and an antagonistic relationship between patient and physician will always result in failure. Furthermore, a single approach to what is essentially a multi-faceted problem is equally non-productive. The physician dealing in chronic pain should have available complete diagnostic facilities and should choose from multiple therapeutic modalities based upon an accurate diagnosis. The diverse nature of the origins and manifestations of chronic pain demand an eclectic approach and those physicians who do not adhere to this tenet are unlikely to provide optimal assistance for their patients.

REFERENCES

ADAMS J.E., HOSOBUCHI Y. & FIELDS H.L. (1974) Stimulation of internal capsule for relief of chronic pain. *Journal of Neurosurgery*, **41**, 740–4.

BION W.R. (1959) *Experiences in Groups and Other Papers*. Basic Books, New York.

BLUMER D. (1975) Psychiatric considerations in pain. In *The Spine* (Eds. Rothman & Simeone), Vol. 2, Chapter 18. W. B. Saunders,

BONICA J.J. (1953) *The Management of Pain*. Lea and Febiger, Philadelphia.

BONICA J.J. (1964) The management of pain of malignant diseases with nerve blocks. *Anaesthesiology*, **15**, 134–45, 280–301.

BRODSKY C.M. (1971) Compensation illness as a retirement channel. *Journal of the American Geriatrics Society*, **19**, 51–60.

CHODOFF P. (1974) The diagnosis of hysteria: an overview. *American Journal of Psychiatry*, **131**, 1073–8.

FORDYCE W. (1973) Behavioural therapy for chronic pain. *Postgraduate Medicine*, **53**, 58–63.

FOX J.L. (1974) Dorsal column stimulation for relief of intractable pain: problems encountered with neuropacemakers. *Surgical Neurology*, **2**, 59–64.

HACKETT T.P. (1971) Pain and prejudice. Why do we doubt that the patient is in pain? *Medical Times*, **99**, 130–9.

HARRIS W. (1940) An analysis of 1,433 cases of paroxysmal trigeminal neuralgia (trigeminal-tic) and the end results of gasserian alcohol injection. *Brain*, **63**, 209–24.

HOSOBUCHI Y., ADAMS J.E. & RUTKIN B. (1973) Chronic thalamic stimulation for the control of facial anesthesia dolorosa. *Archives of Neurology, Chicago*, **19**, 158–61.

JANNETTA P.J. (1975) Microsurgical approach to the trigeminal nerve for Tic Douloureux. *Progress in Neurological Surgery*, Vol. 7, pp. 180–200. Karger, Basel.

KAHN E.A. & PEET M.M. (1948) The techniques of anterolateral cordotomy. *Journal of Neurosurgery*, **5**, 276–83.

LIN P.M., GILDERBERG P.L. & POLAKOFF P.P. (1966) An anterior approach to percutaneous lower cervical cordotomy. *Journal of Neurosurgery*, **25**, 553–60.

LOESER J.D. (1972) Dorsal rhizotomy for relief of chronic pain. *Journal of Neurosurgery*, **36**, 745–50.

LONG D.M. & HAGFORS N. (1973) Electrical stimulation for relief of pain from chronic nerve injury. *Journal of Neurosurgery*, **39**, 718–22.

MAZARS G.L. (1975) Intermittent stimulation of nucleus ventralis posterolateralis for intractable pain. *Surgical Neurology*, **4**, 93–5.

MELZACK R. & WALL P.D. (1965) Pain mechanisms: a new theory. *Science*, **150**, 971–79.

MERSKEY H. & SPEAR F.G. (1967) *Pain, Psychological and Psychiatric Aspects*. Ballière, Tindall & Cassell, London.

MODLIN H.C. (1967) The post-accident anxiety syndrome: psychological aspects. *American Journal of Psychiatry*, **123**, 1008–12.

MULLAN S., HEKMATPANAH J., DOBBEN G. & BECKMAN F. (1968) Percutaneous, intramedullary cordotomy utilizing the unipolar anodal electrolytic lesion. *Journal of Neurosurgery*, **22**, 548–53.

NASHOLD B.S. JR, WILSON W.P. & SLAUGHTER D.G. (1969) Stereotactic midbrain lesions for central dysesthesia and phantom pain. *Journal of Neurosurgery*, **30**, 116–26.

OGLE W.S., FRENCH L.A. & PEYTON W.T. (1956) Experiences with high cervical cordotomy. *Journal of Neurosurgery*, **13**, 81–7.

ONOFRIO B.M. & CAMPA H.K. (1972) Evaluation of rhizotomy: review of 12 years experience. *Journal of Neurosurgery*, **36**, 751–5.

PAPO I. & VISCA A. (1976) Intrathecal phenol in the treatment of pain and spasticity. *Progress in Neurological Surgery*, Vol. 7, pp. 56–130. Karger, Basel.

PEET M.M. & SCHNEIDER R.C. (1952) Trigeminal neuralgia. A review of 689 cases with a follow-up study on 65 per cent of the group. *Journal of Neurosurgery*, **9**, 367–77.

REISER H. (1972) Psychotherapeutic drugs and the alleviation of pain. In *Pain, Basic Principles—Pharmacology-Therapy* (Eds. Payne J.P. *et al.*), pp. 174. Williams & Wilkins, Baltimore.

RICHARDSON D.E. & AKIL H. (1977) Long term results of periventricular gray self-stimulation. *Neurosurgery*, **1**, 199–202.

SHAW R.S. (1964) Pathologic malingering: the painful disabled extremity. *New England Journal of Medicine*, **271**, 22–6.

SIEBENS A.A. (1974) Percutaneous radiofrequency rhizotomy. *Surgical Neurology*, **2**, 319–26.

SIEGFRIED J. (1977) Stereotactic pulvinarotomy in the treatment of intractable pain. *Progress in Neurological Surgery*, Vol. 8, pp. 104–13. Karger, Basel.

SOUREK K. (1977) Mediolongitudinal myelotomy. *Progress in Neurological Surgery*, Vol. 8, pp. 15–34. Karger, Basel.

STERNBACH R.A. (1974) *Pain Patients: Traits and Treatment*. Academic Press, New York.

STERNBACH R.A. (1978) Treatment of the chronic pain patient. *Journal of Human Stress*, **4** (3), 11–15.

STERNBACH R.A., WOLFE S.R., MURPHY R.W. & AKESON W.H. (1973) Traits of pain patients: the low back 'loser'. *Psychosomatics*, **14**, 226–9.

SWEET W.H. (1977) Intracranial electrical stimulation for relief of chronic intractable pain. *Progress in Neurological Surgery*, Vol. 8, pp. 258–69. Karger, Basel.

TIBBITS C. (1954) Retirement problems in American society. *American Journal of Sociology*, **59**, 301–8.

WHITE J.C. (1946) Painful injuries of nerves and their surgical treatment. *American Journal of Surgery*, **72**, 468–88.

WHITE J.C. (1962) Modification of frontal leucotomy for relief of pain and suffering in terminal malignant disease. *Annals of Surgery*, **56**, 394–403.

WHITE J.C. (1976) Role of sympathectomy in relief of pain. *Progress in Neurological Surgery*, Vol. 7, pp. 131–52. Karger, Basel.

WILSON M. & MEYER E. (1965) The doctors' vs. the nurses' view of emotional disturbance. *Canadian Psychiatric Association Journal*, **10** (3), 212–15.

Chapter 11
Rehabilitation of the Patient with Chronic Neuromuscular Disease

Chronic neuromuscular disease may arise in any of the components of the motor unit and in recent years the distinction between primary disorder of muscles (myopathy and dystrophy) and secondary disturbance has become blurred. When any component of a motor unit is involved, biochemically or structurally, muscle weakness is the most obvious feature. Secondary features, such as contractures and scoliosis, may develop with many chronic neuromuscular disorders. Although the contractures and scoliosis may vary considerably from disease to disease, in any one condition the main aims of the rehabilitation team are in overcoming the effect of muscle weakness (i.e. loss of mobility and loss of function) and the prevention, correction and counteraction of deformities (i.e. flexion contractures or scoliosis).

The aim of this chapter is to attempt to outline a philosophy of patient management in chronic neuromuscular disease. Some of the more common conditions will be considered in detail, as examples of rehabilitation problems. Apart from the problems associated with specific disease entities, there are also the wider medical and social implications of severe disability. This, inevitably, leads to mentioning facilities which are available in the National Health Service (UK), and although such facilities are not necessarily universally available, they are described in some detail since they form integral components of management.

In the chronic neuromuscular disorders the diagnosis is often tantamount to issuing a death certificate. The relentless progressive nature of these diseases presents the clinician, nurses and therapists with the insurmountable difficulty of having to face patients with that knowledge. However, whereas terminal care units have been created for cancer patients, there are few facilities to help patients and families cope with the long-drawn-out deterioration of chronic neuromuscular disease. Increasing weakness, incontinence, loss of independence, are often more difficult to manage than the more dramatic problems of pain and cachexia of cancer. There are many symptoms apart from pain which can be helped, for example: spasm, anorexia, nausea and vomiting, dysphagia, dental caries and buccal infection, anxiety and depression, constipation, incontinence, insomnia and decubitus ulcers. Many patients develop a fear of dying and difficulties with breathing and swallowing exacerbate this. Increasing dependence increases the patient's psychological reaction and problems. Uncertainty leads to anxiety, and there is often a reluctance on the part of doctors, therapists and family to discuss frankly the reality so that realistic plans for long-term care and management can be instituted. This 'conspiracy of silence' hinders all aspects of the caring procedure by spoiling relationships, and the compounding dishonesty often prevents the acceptance of adequate plans and prevents the patient from making the most of his deteriorating capabilities. Many clinicians feel that it is not right to tell a patient that he has an incurable disease, but the patient needs to be told what is wrong with him and how it will affect him. It is important to balance the truth with a clear explanation of what can be done to help, and to show the patient that there is an organization and a *person* who will be there to help and guide him and his family.

THE PLACE OF PHYSICAL THERAPY

During the past 20 years there has been a definite and logical swing away from undue reliance on passive and palliative physical treatment. Patients with chronic disability and apparently insuperable problems demand that their doctors do something. For such patients, the provision of aids and appliances, coupled with palliative physiotherapy constitutes the modern placebo therapy, but placebo therapy becomes hazardous if it diverts attention from real needs. Many of the problems and complications of rehabilitation derive from failure to identify the basic problems, and therefore failure to apply the most appropriate treatment.

Physiotherapy in the form of various applications of heat or cold can help to reduce spasm. The main value of this activity is to enable the therapist (or family) to stretch contractures or encourage active exercises. Contractures require frequent stretching of the affected muscles, and maintaining the improvement by splints both by day and at night. Several treatments each day by a relative, and the wearing of corrective splints at night, will achieve more than intermittent attendance at a physiotherapy department. Similarly, strengthening exercises for improving function and coordination must be practised frequently if they are to be effective.

Thus the physiotherapist is much more an 'assessor and teacher' than 'therapist'. She must be fully integrated into the diagnostic and therapeutic team so that she can contribute to the repeated assessments and be quite clear of her role in the overall management. There must be no confusion of advice to the patient.

The occupational therapist is involved in the assessment of actual and potential function, for provision of and instruction in the use of aids and appliances, and for assessing work potential. Her work must overlap and link with that of the physiotherapist, for while the physiotherapist is concentrating on walking and the use of sticks and walking frames, the occupational therapist may be able to demonstrate that safe domestic independence can be better achieved from a wheelchair. The timing of change from walking to wheelchair activity is a matter for discussion between all the members of the clinical team and should include the patient and family, to whom the 'pros and cons' should be clearly explained.

MOBILITY

Physical disability reduces the alternatives from which the individual can choose by limiting the places where he can live, his career, hobbies, friends and even the clothes he wears and the food he eats. It imposes architectural, administrative and financial barriers. The key problem—both indoors and outdoors—is mobility, and much of the long-term management of patients with chronic neuromuscular disease is directed towards maintaining their independence of mobility. Achievement in mobility will determine most of the other problems of management and rehabilitation. As disability progresses it is important to maintain a minimal level of independence for as long as possible. The ability to stand up, take a few steps, turn round and sit down can render a person able to continue with many activities of daily living, including using the toilet. Once a patient becomes confined to a wheelchair, social activities become increasingly difficult and secondary depression may ensue. As mobility deteriorates, whether due to weakness, pain or lack of coordination, simple walking aids such as sticks, crutches, quadruped sticks or walking frames may help considerably.

Walking Aids

A single stick or crutch can be used to relieve weight by patients with unilateral disease, and should be used on the contralateral side. Better weight relief and balance are provided by the use of two sticks. The handle of the stick should be level with the greater trochanter, with the patient standing erect in shoes. The handle of many sticks and crutches is too small and hard for arthritic, wasted or spastic hands. Soft padding, sorbo rubber or 'plastazote' can be used to provide the correct sized handle and make it easier to grip. Strong, lightweight inexpensive metal sticks with suitable moulded left or right handles are available, and these can be cut to the correct length. Some patients prefer a straight handle to the traditional curved handle. The traditional under-arm crutch is rarely suitable or necessary for patients with chronic disease, as they are designed to relieve weight-bearing in one limb.

Elbow crutches are easier to use, but in severe disability a forearm guttercrutch is more suitable, since it demands less of the upper arm joints. The crutch height should always be adjustable and it is preferable to use elbow crutches which have adjustable arm supports.

Aids to walking such as 'quadruped sticks' (sticks with four small legs) provide more support and are particularly useful for those patients who have poor balance. All sticks, crutches and quadrupeds should be fitted with large, renewable rubber ferrules. It is as important to replace worn ferrules as it is to replace worn tyres on motor vehicles.

More severely affected patients are better served by a lightweight walking frame with a wide base. Patients with poor hand function and weak arms cannot manage to lift the walking frame, and a modified version with two small wheels on the leading legs and suitably adjusted arm supports should be provided. However, such aids do not encourage normal walking movement and are very cumbersome in most small-roomed houses.

The use of crutches and other aids in confined spaces is difficult. Carefully positioned furniture is useful as support, but in other cases a small trolley may be preferred, providing both a walking aid and a carrying surface. Easily held, strong rails should be placed beside all stairs and steps, and banisters should be fitted to both sides of the stairs. Rails may also be required outside the house to provide extra support during wet or snowy weather, and this is particularly important if the patient needs to use an outside toilet. For very severely disabled people it may be better to provide a ground-floor bedroom and bathroom and replace all outside steps by suitably inclined ramps. For flat dwellers a change of accommodation may be necessary.

Many patients have difficulty in sitting down and rising from chairs, beds and toilets of normal height and this is particularly so if calipers are used. Although alterations in heights can easily be undertaken, many patients prefer a special chair which is not only of the correct height, but which has firm arms, a high moulded back and a seat of reduced depth.

Alterations to the house and the choice of furniture are quite clearly personal matters. There must be close collaboration between the hospital and local authorities and much of the assessment for the detailed work must be done in the patient's own home, whether by staff based in hospital or by local authority domiciliary workers.

Wheelchairs

A wheelchair is usually regarded as the insignia of disability. Certainly the majority of wheelchair users are elderly and suffering from degenerative disorders and require a wheelchair for use out of doors. However, for younger disabled people a wheelchair should be regarded as an *aid to mobility*. If optimum mobility independence is to be achieved the assessment for an appropriate chair and accessories is of considerable importance. The patient who requires a wheelchair may have it issued through United Kingdom National Health Service (NHS) free of charge, although it will still remain the property of the Department of Health and Social Security. A patient who needs a chair for both indoor and outdoor use may be issued with two chairs when one is not suitable for both purposes.

Wheelchairs may be self-propelled, attendant-propelled or electrically powered. Attendant-propelled chairs usually have small wheels and thus can more easily be stored in the boot of a car. Most chairs are available in standard and lightweight versions, and are made in a range of sizes. There are variations in the recline of the back rest, and in the design of foot and leg rests, and the arm rests, some of which are detachable. There are a number of available accessories such as cushions, trays and extending head rests. The choice of wheelchair depends upon the patient's physical capabilities and the situation in which the chair will be used, and the activities which the user wishes to pursue whilst in the chair. Frequently the choice of chair and its accessories cannot be separated from other decisions regarding the general management of the patient. For this reason, collaborative clinics, sharing the skills of remedial therapists and technical officers, are the best way of achieving improvement in the service to severely handicapped patients, both with regard to prescription, supply and maintenance of the chair, and in training the patient and helping him to use the chair to maximum advantage.

Individually Contoured Seating for the Disabled

Many severely disabled patients present sitting problems, and some of these can only be solved by the manufacture of an individual seat. Some can be made comfortable with cushions and sometimes lateral supports will adequately control a collapsing spine. In recent years a number of centres have described techniques for the construction of individually manufactured seats. These usually depend upon an accurate body cast and vacuum consolidation techniques have been introduced. However, some patients, particularly those with severe collapsing scoliosis, are almost impossible to cast accurately and they can become acutely distressed during the conventional casting procedures. The seats made from these techniques can be used as inserts for wheelchairs, or may be made up as feeding chairs for children, toilet chairs or car seats. It is sometimes possible to use one seat for a number of situations.

It should be emphasized that the more accurate the fitting of a body support, the more restrictive it will be. A number of severely disabled patients, particularly those with progressive disabilities such as muscular dystrophy, may lose their remaining functional activities if their trunks are too closely supported.

Hoists

Many disabled people can be trained to transfer from one seat to another, but as disability increases they become more reliant upon relatives or other attendants. Frequently the attendants themselves find the effort of lifting difficult and dangerous and in these circumstances a hoist can make transfers easier and safer, both for the patient and his helper, but the efficient use of a hoist demands training and experience.

There are a wide variety of hoists, portable or fixed, hydraulic, mechanically or electrically operated. Some are designed for specific purposes such as car hoists or bath hoists. The choice will depend upon the situation in which it will be used, and the space available. The selection of the sling to be used is as important as the type of hoist, to ensure comfort and safety. The choice of hoist and slings is complex, and patient and helper need time, practical trials and training.

Conventional portable hoists with band slings are cumbersome and cannot be easily manoeuvred in the confines of the average lavatory or bathroom. An electrically operated overhead hoist which is either fixed over the toilet or mounted on a gantry or a ceiling track may be suitable for the patient to operate, and certainly its ease of operation will ensure that both attendant and patient will use such a device. The gantry-type hoist requires no structural alterations, and is easily installed, but it is of great importance that the correct sling, usually the hammock type for patients with poor head control, is supplied.

In the UK most hoists are provided through the local authority services. Many authorities have a small stock of hoists so that they can be supplied quickly, or a trial at home can be arranged. Electric hoists for assessment and training are usually found in hospital assessment units.

SEVERE UPPER LIMB WEAKNESS

Lower limb weakness restricts mobility and calls for a response in mechanical terms. Upper limb weakness causes considerable functional loss but is much more difficult to overcome with aids and appliances. The functional capacity of the upper limb in terms of manipulative and sensory skill of the hand, and the ability of the arm to place the hand in space, are extremely difficult to replace with a mechanical device.

For a small number of patients there are two types of device which may help: 'flail arm splints' and 'mobile arm supports'.

Flail Arm Splints

Upper extremity paralysis occasionally calls for management by means of a splint. The basic problem is to substitute for absent shoulder and elbow flexion and extension, and associated pronation and supination, in order to place the hand in a functional position.

The conventional flail arm splints consist of a shoulder cap, upper arm and forearm troughs, and inner and outer steels. These devices are made to casts of the patient's shoulder and arm, and the manufacture, fitting and delivery may take many weeks. A number of designs have been successfully used for patients with brachial plexus lesions, but few devices appear to be successful for patients with chronic neuromuscular disease.

The splints are rejected because of:
1.   the effort required to operate the splint
2.   the splint appears crude and clumsy, and cosmetically unacceptable
3.   the splint is too heavy
4.   complex problems of assembly and maintenance.

The problem in progressive neuromuscular diseases is in making a realistic and accurate prognosis of the condition in relation to the patient's overall functional capability. Some patients will remain ambulant for months and years, but a heavy flail arm splint is inevitably an additional burden to carry, with little gain in function.

Mobility and communication these days can be achieved by many physically disabled people by using electrically powered wheelchairs, environmental control devices, electric typewriters and so on. The increasing flexibility of prescribing and providing these sophisticated devices has therefore overtaken many of the needs for non-powered flail arm splints. Properly fitted mobile arm supports are likely to be much more useful, giving a wider range of mobility than flail arm splints or powered flail arm splints.

Mobile Arm Supports

Mobile arm supports (balanced forearm orthoses, balanced linkage feeders, or ball-bearing arm supports) allow frictionless, gravity-eliminated movement on the horizontal plane, with some vertical movement provided by means of a pivotal trough which supports the forearm. The basic assembly consists of a clamp or bracket fixed to the upright of a chair, two swivel arms which rotate on plastic bearings, and a forearm trough. Considerable adjustments are possible, and other individual requirements can be met by standard or bespoke fittings.

Mobile arm supports are fitted for patients with weakness in their shoulder girdle and upper arm and neck musculature. They are not suitable for patients with much spasticity or gross tremor. They are most useful for patients with poliomyelitis, muscular dystrophy, motoneuron disease and high spinal cord lesions. There are three basic requirements for the fitting of mobile arm supports:
1.   good sitting posture and a stable trunk, so that the patient's arms are free
2.   good range of passive movements in the upper limbs and strength in either the shoulder girdle muscles or the neck and trunk muscles
3.   a suitable chair or wheelchair to which the clamp may be fitted.

Rejection of Aids and Appliances

It is natural to assume that a physical impairment can be compensated for by the provision of suitable aids or appliances. Many engineers, technicians, therapists and doctors enjoy devising a piece of equipment which would appear to supply the patient's need. Such activities have the full approbation of the patient, and the inevitable period of involvement and enthusiasm during which the complex equipment is designed and prototypes are produced is a powerful placebo. The patient will naturally respond with enthusiasm when interest is directed towards him, whether through medicines, physiotherapy or appliances; but the rejection rate for appliances is very high. To be acceptable an appliance must provide an immediate and obvious practical gain without the imposition of too high a penalty of discomfort, awkwardness, mechanical unreliability, restriction of other activities, or unpleasant appearance.

Although many physically disabled people appear to need aids and appliances, only a careful assessment will reveal the true need and the likelihood of acceptance of an appliance, or whether extra home help or admission to residential or warden-supervised accommodation would be more appropriate. However, admission to a residential unit is a second-best solution and there is increasing pressure from physically disabled people themselves to resist relegation to an institution. Thus much of rehabilitation of patients with chronic neuromuscular diseases consists of providing all the necessary support for the patient, the family and helpers to maintain them at home in the community.

MOTIVATION AND PERSONALITY

Although the problem of remunerative employment frequently does not arise with the severely physically disabled, many desire to achieve some creative activity. Indeed, they often prefer to expend their available energy upon creative hobbies or work than activities of daily living, and there are those who work for many hours a day yet are completely dependent upon others for toilet, dressing and feeding.

The conventional psychometric test batteries not only include a large number of irrelevant and inappropriate questions, but they are also fatiguing to physically handicapped people and are not sufficiently discriminating at the higher and lower levels of intelligence. Therefore, psychometric tests for the severely physically handicapped have to be chosen and abbreviated so that they do not fatigue the patient, and yet cover the conventional areas of memory, recall and personality assessment. The variation in cognitive functions and the personality variables follow the pattern expected in the normal population. Variations may occur due to factors such as the time lapse between onset of disability and rehabilitation, the patient's age, lack of education and, in particular, lack of experience. When a relatively mature person becomes disabled, his reaction to the disability must depend upon his premorbid personality. Parental attitudes play a large part in a child's adjustment to disability, and reaction to rehabilitation.

Reactive depression is a common feature in patients with severe physical disability. Unfortunately it is not possible to alter the main cause—the physical disability. Improving the general environmental situation, providing appropriate aids and appliances, and general care and counselling may help. Too frequently, however, it is not possible to affect the depression in this way and pharmacological management may be necessary before the patient can respond to the rehabilitation programme.

Clinical psychologists contribute to the overall assessment of the patient by helping to determine intellectual impairment which might affect the ability to respond to a rehabilitation programme (e.g. memory impairment, perceptual problems). Educational possibilities and intellectual capabilities are important, and interests and aptitudes are relevant for both work and leisure activities. It is also important to determine the extent to which mood and behaviour factors (anxiety and depression) are involved. Serial testing helps to determine the rate of progression. Clinical psychologists can also contribute to the treatment of patients with physical disability. Their approach may be behavioural (based on learning principles) or psychotherapeutic (based on personality dynamics).

The psychological features are often closely interwoven with the social ones, and patients and their relatives require the combined help of clinical psychologists and social workers. In particular, they would be concerned with those having difficulty in responding to the rehabilitation programme; those who are withdrawn or over-talkative; those who demonstrate attention-seeking behaviour, who have marital problems, who have problems with children, who have no visitors; or those with an over-demanding or unsympathetic spouse.

The social worker will also be concerned with the practical problems of employment, housing, finances, holidays and domiciliary services such as home helps or meals on wheels.

MANAGEMENT OF DUCHENNE MUSCULAR DYSTROPHY AND SPINAL MUSCULAR ATROPHY

Appropriate treatment and advice concerning any disease depend upon accurate diagnosis. The importance of diagnosis when considering the difference in prognosis between cases of Duchenne muscular dystrophy and the later onset types of spinal muscular atrophy is clear.

Regular physiotherapy has been considered of vital importance by many authors, but no acceptable controlled trials have yet been published. In practice, management is mainly directed to supportive care for the child and the family.

Management

A frank, open discussion with the parents, the patient and his siblings is usually the best way to start. Often there is initial, understandable, resentment and refusal to believe or accept the truth, and discussions require patience, time and effort. The main features of Duchenne muscular dystrophy requiring physical rehabilitation are the loss of independent mobility, increasing flexion deformities of hips, knees and feet, and collapsing scoliosis. In addition, the progressive weakness brings problems of personal care: dressing, washing, feeding, toileting, and problems of comfort when sitting and lying in bed. Secondary problems relate to education, leisure activities, occupation and general activities of every-day life. These problems are as numerous, but less aggressive in form, in the other dystrophies and spinal muscular atrophies, depending upon the age of onset and rate of progression. In Duchenne muscular dystrophy progression is fairly predictable and almost standardized treatment schedules can be undertaken. The spinal muscular atrophies, by their heterogeneity, demand individual assessment and treatment.

Mobility

Boys with Duchenne muscular dystrophy cease independent walking between the ages of 9 and 13 years. In spinal muscular atrophy the picture may vary considerably. Extensive external support in the form of braces and calipers is often provided to keep these children standing and walking for a period of several hours each day. Such active treatment of this type is said to delay the progression of muscle weakness, delay the scoliosis, and improve the psychological outlook of both child and parents. Once the child ceases walking and resorts to a wheelchair, flexion deformities of the legs rapidly develop and collapsing scoliosis progresses. The problem is whether the immense effort required by the child to cope with the extensive external bracing, and the logistical problems of providing adequate bracing during growth, outweigh the advantage of swift, easy mobility in a wheelchair, self-propelled or powered. Once a child has experienced the relative mobility of a powered chair, he will rarely continue to struggle with calipers and crutches.

Although a wheelchair is often seen as an admission that disability is increasing it should be accepted as a symbol of *mobility*. In Duchenne muscular dystrophy and spinal muscular atrophy the use of self-propelled chairs is limited because of decreasing upper limb power. Lightweight chairs are to be preferred as they weigh approximately 16 kg, compared with standard chairs which weigh in excess of 25 kg. Patients who are unable to sit upright because of impaired balance or respiratory function require a wheelchair with an adjustable back rest or special seat supports.

A suitable, powered wheelchair, modified as necessary, is the most appropriate method of gaining mobility when one of three clinical situations supervenes:

1. when walking is unsafe and can be expected to lead to a fall
2. when walking is possible only with aids which put a detrimental degree of stress on the upper limbs
3   when walking is physically so exhausting that it interferes with the achievement of other activities.

Powered Indoor Wheelchairs

In the UK powered wheelchairs are available on prescription to those who are unable to walk and are also unable, or are medically unfit, to propel themselves in standard wheelchairs. Although initial recommendations may be resisted, the opportunity to use such a chair in an assessment environment demonstrates its effectiveness as a mobility aid, and the energy then available for other activities becomes apparent. A number of different models are available, and prescription depends upon size, manoeuvrability, the controls, the ease with which accessories (e.g. mobile arm supports, leg rests or supportive trunk padding) can be fitted. The environment in which the chair is to be used is also important—slopes, size of doors, distances to be traversed.

The foot rests are important in helping to prevent increasing foot deformities, and the position of the arm rests must also be considered so that access to a table or participation in educational and recreational activities is possible. A practical trial is the most important method of determining the most suitable chair. The child will use the chair all day, every day for many years, and the time spent in getting the right chair with the right modifications is time well spent. As a device it becomes an integral part of the patient's life—like a pair of artificial legs for a double amputee.

Mobile Arm Supports

Mobile arm supports may enable a patient to continue to feed independently, an aspect of independence much cherished by the patient, and writing, reading and appropriate hobbies may be easier to accomplish. Mobile arm supports are difficult to fit properly and require regular adjustment and servicing. The sitting posture must be determined and stable. Without adequate trunk support the device will not function normally, and if a spinal brace or wheelchair trunk support is necessary this must be supplied prior to the fitting of the arm support.

By the use of 'trick' movements some boys are able to overcome many of the manipulative problems presented by their disease, and although mobile arm supports may theoretically provide them with a greater independence, they are not always readily accepted and any aid or appliance will be valueless if the patient does not wish it.

Outdoor Mobility

Lack of outdoor mobility is often a great frustration. There are powered wheel-chairs designed for outdoor use, but in the United Kingdom these are not provided through the Department of Health and Social Security. A mobility allowance is paid in addition to other Social Security benefits to those people within certain age limits who are unable to walk because of persistent dis-ability. This allowance may be used to provide or contribute towards appro-priate outdoor transport—powered chair, adapted motor car, or for the hire of transport.

Some patients find that a 'caravanette' type of van fitted with a powered hoist for entry and exit provides suitable transport. Alternatively, some patients use a specially designed hoist for access to and from a car.

When travelling by road either by car or caravanette it is advisable to use efficient seat belts and clamps to restrain the wheelchair. Many wheelchair users are more safely transported in their chairs rather than using conventional seat-ing, but even a minor accident or an emergency stop can result in major injury to a severely disabled and inadequately harnessed passenger.

Foot Deformity (Duchenne Muscular Dystrophy)

In the early stage of Duchenne muscular dystrophy the foot becomes plantar-flexed. Initially it can be passively corrected to the neutral position, but with increasing age this becomes less possible. When walking ceases there is also increasing inversion of the forefoot and this deformity soon becomes fixed. Numerous attempts have been made to prevent or delay the progression of this deformity, but surgery has a very limited place.

However, if the foot is maintained in a neutral position normal footwear can be worn, a factor often of considerable importance to the patient, and a mobile or plantigrade foot is easier for dressing than a foot fixed in equino varus. Maintaining this position can be attempted initially by the provision of moulded polythene night splints which, if sufficiently comfortable, can be worn during the day as well. An adequate splint worn all night will have greater effect on the position of the foot than brief intermittent periods of physiotherapy. If correc-tion is not possible sheepskin 'bootees' provide warmth and protection.

Foot Deformity (Spinal Muscular Atrophy)

In common with many other features of spinal muscular atrophy the foot deformities are heterogeneous. Calcaneovalgus in patients who are still walking is well recognized, but in more severely affected patients fixed equino varus is often seen. In many of the more mature patients who had early onset of disease the foot adopts a plantigrade position and is passively quite mobile. Management of the foot deformity will depend on whether the patient is still walking and the presence or otherwise of skin ulceration. Treatment includes corrective night-splints and may proceed to surgical correction.

Spinal Deformity (Duchenne Muscular Dystrophy)

Paralytic deformities of the spine are well recognized in Duchenne muscular dystrophy. The more severe forms of spinal deformity start with a slight pelvic tilt to one side and progress to form a gross kyphoscoliosis with rotation of the spinal column. This 'end stage' situation is difficult to manage, and leads to respiratory embarrassment, alveolar hypostasis, and secondary infection. A more benign situation is characterized by an exaggerated lordosis throughout the whole thoraco-lumbar spine, which remains inherently stable. The inference is that the lordotic type of spinal deformity, which possibly starts as the increased lordosis seen in patients whilst still ambulant, should be encouraged.

Many types of spinal brace have been advocated for the collapsing scoliosis of progressive neuromuscular disease and many different materials have been used—plastic, celluloid, fibreglass or block leather. Such a jacket may need to be reviewed at six-monthly or more frequent intervals during growth spurts. A well-made jacket provides considerable support and may well delay the formation of spinal deformity providing that it is worn during the greater part of the day. When scoliosis has progressed beyond 45–60° from the vertical then external bracing of this type is no longer a practical form of treatment. At this stage, external padding attached to the arms of the wheelchair, or fitted within the wheelchair, can support the chest on the convex side of the scoliosis and provide gentle corrective pressure to the concave aspect. In severe cases, where deformity has resulted in the ribs pressing on the iliac crest, much relief has been obtained by using 'cushions' of stockinette filled with polystyrene beads.

Spinal Deformity (Spinal Muscular Atrophy)

In the severe forms of spinal muscular atrophy weakness of the paraspinal musculature will also lead to a progressive spinal deformity. As with patients with Duchenne muscular dystrophy attempts can be made to control early scoliosis by the use of spinal jackets, continuing into late adolescence. Because of the better prognosis surgical correction for scoliosis in spinal muscular atrophy has been attempted in a number of patients, but with varying results, the operation often leading to loss of a basic function such as balance or the ability to roll in bed. Operative complications can be kept to a minimum by careful preoperative assessment of cardiac and respiratory function, and by selecting before gross deformity embarrasses respiratory function. Unfortunately, the scoliosis of spinal muscular atrophy often goes untreated because the relatively favourable prognosis in some patients is not appreciated. Thus part of the organization for caring for these patients requires the facility for early diagnosis, effective follow-up, good preoperative assessment and correct conservative management and close liaison with orthopaedic surgeons. Given these conditions it should be possible to prevent many scolioses. Patients with advanced fixed spinal deformity, where corrective surgery is not contemplated, can be offered external support using padding inside their wheelchairs.

Flexion Contractures

In spite of active therapy, flexion deformities develop at many joints, particularly the hips and knees. A period of enforced bed rest will often, apparently, start the problem in previously mobile joints or exacerbate the deformity in affected joints. There does not appear to be a satisfactory reason offered for the aggressive development of these deformities. Passive stretching undertaken by physiotherapists or by parents is usually recommended. Numerous surgical procedures have been recommended to overcome some of these problems and maintain an upright posture to enable caliper walking. Posterior tibial tendon transfer, iliotibial band release and hamstring release have all been advocated, but postoperative management involving bed rest and splinting is liable to undo much of the benefit resulting from surgery. Respiratory impairment and cardiac disease make anaesthesia difficult and potentially dangerous.

Respiration

Cardio-respiratory failure and respiratory tract infections are the most common cause of death in Duchenne muscular dystrophy. In advanced Duchenne muscular dystrophy the vital capacity drops considerably below one litre and accurate measurement becomes difficult with conventional equipment. Estimation of peak flow rates is similarly difficult. The severe deformity seen in the late stages of Duchenne muscular dystrophy is usually associated with recurrent chest infections and impairment of gaseous exchange. When recurrent infection becomes a problem, especially during the winter months, it seems very reasonable to suggest that the early use of broad spectrum antibiotics and active physiotherapy consisting of assisted coughing and postural drainage should be considered. Prophylactic influenza vaccination is often used, but many feel that this is unjustified in the context of this disease. The use of positive pressure ventilation in association with a cuffed endotracheal tube or a tracheostomy has been suggested, but such heroic measures in the late stages of a progressive disease are, in the opinion of many clinicians, unjustifiable.

Comfort and Immobility

In Duchenne muscular dystrophy and spinal muscular atrophy motor impairment is not accompanied by a sensory defect and development of pressure sores is rare. The patient will indicate discomfort, and frequent requests for a change of position become trying for both patient and attendant, so any measure which reduces discomfort and movement is helpful.

Any clothing material which rucks or wrinkles over pressure points must be avoided and clothes should be designed so that seams are not over points of pressure. Medical sheepskins are effective, relatively cheap and easily washed, and their prolonged use has stood the test of time. Synthetic substitutes are cheaper, but do not have the same water vapour absorbing properties. Numerous mechanical devices are available to supplement the sheepskin when necessary. Alternating compartment air-filled cushions of the 'ripple' type are available for wheelchair use, and are run by a portable and rechargeable battery. Various types of gel-filled cushions are also available, but are often of limited value. The best cushions for use in any particular case can only be decided by trial and error.

Individually moulded body shells have been devised to overcome the problem of providing a comfortable sitting position. However, many very severely disabled patients make use of 'trick' trunk movements. These movements, although minimal, are often very valuable, and may be lost if an individually moulded body shell is provided. Often a 'wheelchair insert', built up by using plywood on which polyester foam is placed to support those weight-bearing points which are under greatest stress, is the most effective body support. By trial and error, a completed insert can be produced, consisting of several separate cushions which are positioned individually once the patient is seated in the wheelchair. All cushions should be covered in a material which is easily washed and not easily creased. Dependent, paralysed lower limbs will rapidly become oedematous and prejudice the peripheral circulation. Diuretics are of little use in this situation and long-term usage may precipitate electrolyte imbalance. The use of supportive bandages or stockings with elevating leg rests on the wheelchair will control oedema but usually interfere with wheelchair mobility. Chilblains may be helped by the use of sheepskin 'bootees'.

Nocturnal discomfort is a common feature in many neuromuscular diseases, often necessitating change in position many times each night. Some patients in the advanced stage of the disease find an 'electric' bed helpful in altering position. Various types of electric bed, controlled by a variety of switching devices, are available. Most manufacturers are prepared to allow a short period 'on approval' in the patient's own home.

Obesity

A tendency to obesity occurs in some patients who are severely disabled and particularly in Duchenne muscular dystrophy. When a heavy child can no longer be lifted by a parent, toileting and personal hygiene may present considerable problems. The parents accept that their child needs less food to meet his lessening energy requirements, but dieting in a family context is often difficult.

Personal Care

Inability to feed independently is not only frustrating but increases the patient's dependence on others. Impaired motor power in the upper limbs leads to an inability to cut food, particularly meat, and weak grip interferes with the handling of cutlery. Each patient's difficulties must be assessed by an experienced therapist.

Drinking may be even more difficult because of the need to lift and balance a container of liquid. If standard crockery proves unsuitable a lightweight mug or cup with a large, conveniently shaped handle may be grasped more easily, but many severely disabled people find a straw or polythene tube the most satisfactory solution. Mobile arm supports were originally developed for patients disabled by paralytic poliomyelitis, who often maintained trunk stability, and their provision requires careful assessment of posture, especially if sitting balance is poor, and fitting is often a time-consuming activity. However, the ability to feed independently is cherished by most patients, and these supports deserve to be considered more frequently as an aid for this.

Those who are dependent upon a wheelchair for mobility, especially when an upper limb weakness is present, will have considerable difficulty in washing, particularly the lower half of their bodies. Most patients who are severely disabled will require some help with washing and bathing. The disabled person who is ambulant or wheelchair bound but retains reasonable upper limb function, and sitting stability, may find it possible to bath with the aid of a bath board or a bath seat. For the more severely disabled a hoist may prove useful. Patients who are unable to bath themselves have four practical alternatives:
1. to take a bath with the aid of a helper
2. to take a bath with the aid of a helper and a hoist
3. to take a shower
4. to be given a bed bath.

Long-handled combs, long-handled make-up appliances to hold cosmetics, and electric toothbrushes are all readily available and are not obvious symbols of disability.

However physically disabled they may be, people like to dress in clothes which are currently fashionable. In general, even minor clothing alterations are often resisted although they would lead to a greater degree of independence—the wish to look 'normal' is paramount. Simple, unobtrusive measures such as the substitution of 'Velcro' for shirt buttons, and the insertion of zip fasteners in the inside leg seam of trousers so that calipers or urine collecting bags are covered, whilst still retaining ease of access to the appliances, are often helpful.

Many patients find dressing difficult, tiring and time-consuming and for many, in the later stages, it may be more sensible to advise them to accept help with dressing so that they have more energy to enjoy educational and recreational activities.

Toileting

It is very helpful if all severely disabled patients can be trained so that bowel actions will occur at regular and predictable times, usually based on the natural gastro-entero-colic reflex, coupled if necessary with the use of senna derivatives or bran. Thus the bowels may be opened reliably at a convenient time (usually before dressing in the morning) on two or three occasions each week. If a satisfactory bowel routine is not established, faecal retention will almost inevitably occur with consequent spurious diarrhoea. Although bedpans and commodes are frequently supplied, these devices are not generally acceptable to either patient or family, and, if at all possible, the bowels should be opened in the lavatory. With suitable training, equipment, and perhaps some modification to the home, this should be possible for most patients. A lavatory compartment large enough to allow transfer from wheelchair to toilet seat, with suitably sited grab rails, may be all that is required.

Where access is restricted, a commode wheelchair to which the patient can be transferred outside the lavatory, and which can then be placed into position over the lavatory pedestal, may solve the problem. For those patients who are severely hypotonic or who have severe spinal deformity it may be more appropriate to use a hoist with slings, with a specifically designed toilet aperture. Perineal cleansing following defaecation commonly presents difficulties. Although a small number of patients are able to manage this by holding the toilet paper with a pair of long-handled tongs, the majority require an attendant's assistance.

Micturition rarely presents difficulties for ambulant patients, except where severe impairment of upper limb function leads to difficulty in managing clothing. Usually an experienced therapist will be able to help with such problems. Most patients desperately wish to be as independent as possible for toileting, and most, even those with severe disease, will be able to remain at least partially independent for some considerable time if they are provided with adapted clothing and an appropriate urinal. If adequate provision is not made for independent micturition patients often solve the problem themselves by voluntarily restricting their fluid intake. Such a policy must be discouraged, for it may precipitate urinary infection and renal stone formation.

Home Management

Duchenne muscular dystrophy and spinal muscular atrophy lead to functional impairment in childhood and adolescence, and it is incumbent upon the parents to decide whether to undertake the responsibility of providing care themselves, or whether to gradually transfer responsibility, firstly to a school for the physically handicapped, and later to a residential establishment. The choice of domestic or institutional care depends upon many interdependent factors, mostly social and environmental. Most parents, provided that they are given moral and practical support, prefer to care for their children at home, even when the disease has resulted in severe deformity and gross weakness. Similarly, children come to rely on their parents' practised understanding of their needs and resent the sometimes clumsy and less accomplished efforts of others.

For those with disease onset in childhood who survive into adult life and for those developing chronic neuromuscular disease in later years, similar problems will develop, but they will be compounded by the likelihood that those family members who could be expected to provide care may themselves become frail and disabled with increasing age. Although many patients are so disabled as to be dependent upon others for help with dressing, washing and toileting, only a few require institutional care, but if long-term care at home is to be a practical proposition, the family will need much help and support.

Under the United Kingdom Chronic Sick and Disabled Persons Act (1970) the identification of need and the provision of equipment to ease the caring problems is within the mandate of the Social Services.

The provision of suitable housing and adaptation of the environment are essential if the full potential of disabled people is to be realized. If it is impossible to adapt the patient's home, then re-housing to purpose-built accommodation should be considered so that the disabled person may live with his family or have access to warden supervision. In recent years a number of special units for the young disabled have been built. Often they are sited well away from the communities they serve and such isolation has led to problems for both staff and residents, and the philosophy of creating such units has been challenged. There is a need for small units, accommodating perhaps five or six people, adjacent to areas in which they have always lived, and in situations providing easy access for shops, recreational facilities and possible remunerative employment, provided that adequate support is given by local community and social services.

Intellectual and Psychological Problems

Studies of the intellectual abilities of patients with neuromuscular disorders have mainly concentrated on Duchenne muscular dystrophy. Considerable variation in the incidence of retardation and subnormality has been reported, partly because of differences in the assessment techniques and in the definitions of subnormality. Intellectual impairment in verbal skills seems to be present in some patients with Duchenne muscular dystrophy, which may lead to them being labelled 'subnormal' or 'retarded', but in the more severely disabled children this may not be a true reflection of their ability, as non-verbal testing at this stage is affected by their physical disability. Any child with muscular dystrophy should therefore receive a very careful assessment of his intellectual capabilities as soon as the disease is diagnosed. Children with spinal muscular atrophy, because they show no intellectual deficits and have a much longer life expectancy, do not present such educational problems. In general, both disabled adults and children tend to be more introverted than the general population but no more neurotic, and adults tend to adjust their replies, making them more socially acceptable. There appears to be a significantly higher frequency of potential minor psychiatric disturbance in disabled adults than would be expected in the general population.

Emotional problems occur, but on the whole these patients cope with them, and the more emotionally disturbed patients seem to come from families with marked conflicts and recorded disturbances from childhood. It is most likely that the behaviour of the parents and siblings will influence that of the disabled child. Management of the children should therefore include counselling the parents and exploring such areas of difficulty as their inevitable guilt feelings, inability to accept the diagnosis and its sad outcome, the increasing amount of time to be spent with the child and the reduced attention available for non-handicapped siblings, the rejection or hostility to the child, over-protection or over-expectations of the child's ability in other areas such as scholastic success, especially if an intellectual deficit is present. The disabled patient needs to learn to handle his aggression, especially if his verbal and physical limitations prevent normal expression through physical activities (e.g. play). He has to handle his knowledge of early death, and how to cope with the difficulties of sexual development and the natural adolescent urge to leave the parental home. Many disabled adolescents find the lack of sexual experience more distressing than the concept of premature death.

Education and Occupation

For most children with severe physical handicap, education in terms of formal teaching and the definition of fields best suited for academic endeavour is sadly neglected, to a degree that would not be tolerated for any other group of children. The majority of children diagnosed as muscular dystrophy receive tuition at schools for the physically handicapped. But the academic standards in many schools for the physically handicapped are low, mainly because a large proportion of children attending are slow learners or are multiply handicapped, thus the child may leave such a school inadequate in reading, writing and numeracy, and having achieved little in the way of formal training in any occupation.

The policy of integrating disabled children into normal schools presents many problems, largely associated with the physical environment and the additional help the children require in the classroom, for toiletry and for meals. Poor prognosis is often used as the excuse for not attempting to overcome these difficulties. Many clinicians, administrators and parents feel that schools for the physically handicapped have many benefits to offer their child, particularly in the availability of regular physiotherapy or hydrotherapy. However, an increasing number of children are attending conventional schools or have some form of integrated education and achieving examination results which truly reflect their intellectual potential. The effect on a child whose intellect is repressed on the grounds of reduced life expectancy is devastating, and when the prognosis is good such restriction is indefensible. As with normal children, a disabled child should be educated to the limit of his intellectual potential. However, achieving an occupational outlet is difficult in the present economic and employment climate.

FACIO-SCAPULO-HUMERAL MUSCULAR DYSTROPHY

Facio-scapulo-humeral muscular dystrophy is usually inherited as an autosomal dominant characteristic. A wide range of clinical expression may be found and it is likely that many affected persons are not recognized for they may exhibit only minimal facial weakness throughout their lives, whereas in other members of the family, the disease may run an aggressive course. The most severely disabled are those in whom the disease onset has been in early childhood, and it is common to find that in such patients the disease is sporadic rather than being associated with a typical family history.

Most patients come to rely on a wheelchair for indoor mobility at ages ranging from their late teens to middle age. They usually exhibit a reluctance to give up walking even when it is manifestly unsafe, as with patients with limb girdle muscular dystrophy. Sometimes patients cease to walk after a relatively minor trauma or an intermittent illness rendering them temporarily bedfast. By the time that walking ceases most patients have such impairment of upper limb function that it is only with great difficulty that they are able to propel themsleves in standard wheelchairs.

A significant proportion of patients develop spinal deformity. Although there is little published experience of the use of early bracing techniques in such patients, it seems logical to resort to the provision of a suitable orthosis if, during adolescence, a patient is seen to be developing spinal deformity. If, despite adequate bracing, deformity progressed we could consider undertaking spinal surgery and encouraging results have been reported. The slow progression of this disorder gives many patients a normal or near normal life expectancy, and means that great benefit may be obtained from other carefully chosen surgical procedures. Tarsorrhaphy may be needed to enable a patient to close his eyelids fully and thereby protect the cornea.

Some workers have described a technique to anchor the scapulae to ribs or to the thoracic vertebrae or attach one scapula to the other with strips of tensor fascia lata, but the results do not appear to be helpful.

LIMB GIRDLE MUSCULAR DYSTROPHY

This group of patients, by no means homogeneous, exhibit proximal muscular weakness of gradually increasing severity. Disease inheritance is most commonly an autosomal recessive characteristic, so that in most patients there is no relevant family history. Such patients present with problems due to weak musculature around the pelvic girdle which spreads later to involve the musculature of the pectoral girdle. Increasing difficulty with walking is the major feature, but some patients remain ambulant for many years after disease onset, and continue walking with the aid of calipers and walking aids until they begin to suffer more frequent falls, or perhaps a limb fracture. Most patients have great difficulty in accepting that the use of a wheelchair could be both safer and less exhausting. Many ask to have a device by which they can be helped to their feet so that they can continue to walk. Occasionally patients can operate an overhead electrically controlled hoist, and with this device pull themselves from a sitting to an upright position. Unfortunately, once erect their walking is so potentially dangerous that it is questionable whether a hoist should be supplied for this purpose. When a patient is finding walking troublesome, it is better that this activity should be performed only when there is an able-bodied helper to assist.

Once patients accept a wheelchair they are rarely able to propel themselves for more than a few metres, and they rapidly become exhausted. Such patients should be offered an electrically powered wheelchair for safety, and in order to preserve energy. Acceptance of such a wheelchair will improve function and morale and will often obviate the need for a number of aids and appliances.

Patients no longer ambulant are also usually totally dependent on others for washing, dressing and toileting. Despite this, only a few are in institutional care: such admissions usually being for social reasons. It is all too easy for the patient with limb girdle muscular dystrophy, especially if he has received an inadequate education, or if he is of low intelligence, to drift from one job to another because he is unable to cope with the physical demands made upon him. Those patients who are unemployed have usually been so for many years, but had an appropriate training scheme been provided during adolescence, or early adult life, it is likely that some could have remained in remunerative employment for many years. Clerical duties or light bench work are the most suitable forms of employment, and as disability progresses it should be possible to continue with these activities from a wheelchair.

Undoubtedly, the most helpful asset is the attention of a loving spouse; with the help assured at home the patient will not need to worry unduly about the prospects of being relegated to institutional care. The course of this heterogeneous group of disorders is almost invariably slowly progressive, with death from intercurrent infection and general inanition commonly 30 years or more after the disease onset.

BENIGN X-LINKED MUSCULAR DYSTROPHY

Benign X-linked muscular dystrophy exhibits many of the clinical features of Duchenne muscular dystrophy, with a slower disease progression; the child remains ambulant into late adolescence or early adult life, and spinal deformity is not usually a problem. Many patients remain ambulant into their fifth or sixth decades, and even when walking is no longer possible, self-propulsion in a wheelchair may be possible for many years. They rarely develop peripheral joint contractures unless they become wheelchair-bound. Patients who are most severely affected benefit in later years from electrically powered wheelchairs, and from other devices such as hoists and environmental control systems.

As debility and age increase it is inevitable that those with benign X-linked muscular dystrophy should become more susceptible to respiratory tract infections. Such a wide range of disease severity is encountered that no firm guidelines as to prognosis can be given, but it is of interest that a large proportion of severely disabled patients with this disease exhibit electrocardiographic abnormalities similar to those encountered in Duchenne muscular dystrophy, although it is rare to record any clinical evidence of cardiac embarrassment.

MOTOR NEURONE DISEASE

Clinically, cases of motor neurone disease are capable of great variety but all fall within the three clinical types: amyotrophic lateral sclerosis, progressive bulbar palsy and progressive muscular atrophy. Transitions between these types and combinations, particularly of amyotrophic lateral sclerosis and progressive bulbar palsy, are common.

Although the disease is progressive and patients become dependent for washing, dressing and toileting, about a quarter retain sufficient power and control of their leg musculature to continue to walk indoors for a year or two after onset, and some patients with amyotrophic lateral sclerosis or progressive muscular atrophy may still remain ambulant three years after disease onset. But it is almost inevitable that within three years of the disease onset, most affected patients will only be mobile and comfortable in a wheelchair, whose back rest can provide full-length support in a reclining position. Such a wheelchair provides an obvious symbol of disability for those who have difficulty in accepting their increasing dependence upon others, and it is so bulky that it may not fit easily into the patient's home. For all these reasons it is often expedient to provide a smaller, cheaper and more readily available car transit wheelchair whilst the patient is still ambulant, and explain that the fitting of mobile arm supports is more practical on such a chair than on a domestic chair, and that it may be of use also for outdoor activities.

The provision of mobile arm supports can exert a morale-boosting effect upon these patients, facilitating such everyday activities as feeding, writing or turning the pages of a book. They will also reduce the problem of hand swelling as a result of immobility, and relieve dramatically the dragging sensation across the shoulders which many patients experience.

Increasing dependence, although causing great psychological stress for the patient, can lead to almost intolerable psychological and physical stresses on the patient's helpers or relatives. As the disease progresses so dependency will increase and it is important to consider the provision of any equipment which will help to ease the formidable task of providing care. Electric hoists and beds, page turners, and environmental control devices should be considered as soon as the diagnosis is clear, for problems of supply will commonly occur and it is important to capitalize on the morale-boosting effect of having equipment available as soon as the patient will accept it. It is important, however, not to overload either the patient or the family with too much equipment too quickly. Early on in the disease the patient experiences difficulty in swallowing. Dribbling may be reduced by using anticholinergic drugs. Swallowing may be improved with crico-pharyngeal myotomy—a comparatively minor operation.

Although potency is commonly retained, sexual relationships are often a problem because of physical weakness, and sexual counselling of both partners can often help mutual understanding and the marital relationship. The increasing physical dependence, the natural reaction to frustration—including emotional outbursts and depression—all throw increasing strain upon the patient's spouse. Pharmacological measures often fail to help, and supportive measures for the married partner, including holiday admission to an appropriate unit, may help the domestic situation.

Terminally, the patient becomes bedridden, and the help of a terminal care unit is sometimes appropriate. Opiates in small regular doses are often necessary to suppress coughing and to relieve general distress. As with the terminal phase of most chronic neuromuscular diseases, regular attendance by a caring physician helps both patient and partner. A severe choking attack is frightening and reassurance that care is at hand is of great importance.

The average duration of amyotrophic lateral sclerosis from onset to death is about three years, whereas with progressive muscular atrophy it is about eight years. Disease progression in both of these clinical forms of motor neurone disease is relentless and invariably the patient's death comes as a happy release for both him and his family. Death is usually from aspiration pneumonitis or hypostatic bronchopneumonia for which, in these circumstances, antibiotics are inappropriate.

MULTIPLE SCLEROSIS

The exact number of patients who suffer from multiple sclerosis is not known (about 50 000 in the UK), but the number of people severely disabled by this disease is a relatively small proportion, many living a normal life and experienc-

ing a full and normal life span. The physical features of MS which are particularly pertinent to the problem of rehabilitation are:
1. the onset is usually between 20 and 40 years of age
2. the high incidence of spasticity and spasms and tremor
3. the high incidence of incontinence.

Spasticity

The spasms and spasticity are disabling in their own right and often predispose to even more disabling contractures.

Drugs such as Diazepam, Chlordiazepoxide, Baclofen and Dantrolene are widely used to reduce the spasm and are a useful supplement to physical therapy.

Ice packs will often reduce spasm and enable the physiotherapist to obtain a greater degree of mobility and, by passive and active movements, to help the patient to gain more active control of movements, and to prevent the development of contractures. In the longer term, injection of 42% alcohol into the motor points of muscles may be of considerable value, particularly in enabling the thighs to be abducted for toilet purposes. Patients with multiple sclerosis often react badly to surgical procedures for contractures such as adductor tenotomy, or obturator neurectomy; whether this is associated with the surgery or anaesthetic, or to the enforced immobilization in bed, is difficult to analyse, but simple procedures are preferable.

Tremor

Tremor of the upper limbs makes for many difficulties of daily living—writing and feeding in particular. Adapted aids—special spoons, felt-tipped pens, etc.—may be of value, and some patients can be helped by weighted arm cuffs, but there is little that can be done to damp down *marked* tremor.

Head tremor can also be very distressing. Sometimes a collar, plastazote or felt, or head rests on the wheelchair, may help to control the tremor enough for a patient to be fed more easily or to enable him to read or write. The effect of nystagmus and head tremor can sometimes be reduced by the use of an eye patch or 'blinkers' restricting sideways vision. The combined tremor of head and upper limbs is almost unmanageable.

Tremor and spasm of the legs can prevent a patient walking. A weighted walking frame may give stability, and careful attention to achieving an optimum height for the chair seat may reduce the provocation of tremors as the patient strives to stand up.

Incontinence

Frequency and urgency of micturition are symptoms which the patient may volunteer, but he rarely admits to incontinence. One of the advantages of residential accommodation in a rehabilitation unit is that many of the inconsistencies in the patients' opinion of themselves become apparent. Although denying incontinence, the female patient in particular will frequently accept the need for, and appreciate the social benefit of, an indwelling catheter.

Management of incontinence is described in Chapter 8.

Aids and Appliances

Most patients with MS have mobility problems but are often reluctant to accept many aids and appliances. Wheelchair hoists and electric beds are often more aids for the relatives than for the patient. One of the most important aspects of rehabilitation of patients with progressive or permanent disability is the acceptance of their disability. Only when the disability is accepted can alternative methods of function be achieved. MS patients rarely develop trick movements and rarely become skilful with appliances. It is their lack of adaptability which underlies the difficulties of rehabilitation in multiple sclerosis.

Psychological Features

The rehabilitation of most severely disabled patients depends on the patient's personality, financial incentives and the degree of disability: *in that order*.

Many MS patients appear to be euphoric and this is often regarded as evidence of high morale. However, there is evidence that this is a pathological phenomenon strongly associated with intellectual deterioration. Many suffer from a patchy dementia with impairment of conceptual thinking and preseveration. The onset of intellectual damage is insidious and often undetected, and may precede obvious gross physical disability. Furthermore, a number of patients are depressed. In addition to the depression a number demonstrate a mood of cheerful complacency out of context with their total situation. The patient's apparently cheerful description can be very misleading, and as the contact with hospital staff can only be on a casual, intermittent out-patient basis, only a domestic assessment by trained personnel may reveal the real situation. It is important to try to uncover the depression so often underlying the euphoria because it can be improved by the use of drugs.

CONCLUSION

Patients with chronic neuromuscular disease are amongst the most severely disabled members of the community. Many, until recently, could not have expected to survive an intercurrent infection, but as a result of advances in medical care their life expectancy, and with it their expectations of life, has increased. Such an increase in the life-span of the patient has unleashed many problems. The majority of these patients are dependent on others for help with personal care activities. The contributions of medical and paramedical workers often appear to be limited, but nevertheless can transform the lives not only of the patients but also of their families and friends. To be meaningful, such assistance must be based on accurate medical diagnosis, for without this, disease progression and the patient's prognosis cannot be predicted.

Effective management of the severely physically handicapped can only be accomplished by a close collaboration between clinician, therapists, social workers, psychologists, and education and disablement resettlement officers who are experienced in assessment of the severely disabled in their homes, at school and at work. Voluntary workers and supportive organizations, whether concerned with specific disease or of a general nature, have a valuable part to play.

Education is particularly important when physical disability will clearly restrict employment potential. The development of creative leisure activities can be a useful substitute for work as disability worsens.

Rehabilitation embraces the many physical, social and organizational aspects of patient care. In the case of chronic neuromuscular disease the social and organizational aspects are more important than conventional physical rehabilitation.

REFERENCES

General

GOLDSMITH S. (1977) *Designing for the Disabled*, 3e. RIBA, London.
LENMAN J.A.R. (1959) A clinical and experimental study of the effect of exercise on motor weakness in neurological disease. *Journal of Neurology, Neurosurgery and Psychiatry*, **22**, 182–94.
NICHOLS P.J.R. (1972) *Rehabilitation of the Severely Disabled*. Butterworths, London.
OFFICE OF HEALTH ECONOMICS, prepared by David Taylor (1977) Studies of Current Health Problems. No. 60. *Physical Impairment: Social Handicap*. OHE, London.

Motor neurone Disease

SINAKI M. & MULDER D.M. (1978) Rehabilitation techniques for patients with amyotrophic lateral sclerosis. *Mayo Clinic Proceedings*, **53**, 173–8.
SMITH R.A. & NORRIS F.H. (1975) Symptomatic care of patients with amyotrophic lateral sclerosis. *Journal of the American Medical Association*, **234**, 715–17.

Multiple Sclerosis

MATTHEWS B. (1978) *Multiple Sclerosis: The Facts*. Oxford University Press.
RITCHIE RUSSELL W. & PALFREY G. (1969) Disseminated sclerosis rest-exercise therapy—a progress report. *Physiotherapy*, **55**, 306–10.

Muscular Dystrophy and Spinal Muscular Atrophy

BOSSINGHAM D., NICHOLS P.J.R. & WILLIAMS E.W. (1979) *Severe Childhood Neuromuscular Disease.* Muscular Dystrophy Group of Great Britain, London.

GIBSON D.A. & WILKINS K. (1975) The management of spinal deformities in Duchenne muscular dystrophy. *Clinical Orthopaedics and Related Research*, **108**, 41–51.

LEVITT R. (1973) The role of foot surgery in progressive neuromuscular disorders of children. *Journal of Bone and Joint Surgery*, **55A**, 1396–410.

SCHWENKER E.P. & GIBSON D.A. (1976) The orthopaedic aspects of spinal muscular atrophy. *Journal of Bone and Joint Surgery*, **58A**, 32–8.

WINTER R.B. & MOE J.H. (1974) Orthotics for spinal deformity. *Clinical Orthopaedics and Related Research*, **102**, 72–91.

WILKINS K.E. & GIBSON D.A. (1976) The patterns of spinal deformity in Duchenne muscular dystrophy. *Journal of Bone and Joint Surgery*, **58A**, 24–32.

Psychological Aspects

JAMBOR K.L. (1969) Cognitive functioning in multiple sclerosis. *British Journal of Psychiatry*, **115**, 765–75.

KAHANA E., LEIBOWITZ V. & ACTER M. (1971) Cerebral multiple sclerosis. *Neurology*, **21** (12), 1179–85.

LINCOLN N.B. & STAPLES D.J. (1977) Psychological aspects of some chronic progressive neuromuscular disorders. *Journal of Chronic Diseases*, **30**, 207–15.

NICHOLS P.J.R. (1975) Some psychological aspects of rehabilitation and their implications in research. *Proceedings of the Royal Society of Medicine*, **68**, 537–44.

REITAN R.M. (1971) Cognitive motor and psychomotor correlates of multiple sclerosis. *Journal of Nervous and Mental Disease*, **153** (3), 218–24.

SURRIDGE D. (1969) An investigation into some psychiatric aspects of multiple sclerosis. *British Journal of Psychiatry*, **115**, 749–64.

WEINSTEIN E.A. (1970) Behavioural aspects of multiple sclerosis. *Modern Treatment*, 7, 961–8.

YOUNG A.C., SAUNDERS J. & PONSFORD J.R. (1976) Mental change as an early feature of multiple sclerosis. *Journal of Neurology, Neurosurgery and Psychiatry*, **39**, 1008–13.

Sexual Aspects

GREENGROSS W. (1976) *Entitled to Love*. Malaby Press Ltd, London.

HESLINGA K. (1974) *Not Made of Stone*. Stephen Nordquist Int., Leyden, Holland.

MILLER E.J. & GWYNNE G.V. (1972) *A Life Apart*. Tavistock Press, London.

Spasticity

COCKIN J., HAMILTON E.A., NICHOLS P.J.R. & PRICE D.A. (1971) Preliminary report on the treatment of spasticity with 45% ethyl alcohol injection into muscles. *British Journal of Clinical Practice*, **25**, 73–5.

Special Seating

DENNE W. (1979) An objective assessment of sheepskins used for decubitus sore prophylaxis. *Rheumatology and Rehabilitation*, **18**, 23–9.

NELHAM R.L. (1975) Manufacture of moulded supportive seating for the handicapped. *Biomedical Engineering*, **10**, 379–81.

STRANGE T.V., HARRIS J.D. & NICHOLS P.J.R. (1978) Individually contoured seating for the disabled. *Rheumatology and Rehabilitation*, **17**, 86–90.

Special Splints

HAWORTH R., BUNSCOMBE S. & NICHOLS P.J.R. (1978) Mobile arm supports—an evaluation. *Rheumatology and Rehabilitation*, **17**, 240–4.

NICHOLS P.J.R., DAY H.J.B., WELCH D.C., WILLIS L.A. & STRANGE T.V. (1975) Flail arm splints. *Rheumatology and Rehabilitation*, **14**, 253–9.

NICHOLS P.J.R., PEACH S.L., HAWORTH R.J. & ENNIS J. (1978) The value of flexor hinge hand splints. *Prosthetics and Orthotics International*, **2**, 86–94.

Terminal Care

MOUNT B.M. (1978) *Palliative Care of the Terminally Ill.* Royal College Lecture. Royal College of Physicians and Surgeons, Canada.

TWYCROSS R.G. (1975) *The Dying Patient.* The Christian Medical Fellowship, London.

Wheelchairs

DEPARTMENT OF HEALTH AND SOCIAL SECURITY (1970) *Handbook of Invalid Chairs and Hand Propelled Tricycles* (MHM 408). HMSO, London.

FENWICK D. (1977) *Wheelchairs and their Users.* HMSO, London.

PLATTS E.A. (1974) Wheelchair design—a survey of users' items. *Proceedings of the Royal Society of Medicine*, **67**, 414.

WINYARD G.P.A., LUKER C. & NICHOLS P.J.R. (1976) The uses and usefulness of electrically powered indoor wheelchairs. *Rheumatology and Rehabilitation*, **15**, 254–63.

Young Disabled Units

SYMONS J. (1974) *Residential Accommodation for Disabled People.* CEH Design Guide 2. Centre on Environment for the Handicapped, London.

Organizations Specifically Concerned with Patients with Chronic Neuromuscular Disease

Friedreich's Ataxia Association,
5/6 Clipstone Street,
London W1.

Multiple Sclerosis Society,
4 Tachbrook Street,
London SW1V 1SJ.

Muscular Dystrophy Group of Great Britain,
Nattrass House,
35 Macauley Road,
Clapham,
London SW4 0QP.

General Information for Physically Handicapped People

Royal Association for Disability and Rehabilitation (RADAR),
25 Mortimer Street,
London W1N 8AB.

Disabled Living Foundation,
346 Kensington High Street,
London W14 8NS.

Equipment for the Disabled

Published by the Oxford Regional Health Authority on behalf of the Department of Health and Social Security, UK:

1. Outdoor transport
2. Communication
3. Wheelchairs
4. Hoists and walking aids
5. Housing and furniture
6. Home management
7. Clothing and dressing for adults
8. Leisure and gardening
9. Personal care
10. Disabled mother
11. Disabled child.

PART III
FUTURE POSSIBILITIES
IN NEUROLOGICAL
REHABILITATION

The final three chapters review novel approaches to rehabilitation. It is intended that these should be read as guides rather than established procedures. Engineers now have a framework of how to design a machine to undertake complex functions and yet still be under total volitional control without taxing the attention and concentration of the user. Alternative sensory channels can be exploited by modern technology, but the important outcome is that the brain can integrate the substituted sensory information with natural sensation. Stimulation of the nervous system offers a possibility of modifying its function and possibly the plastic processes within it. Technological innovation will play an important role in rehabilitation but, as these chapters illustrate, a deep understanding of the man–machine interface is the cornerstone of success.

Chapter 12

Trends in Engineering Aids for Neurological Disability

The provision of physical aids for the disabled generally involves some engineering design. However, at present, it is likely that the traditional technologies of mechanical engineering, concerned with structures and machines, or basic electrical or electronic engineering devices will be employed. Recent advances in the fields of communication, data processing and control have, as yet, had little impact in the field of rehabilitation. There are, however, good reasons to suppose that these developments have great potential for advance in the rehabilitation of neurological disorders. One obvious reason is the considerable reduction in the size and weight of electronic systems which allows complex apparatus to be easily carried about the person. There has been a strengthening of the conceptual relationships between the processes of the central nervous system and signal processing in modern computer and control systems. Our present state of knowledge does not allow direct electronic replacement of damaged sections of the nervous system and it is probably more meaningful to think of engineering systems which complement and augment the existing central nervous system. Such engineering systems are of increasing complexity: at a basic level they can regulate movement automatically and thus provide reflex responses. At a more intellectual level they can monitor and assess their own performance and can modify their responses or even their intrinsic structure to bring about more consistent or improved performance. This *adaptive* and *learning* behaviour is displayed by all living organisms and the extent of such facilities within the human nervous system reflects the success of the species. Machines displaying a similar virtuosity are finding increased application in industry where they are designed to extend or even replace human skills. Whether they possess real intelligence is an argument best left to philosophers while engineers exploit their considerable benefits in a practical way. Major problems could arise in rehabilitation through incompatibility between the user and the machine. The concept of *integration of control* may be stated as allowing the wearer complete volitional control over all phases of machine action through a simple and natural *command structure*, but detailed control over the many freedoms which make up a complete action should involve little more conscious effort and activity than in the normal performance of such a task. The implementation of these requirements presents extreme paradoxes in the design specifications of devices. Whereas solutions to these problems exist within our own neurological systems we must not assume that an engineering solution in the form of a replica is feasible or desirable. A dangerous, although well-meaning, principle states that to achieve simple control of function, devices must be mechanically simple. Fortunately the converse is not necessarily valid, but an outcome of modern technology is that providing a mechanism with its own autonomous internal control structure may allow a simple mode of control from the outside world.

' Design of aids for those with impaired limb function due to neurological or other disabilities poses some problems which are predominantly engineering in nature. These concern the size, weight, strength, flexibility, appearance and power requirement of any apparatus to be given to the patient. Such aspects rightly receive much attention and, since the objectives are generally well defined, progress is steady if not always spectacular. Another area where engineering effort is required concerns assessment of degrees of disability, measurement of residual function and, possibly, apparatus and programmes for retraining the disabled person. Here again constructive engineering design coupled with clinical investigation is beginning to lead to a rational approach to the selection of those variables which are significant from a functional viewpoint, how they may be measured reliably and the use to which these measurements may be put. Ideally such measurements should lead to specification of aids which are optimum for a particular patient. However, the present state of biological engineering together with the intrinsic difficulties of many rehabilitation problems tends to produce solutions involving compromises which are often far from satisfactory.

If engineers are to contribute significantly to progress in rehabilitation, their work should be methodical and systematic. One approach which can open up the way for progress is the investigation of the mechanics of locomotion and manipulation and the limitations imposed by disability. There are some inherent problems of a dynamic nature which, quite apart from any clinical considerations, make certain device proposals quite unrealistic, and it is important to realize that these are impractical on a purely engineering basis, thus preventing fruitless attempts to overcome the problems.

Once the nature of the mechanical problems to be overcome has been established, the achievement of functional responses through a suitable control system depends largely on the facilities for two-way communication between the patient and his aid since the rate at which information can be transferred consciously through any communication channel, even by a normal subject, is quite restricted. Simultaneous transmission through several channels does not improve the information capacity and, in practice, often worsens the overall performance by introducing errors. Apparently the information required to perform quite simple manual tasks with the hands, for example, is enormous and well beyond the signal-capacity of a single channel. However, investigation of the extent to which information to the peripheral actuators can be generated autonomously and how command sequences can be produced from simple codes suggests that in practice considerable reductions in consciously transmitted information can be made. In this way complex mechanical aids can be driven by simple and robust command signals.

The contents of this chapter are largely speculative and discuss the application of the foregoing ideas in the field of neurological rehabilitation. It does not catalogue devices or systems since it is felt that the basic principles are largely independent of the means of implementation. However, some practical examples are cited and, although these relate mostly to work undertaken on prosthetic upper limbs, it is felt that they still demonstrate the feasibility of the design concepts generally.

AN ENGINEER'S VIEW OF LIMB FUNCTION

It may be argued that it is less than valid to consider any aspect of human function in mechanistic terms. However, while such an approach can in no way predict how individuals may perform the wide variety of tasks encountered in everyday life it can at least provide an accurate description of the apparatus available to perform these tasks. Further, when disability occurs, it is possible to quantify the loss of mechanical freedom.

Performance of tasks requires the acquisition of intellectual and manual skills and here there is a wide diversity of achievement among individuals. Factors such as motivation, fatigue, frustration, fear etc., produce wide fluctuations in individual performance which are emphasized in disability. Thus attempts to form causal models or descriptions of the processes by which we control our limbs, while of great value to the neurologist, are of only limited help to the engineer attempting to devise mechanical aids. An alternative approach seeks to describe the performance of tasks in terms of the mechanics of the interactions which must occur between the limbs and the external environment. These interactions involve coordinated action in the sets of muscles, which must be represented by a logical description, and energy exchanges between the mechanical structures involved. It is then possible, at least in principle, to devise a minimal control structure which can achieve an acceptable performance of the task. In normal engineering practice this represents the complete problem, but here it is really only a starting point. One is then faced with the major problem of determining how much of the required control structure resides in the patient *and is accessible*, then to design a complementary external control system which will meet the overall performance requirements while satisfying the previously mentioned conflicting needs of autonomy and compatibility. Finally this theoretical system specification must be realized in hardware of a realistic design which also satisfies any economic constraint which may be imposed.

Limbs are constructed of hinged levers driven by opposing muscle pairs which apply differential torque about the hinges. If the resulting tension is not balanced by a load reaction the muscles contract and cause rotation of the joints. However, position feedback signals from muscle spindle receptors act to cancel the excitatory neuron activity and so allow a continuous range of displacements to be achieved. Groups of muscles act together to give patterns of movement to the related skeletal members, resulting in what we recognize as coordinated movement such as walking, gesturing, etc. It is possible to classify the resulting patterns of movements into the following broad categories:

1. ballistic movements
2. stereotype rhythmic patterns which are often involuntary with only the general pattern important and the exact timing of little consequence
3. precise voluntary movements where pattern, sequence and timing are of critical importance
4. voluntary control of forces involving limited and constrained limb movements, for example when handling and manipulating objects.

Ideally all of these components should be present when a rehabilitation aid is proposed since they allow normal functions to be performed in a natural way. Clearly, however, to achieve this may call for extreme flexibility in the resulting mechanical system. These conflicting requirements are most severe in the upper limb, where movements are seldom repetitive and where an extreme range of environmental conditions is encountered. Most of the subsequent discussion relates to the upper limb, where it is important to recognize *movement* and *prehension* as two distinct problems.

The role of the muscle *spindle* feedback mechanisms in the control of muscle contraction has long been recognized by physiologists. Other peripheral feedback loops involving the Golgi tendon organ and other sensory units are also known to be important in the control of muscle activity. However, simple feedback concepts fall far short in explaining the variable behaviour of the skeletal muscles. These muscles have a remarkable performance specification which may be summarized as follows.

Movements can be controlled to an accuracy of a few minutes of arc at the joints. Speed of response up to several cycles per second for small movements can be achieved. Response characteristics are independent of load in spite of wide variations. There appears to be a strong predictive component of response which allows stable grips to be maintained in adverse dynamic conditions.

Force characteristics are variable. They allow either *hard* or *soft* grips to match the compliancy of an object being handled. Further, the posture of an object within the grip may be changed by controlling the frictional forces between the hand and the object.

To achieve this kind of flexibility in a mechanical replacement it seems essential to incorporate two modes of feedback, *position* and *force*, which can be interchanged at an appropriate threshold. In addition the force sensitivity should be variable to accommodate light or heavy objects. All these features are known to exist in the peripheral CNS and are believed to be essential to manipulation. Whilst apparently adding to the mechanical complexity, these features are comparatively simple to incorporate, and in a hand prosthesis (Codd, 1974) considerable functional flexibility was achieved. Feedback is provided by sensors having the characteristics shown in Fig. 12.1. Displacement D and force F represent the lowest threshold at which the characteristics change from position to force control and they determine the ultimate sensitivity of the device if it is to handle small, light objects. Ideally the threshold should be variable and there is some evidence that this occurs in normal limbs. Dual feedback in the form we have described allows the position of a limb member to be controlled in the absence of any opposing reaction forces. However, when an object is encountered which produces a reaction, detected by the force sensors, which is greater than F then the force feedback mechanism dominates and the limb member is able to exert a controlled force on the object even if there is no displacement.

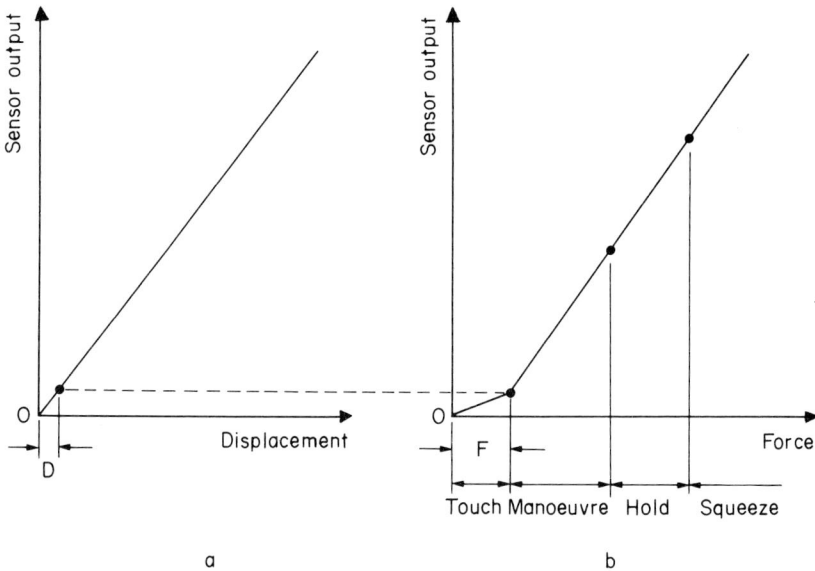

Fig. 12.1 Displacement and force sensor characteristics.

Attempts have been made to incorporate similar displacement/force sensory feedback in prosthetic and orthotic devices in the past. Traditionally the command signals for controlling the drive motors have been obtained directly from residual muscle activity, either mechanical or electrical (EMG). If the two feedback signals are supplied directly to the wearer he has little or no means of knowing which mode should be dominant and consequently little facility for manipulation. Displacement feedback is of course inherent through vision, but this alone is a poor substitute for proprioceptive feedback and presents difficulties which will be discussed in some detail further on. Force sensory feedback presents even more difficulties since the information has to be transmitted in the form of a sensation. Various techniques have been tried including steady and vibrating pressure, electrical excitation and auditory signals, but in general they have been unsuccessful. Even if a reliable measure of force is obtained in this way, problems of interpretation and translation into appropriate actions are extremely difficult and the resulting control of the limb is largely static. One of the greatest difficulties is attaining sufficient sensitivity to differentiate light and pliable objects and thus to manipulate them without damage. Direct control of manipulative aids requires not only the intellectual capacity of the brain, which is often unimpaired, but a good manipulative skill which can be harnessed through a residual muscle activity. The required dexterity is often well beyond even normal subjects under very favourable conditions when trying to operate a manipulator in this way. Manipulative tasks are essentially dynamic and the acquisition of sensory information, making command decisions and taking effector action must all occur within a time interval which is short (of the order of milliseconds) if an object is not to slip from the grasp. This probably presents the biggest single limitation in the development of satisfactory mechanical aids for rehabilitation. In the Control Engineering laboratories at the University of Southampton research has been undertaken to overcome this limitation, and the first positive outcome was to feed the sensory displacement and force signals directly to the motor driving each member so that each tends to cancel the command excitation (negative feedback). Both signals are electrical outputs from transducers and therefore are precise and accurate. The response of the overall mechanism, since it does not involve human intervention and judgement, is rapid enough to deal with problems of manipulative stability.

A Control Hierarchy for Prehension

Very little work appears to have been done to date on the problem of providing a tactile handling device with the necessary combinations of grip properties that make up human hand function. Even in industrial applications this problem is side-stepped by fitting robot arms with specialized terminal equipment for each particular task. However, such a solution lacks the essential flexibility of the human hand and is a poor substitute in rehabilitation. The aim, perhaps an idealized one, should be a hand which can operate any tool or implement encountered in everyday life. The essential basic grips from which such compound functions are built can be specified as follows in terms of the level of applied force:
1. *light* touch forces
2. *medium* forces for holding an object
3. *large* forces for squeezing and deforming an object
4. *fluctuating* forces for manoeuvring an object within the grip.
The ranges of these forces are shown in Fig. 12.1, but they are by no means absolute values. Each level must be quantified for an individual object, the relevant properties being weight, surface texture, shape, etc. There are many ways in which humans assess and measure these properties; indeed, through

experience, we can form estimates merely by visual inspection before touch contact is made. Subsequently we have the inherent ability to adapt our grip if our estimates prove incorrect. This entire process is performed subconsciously and any similar feature built into an aid should not tax the conscious processes of the wearer. The basis of a force level classification system incorporated in the Southampton devices has depended on an indirect measure of the weight of the object. Small sensors* mounted at appropriate points (thumb and palm in a full hand prosthesis) detect the onset of lateral slip between the object and the surface of the hand. The weight of the object is 'determined' by increasing the excitation and hence the applied force until the object just ceases to slip. The range of holding forces is then set from 1.0 to 1.5 times the force needed to balance the weight. Several practical refinements are necessary, including a *refractory* period in the sensor response to inhibit gripping following accidental contact and a *hold-on* period after which the grip is automatically maintained without further input stimulus. Both features help to produce 'natural' behaviour and to reduce fatigue caused by excessive conscious intervention. They can be achieved with little extra circuitry.

In the range of force shown as the *squeeze* range in Fig. 12.1, it is possible for the applied force to be set at an arbitrary level considerably above that needed to just hold an object. An ability to *manipulate* and *manoeuvre* the object being gripped is, of course, an essential function in man. Its absence is, perhaps, one of the main reasons for the rejection of rehabilitation aids. It is probably that the range of manipulations which can be achieved by a mechanism will always be greatly inferior to that of the human hand and at the moment we have only aimed at producing a controlled sliding motion by which an object can move through the fingers under the action of gravity or when the object is pushed against a fixture. This is achieved, once the weight–balance condition has been set, by allowing the applied force to relax until slip just occurs. The applied force is then restored and then relaxed again and so on. The ideal frequency of the resulting oscillation is about 100 cycles per second, allowing smooth slip velocities of a few millimetres per second for typical objects. Rolling motion of objects within a grip is perhaps of more use than sliding motion, however; not only is it difficult to obtain the required mechanical flexibility, but the fine spatial sensor resolution needed to detect such motion is impractical in present designs. Also rolling motion is beset with stability problems which are best avoided. Another stability problem occurs when we grip smooth tapered objects where increasing the gripping force can lead to the object sliding from the hand. This condition can be detected by a logic operation on the sensor signals but, while it is a desirable feature, it requires rather better performance from the sensors than can be maintained with ease. A further modification in the system which regulates

---

*A range of sensors have been used. The simplest are microphonic vibration sensors which are 'all or nothing' devices. More elaborate sensors, based on balanced transformer principles, measure direction and velocity of slip. They are, however, more costly in terms of associated electronic circuitry.

the applied force is the ability to change adaptively the sensitivity of the force feedback loop according to the mass of the object, thus avoiding jerking movements when heavy objects are being manipulated. Again this is an automatic function which may be programmed into the mechanism.

Control of Grip Configuration

The system described so far has two levels of control. Peripheral or reflex loops produce fixed responses of displacement or force in the individual members of the gripping structure. These loops have rapid responses and must therefore be largely automatic, since the speed of variation in inputs for typical manipulative tasks is well beyond the capability of the wearer to produce by conscious variation in residual muscle contraction. The inputs to these peripheral loops are therefore obtained from a higher level in the control hierarchy where functional requirements determine the level and variation in the forces applied to objects being gripped and manipulated. This force-determining system is also largely autonomous and depends on measures of object properties derived from contact sensors mounted on the surface of the gripping device. The essential practical limitation on the availability of sufficient and reliable data is the density with which sensors can be mounted on the structure. Complexity in the signal processing necessary to generate functional decisions from this sensory data is reflected in the associated electronic control circuitry. Since this data processing is essentially programmable and should be adapted to the special needs and abilities of each wearer, it would seem that the microprocessor is ideally suited to this task and this has been confirmed by preliminary experiments.

One aspect not so far discussed in relation to the design of a prehensile gripping device and manipulator is the way that the structural members are configured to form a shape appropriate to a given object and the functional objectives desired by the user. Existing prostheses and orthoses tend to be rather simple mechanically with at most two degrees of freedom in the terminal gripping device, giving a simple clamping hand with perhaps some flexure at the wrist. This has obvious limitations, partly on cosmetic grounds, but more seriously for functional reasons, since the majority of implements and tools are designed for use by normal hands. Essential in normal hand function is the ability to rotate and flex the thumb so that a precision grip may be formed by opposition to the finger tips or so that it may be adducted or abducted when palmar or side grips are performed. Investigation of essential hand movements suggests that in a prehensile hand replacement it is desirable to have a thumb with two independent degrees of freedom and also to have independent drives for the first and second digits (see Fig. 12.2). Thus, the proposed manipulator has four degrees of freedom, each to be powered and controlled, in addition to any extra drives required for movement of the supporting arm or frame. Assuming that it is feasible to incorporate these drives within the device one is then faced with the

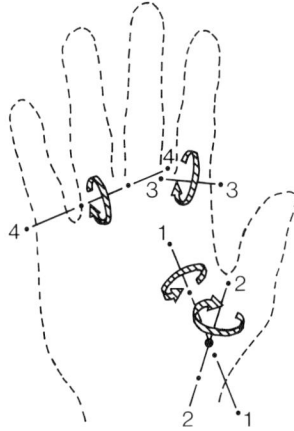

Fig. 12.2 Degrees-of-freedom in Southampton hand prosthesis.

problem of providing input signals to drive and coordinate each movement and to produce useful and, if possible, life-like responses. The direct mode of control favoured in conventional prostheses requires an independent signal channel for each mechanical degree-of-freedom. Where the input signals have been derived as EMG potentials from residual or other muscles the Southampton group believes that simultaneous independent control of several channels is at best a demanding skill and that, generally, the degree of coordination which may be achieved is very poor indeed. Where multiple-site inputs have been used to control wrist and clamping actions, movements appear to occur sequentially and very slowly. This slowness of operation is thought to be inherent in the method of control rather than to be due to inadequacies in the drive motors. Several factors are believed to contribute to this slowness:

1. The EMG signal is basically a noise process associated with the random firing of neural motor units. Only when smoothed, by averaging over a period of the order of a second, does it give a reliable control signal with the precision necessary for positioning digits. This smoothing introduces a delay in the dynamic response of the system.

2. If the resulting movements are controlled by visual monitoring then this involves conscious activity from the user. All decisions and changes are therefore subject to the human reaction time, thus introducing a further delay which is unlikely to be less than 0.2 second.

3. Coordination of the individual muscle groups involved in limb activity, particularly when making small corrective adjustments during the performance of a task, is largely subconscious and depends heavily on proprioceptive feedback. If a wearer has to control consciously similar activities given only visual information he will be very prone to error and his involvement will be such as to cause him fatigue and frustration.

Given the practical limitation of single-channel input from the user the approach

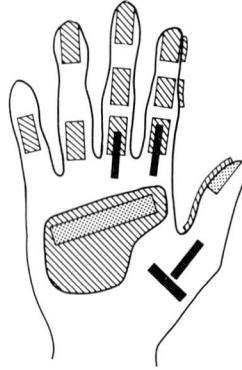

Contact sensors
Slip sensors
Position sensors

Fig. 12.3 Distribution of sensors in Southampton hand prosthesis.

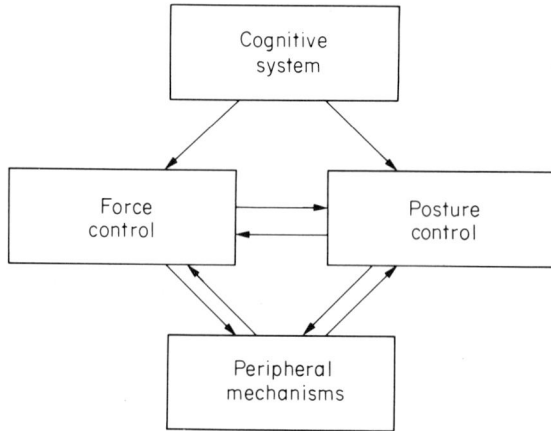

Cognitive
system

Force
control

Posture
control

Peripheral
mechanisms

Fig. 12.4 Control hierarchy.

we have adopted is to select the hand configuration from sensory feedback information obtained from a set of contact pressure transducers mounted on the hand (Fig. 12.3). The various drives are activated or inhibited dependent on a programmed pattern of sensor activity and a wide range of grips is available in our full hand prostheses including side grips, precision finger-tip grips, palmar and full fist grips. The decisions can be expressed as simple logic statements when binary values are assigned for activity or non-activity of the individual sensors. Implementation by digital circuits or microprocessor is simple.

The *force* and *posture* control systems form the intermediate level of the control hierarchy (Fig. 12.4). They are not completely independent as shown, but changes in one system can be made conditional upon the states of the other. This leads to more natural action sequences and avoids accidental release or mishandling. Once again it must be stressed that, since their function is essentially programmable, great flexibility is available to meet the demands of a given patient. It is therefore much better from a design point of view to have a very flexible device and to inhibit unwanted responses rather than to begin with a primitive mechanical device capable only of limited function. The latent skills which the user then develops are very much properties of the mechanisms and do not require him to develop inordinate intellectual and manual skills.

Overall Control: the Cognitive Level

Previous sections have discussed the design philosophy for mechanisms with in-built 'intelligence' which can adapt to the shape, weight and surface characteristics of an object without instructions from the user. A primitive kind of manipulation is possible and may be selected and controlled by a simple input instruction. Manipulative functions can be built up by selection from a small set of discrete instructions which we have called *touch, hold, squeeze, manoeuvre, release* and *relax*. The two latter regimes are essential and, respectively, they allow an object to be released from the grip and, when necessary, the stored information concerning its weight etc. to be wiped from the memory of the control logic systems.

It is now necessary to consider an interface system by means of which the user can communicate his conscious commands to the prehensile manipulator. Although this part of the system is discussed last this aspect of the entire system was actually the first to be considered in the development of the Southampton system. Indeed in any problem concerning complete or partial replacement of limb function by a mechanical aid, it is essential to consider first what signals are actually available from the wearer and the real limitations in terms of information transmission. In considering the suitability of command signal sources the following strategic requirements need to be considered.

1. Control must be easy to apply physically.
2. Training programmes involving the development of unusual skills should be avoided if possible.
3. The amount of conscious control effort should be minimized and should be as near normal as possible.
4. The user should not feel he is in competition with another intelligence and should feel in control of all phases of an action.
5. Transitions from one phase to another and the moderation of an action, such as increasing the squeeze force, should result from similar physical activity, e.g. increased tension in a residual muscle.
6. The wearer should be able to over-ride the responses of the mechanism and suddenly to increase greatly the force or to release the object with a natural response, perhaps a reflex.

7.   It should be possible to inhibit certain responses thus making the device simpler to use, so that increased functional complexity can be built up as each phase is learned.

8.   Performance should not depend critically on visual information and it should be possible to hold and manipulate objects 'in the dark'.

9.   Unlikely sequences of actions should be inhibited to prevent untimely release or damage of objects.

Since the lower systems in the control hierarchy are purely mechanical they are subject to the laws of mechanics and thus normal engineering methods can be used to produce optimum designs. However, the *cognitive* system which must interpret the user commands and transmit appropriate signals to the lower structure is very much concerned with human response and skills. Design here can only be based on observation and intuition and a number of arbitrary design choices must be made. If there is a single design criterion it is probably best summed up by Tomovic's Principle of Maximum Autonomy (1970), which is a therorem which embodies many of the practical requirements just outlined.

Among the possible command signals the most useful are probably residual body movement and electrical signals (EMG) from muscles. The author's view is that body movements are best used to control the overall posture of the limb through shoulder, elbow and wrist joints, particularly if kinaesthetic relationships can be utilized, while EMG signals are best suited for the control of prehension in the gripping mechanism.

It is in the conditioning and use of EMG signals for control that the Southampton work differs most from other prosthetic and orthotic applications. Our view, that EMG signals are unsatisfactory as fine control inputs, is confirmed by Toroq (1978), who considers the information rate in experiments on the control of single motor units. The information available is consistent with our decision to use the EMG signal for discrete level selection rather than as a continuous controller. As we have seen, control of our device requires six independent levels. The actual relationship between control mode and EMG input is shown in Fig. 12.5, and it will be seen that the number of levels has

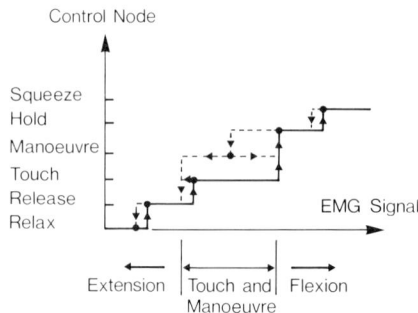

Fig. 12.5   Relationship between selected control mode and EMG input potential.

actually been reduced to five since the *touch* and *manoeuvre* levels are coincident, selection of either one depending on the immediately previous state. The diagram also shows the hysteresis built into the decision logic to prevent unwanted transitions due to random fluctuations in the EMG signal.

Only when the manipulator digits are closing on to an object is the device under continuous direct control from the wearer, but here there are no problems of dynamic stability so that limitations in his speed of response are not critical. It is interesting to compare a signal flow diagram of the complete system (Fig. 12.6a) with a diagram showing the mechanisms involved in the neural control of a pair of antagonist muscles (Fig. 12.6b). It almost looks as if the control structure of the manipulator had been deliberately modelled on the CNS mechanisms.

Another feature is worth mentioning: the EMG signals are obtained from two pairs of surface electrodes, placed over flexor and extensor muscle groups in the

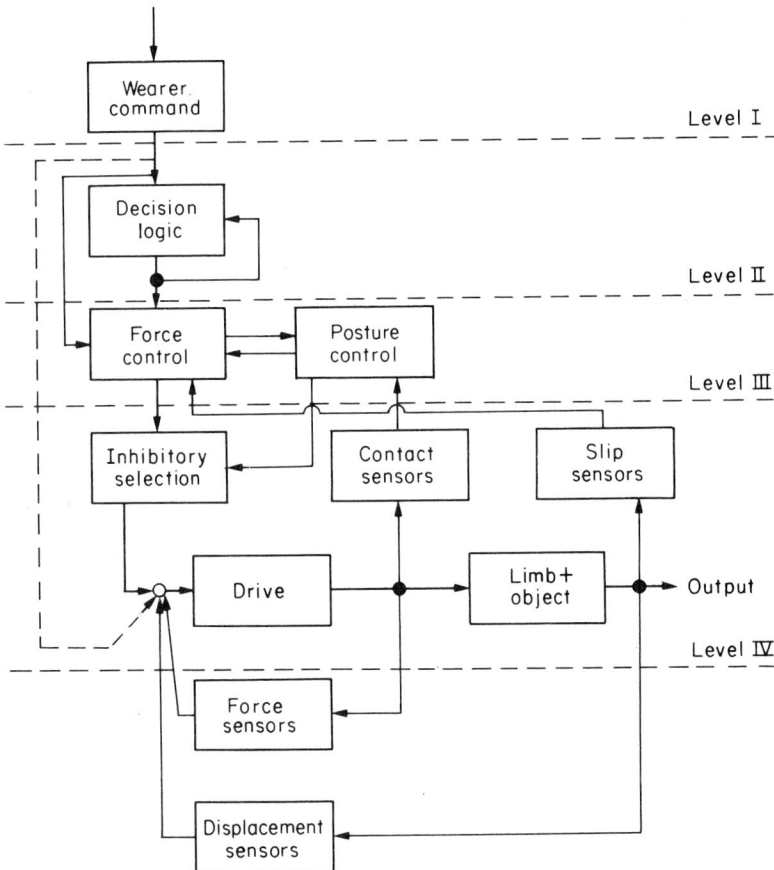

Fig. 12.6a   Signal flows in the prosthesis control hierarchy.

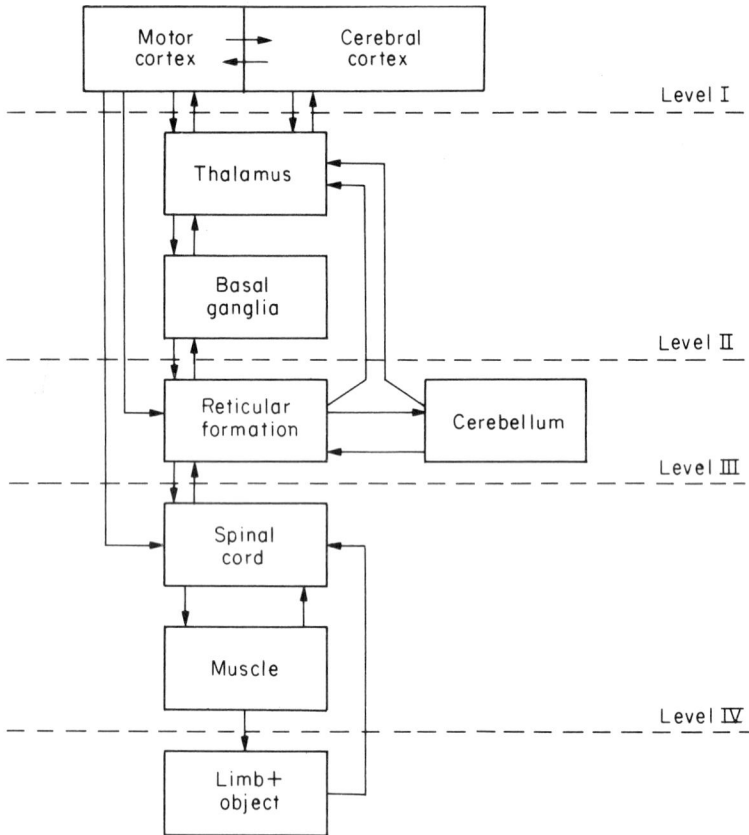

Fig. 12.6b Principal interconnections of anatomical regions of CNS responsible for control of movement.

forearm in our below-elbow prosthesis. A differential signal is obtained by subtraction of the two EMG components and this is normally used to select the appropriate grip function. However, if the two components are added,* when the opposing muscles are contracted simultaneously another command signal is produced and we have used this to select precision grips in which the thumb opposes the finger tips. This seems to be a 'natural' response and it has certainly proved simple for subjects to select and maintain this grip. Whilst in this posture all of the grip functions can be selected by the same discrete level selection logic.

To facilitate training a light-emitting diode display is available which indicates the current force command level and the precision grip state. This could be made available as a permanent display on the back of the hand but, while this is a help

---

* The actual logic combination is slightly more complex than pure addition.

initially, it is felt that it would ultimately hinder progress toward subconscious use of many of the features.

A number of hand prostheses based on these design principles have been contructed and limited laboratory and clinical trials undertaken. These seem to completely justify the control principles and where there have been problems they have been of a purely mechanical nature. The greatest limitation lies in the reliability and robustness of the sensors and much still needs doing to improve their design. However, the current device, with all its drives contained internally within the hand shell and some 30 sensors, weighs only 500 g and, apart from its sensors, it is mechanically reliable.

Control of Arm Posture

When disability involves the loss of wrist, elbow or shoulder joint movement, powered mechanical replacements are possible and a number of systems have been constructed. However, the power requirements due to the comparatively large inertial forces make it extremely difficult to approach the performance of a real arm. Again there are severe control problems since the desirable mechanical degrees of freedom exceed the number of useful signals available as wearer commands. Also motion is generated by rotation at the joint hinges and the desired arm coordinates must be expressed in terms of joint rotation angles, which normally involves extensive computation. The most acceptable arms are likely to be those whose geometry is similar to the human arm although the possibility of mobile robot manipulators is certainly feasible for the severely disabled.

A feasibility study of a full arm prosthesis has been undertaken at Southampton University (Nightingale & Swain, 1978) to verify a control strategy, although the resulting design is not yet easily realizable as an acceptable device. However, the limitations are mainly in the mechanical drive components and this is an area where there are likely to be significant advances. Body movements were chosen as the source of input since residual proprioception provides valuable feedback. From a body harness it was found that three reliable independent signals could be obtained which could be related to the demanded position of the wrist. However, it was necessary to impose a constraint on elbow motion since there are insufficient command signals for complete flexibility. The constraint is that the vertical elbow coordinate relative to the shoulder is half that of the wrist and, although not a natural restriction, the resulting motion seems tolerable.

Besides positioning the wrist, it is of course necessary to orient the hand. Effectively this requires two more command signals to control forearm rotation and wrist flexion. This presents an extremely difficult problem for which the following two-part solution has been investigated.

1.   Wrist and forearm motions controlled, prior to contact, by continuous

control of two drives in the lower part of the arm from estimates of the curvature (convex and concave) of the wrist trajectory resolved in two orthogonal planes.

2.   Corrective manoeuvring of the hand when the object is touched using tactile sensory feedback from the hand control system. Index finger contact causing clockwise rotation of the wrist and little finger contact causing anti-clockwise rotation. The sensors should be insensitive to spurious vibration.

Experiments performed under somewhat contrived conditions at least indicate that such a control scheme is feasible. The problems encountered physically in moving the arm linkage are not dissimilar to those met in industrial robotics. There are some difficulties when the arm takes one of several singular configurations where there are various alternatives through which a desired position may be approached. A simple controller would be unable to choose and probably would develop a tremor. However, a controller with an in-built decision-making ability could be programmed to choose one particular motion even if on an arbitrary basis.

One control aspect of human arm–hand function which is difficult to incorporate is our ability to maintain the hand as a stabilized platform, that is relatively fixed spatially despite gross body movements. Ideally some form of intertial sensing system could solve this problem, but such solutions seem a long way from feasibility at present.

OTHER APPLICATIONS: FUNCTIONAL STIMULATION

This chapter has considered the possible application of advanced feedback systems in problems of limb function and mechanical replacement. Wherever sensory signals and effector inputs are available some form of feedback loop can be established. Whereas simple feedback loops offer accuracy and insensitivity to change, we have considered possible multi-level control structures possessing adaptive behaviour and some primitive forms of self-organization and learning. Since limb prostheses and orthoses are entirely mechanistic, implementation of these schemes is not difficult, particularly since microprocessors are available to perform complex signal processing. It is, however, more difficult to envisage similar applications directly involving physiological processes owing to the much greater uncertainty in their function. It is certainly very difficult to form quantitative models of such processes and without these the design of adaptive or self-organizing control systems is very speculative. One area where some limited investigation has been carried out is functional stimulation.

Chandler and Sedgwick (1972) describe an EMG feedback system in which the integrated M-response is used as a feedback signal to a muscle stimulator (Fig. 12.7). Despite non-linearity in stimulator response the loop is found to give good control of displacement. This result encouraged further study to see if a control scheme, similar to that proposed for the manipulator, could be used

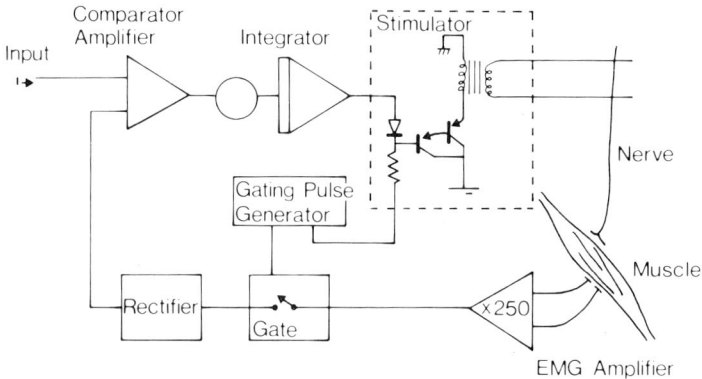

Fig. 12.7 Closed-loop stimulator in which feedback signal is derived from an EMG signal.

for multi-channel stimulation of a hand. Four stimulator channels were used (Fig. 12.8), and inductive sensors mounted on a light glove gave measures of wrist, thumb and finger flexion. Despite sensor interaction the various hand movements could be reasonably controlled by external signals. Later experiments (Chandler & Sedgwick, 1972; Beresford, 1978) considered how excitatory signals could be generated from touch contact sensors as in the manipulator

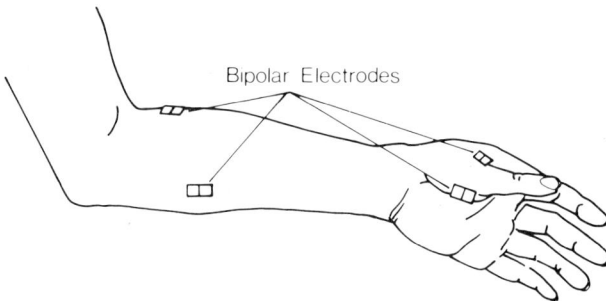

Fig. 12.8 Location of stimulation electrodes in the multi-channel stimulation experiments.

control system. Although this work was encouraging provided the hand was passive, little progress was made with hands subject to tremor or rigidity. One of the major difficulties in the use of surface electrode stimulation is movement of electrodes and change in the impedance characteristics of the skin. Beresford (1978) has described a method of self-adjustment which can compensate for these changes using a multi-segment electrode. His system automatically maps response contours and organizes a search routine for the optimum point of stimulation. His algorithms can easily be incorporated in a microprocessor.

CONCLUSION

In disability the brain is often unimpaired, at least as far as the control of manual tasks is concerned, and it seems logical if the chosen mechanical aid or replacement is able to make use of the intellectual and organizational power of the brain for control of these devices. However, there is a serious limitation in our ability to communicate conscious desires through residual muscular activity or, indeed, through any channel. This drastically limits the useful function which can be achieved through direct control by the patient. An alternative is to build into the mechanical aid similar characteristics of adaptability and organization as well as mechanical flexibility approaching that of the limb whose function is to be replaced. Although engineering systems to achieve this are necessarily complex, the complexity lies within their control systems and if anything their mechanical construction can actually be simplified by this approach. Much of the decision-making required by such systems is programmable and so lends itself to implementation by microprocessor. An added attraction of the programming approach is that the response characteristics of the aid can be tailored to meet the needs of each patient. Before this approach is established generally much work needs to be done, particularly in the development of sensors. Not only does the relationship between sensory feedback and limb function need to be fully investigated, but the realization of small, reliable and robust transducers for measuring all aspects of contact, proprioception, balance, etc., is paramount in all fields of rehabilitation.

REFERENCES

BERESFORD R. (1978) Development of functional stimulation using an adaptive electrode. Ph.D. Thesis, University of Southampton.

CHANDLER S.G. & SEDGWICK E.M. (1972) A proportional stimulator for functional electrical stimulation. *Proceedings of the Fourth International Symposium on External Control of Human Extremities.* Dubrovnik.

CODD R.D. (1976) Development and evaluation of adaptive control for a hand prosthesis. Ph.D. Thesis, University of Southampton.

NIGHTINGALE J.M. & SWAIN I.D. (1978) Adaptive control of an artificial arm. *Sixth International Symposium on External Control of Human Extremities.* Dubrovnik.

TOMOVIC R. (1970) A system approach to muscle control. *Mathematical Biosciences, USA,* **8** (3/4), 265–77.

TOROQ Z. (1978) Control and independence of motor units in human arm muscles. Ph.D. Thesis, University of London.

Chapter 13

Sensory Substitution in Rehabilitation

The human brain has been shown to be capable of adapting to a sensory loss (e.g. blindness or deafness) by (1) developing alternative strategies for obtaining the information usually mediated by the lost sensory system, such as the use of a long cane for mobility by blind persons, and (2) by learning to use the information provided by a sensory substitution system, such as the Tactile Vision Substitution System (TVSS) by blind persons (Bach-y-Rita, 1972). This chapter is primarily concerned with the second means of adaptation. The question posed is: are sensory substitution systems practical means of compensating for sensory losses?

VISION SUBSTITUTION

Tactile Vision Substitution System (TVSS)

When a person becomes blind, he does not necessarily lose the capacity to 'see'. Rather, he loses the use of the sensory end-organ (the eye) normally capable of transducing optical signals into patterns of neural activity which are sent to the central nervous system for processing into a visual percept. However, a substitute end-organ, such as a miniature television camera, can be placed under the motor control of the blind person, and the optical signals received by the camera can be transduced into stimuli applied to another sensory system (such as the tactile sensory system) for relay to the brain (Fig. 13.1). Under these conditions a blind person can be trained to use the information as 'visual'. In fact, even congenitally blind persons develop the ability to use visual means of analysis for adequate processing of the information.

Systems designed to relay optical information to the brain through the skin of blind persons have been developed in several laboratories. Each of these systems utilizes a matrix of artificial photoreceptors connected point-to-point with a matrix of skin stimulators. One of the most sensitive areas of skin is found on the finger tips; Bliss (1971) has utilized this sensitivity in developing a reading aid, the Optacon, for the blind.

The ability of one sensory system to convey information normally mediated

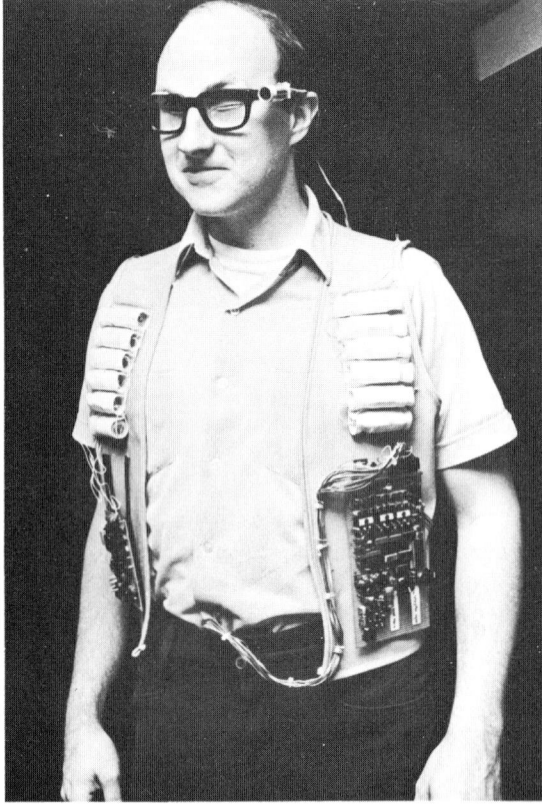

Fig. 13.1   A blind subject is shown using a portable tactile vision substitution system. The television camera is mounted on the frame of a pair of spectacles. The image is led to an electronic commutator (mounted on his vest) which converts it into a tactile image delivered to the skin of his abdomen by an array of electrical stimulators (under his shirt). The batteries are mounted bandolier-style on the vest.

by another (lost) sensory system is dependent on the existence of plastic neural mechanisms. Evidence that brain pathways are not fixed and immutable is available from many sources. These include studies of recovery of function following brain lesions, of changes in individual neurons during learning, of alterations in evoked potentials, and of assessment of cortical structure and chemistry during sensory deprivation or enrichment. With advances in modern technology, the plastic mechanisms which permit the brain to respond to new functional requirements and to training may provide the adaptability necessary for compensating for sensory losses.

With training, the blind subjects using the TVSS can identify and correctly locate in space complex forms, objects, figures and faces. Perspective, parallax, size constancy, including looming and zooming and depth cues, are correctly utilized. The subjective localization of the information obtained through the television camera is not on the skin; it is accurately located in the three-dimensional space in front of the camera, whether the skin stimulation matrix is placed on the back, on the abdomen, on the thigh, or changed from one of these body locations to another.

The equipment developed for these studies and the sensory substitution experiments have been extensively reported elsewhere (e.g. Bach-y-Rita, 1967; 1971; 1972; 1979; 1980a, b; Bach-y-Rita *et al.*, 1969; Collins & Bach-y-Rita, 1973; Scadden, 1974; White *et al.*, 1970). In this chapter I quote extensively from those reports.

The sensory substitution capabilities of the TVSS can best be conveyed by quoting from a report published (Guarniero, 1977) by one of our blind TVSS subjects, who was trained during two periods of three weeks each.

'Inasmuch as I am congenitally blind, I hoped that the System might help to satisfy my curiosity about the visual world. I am currently writing my doctoral dissertation on space perception and one of the subjects I am treating is the organization of the spaces that are perceived by the various senses. In my use of the System, as will become apparent below, I was primarily interested in acquiring visual concepts. However, gaining access to this new source of spatial awareness has also proved to be of great philosophical value.

'The two training programs differed as to their subject matter and the amount of control I had in the selection of activities. The first period of training was designed to enable me to use the System competently. The visual concepts in which I was interested could not be explored until I had mastered the working of the System itself, which occupied a large part of the first training period (Guarniero, 1974). During the second period of training, however, I spent little time in regaining my skill with the System. I was able to devote myself to the acquisition of as many new concepts as my ingenuity and that of the staff could allow. Before turning my attention to the conceptual part of the work, I should like to give a brief account of the training I received in order to make use of the System.

'Throughout my first period the only System we used was a 400-point electromechanical TVSS mounted on a dental chair, though we did make use of two different kinds of cameras—one of which was mounted on spectacle frames, while the other was mounted on a boom and had to be operated manually. This difference made it necessary to learn two entirely different types of scanning techniques. But the chief difference was that the hand-held camera had a zoom lens, a most important part of the apparatus.

'*Spectacle-mounted camera.* For the early part of my training I used the spectacle-mounted camera, because I had vestibular, as well as kinesthetic control over its movement. After a short time I was able to tell whether it was the object or the camera that was moving. An important adaptation I quickly made involved not noticing that the images appeared to move in a direction opposite to that in which I was moving the camera; I had to learn to "see" them as stationary. Recognizing the orientation of straight lines taught me how to orient the camera and to know whether it was straight and level, or, if not, how much and in which direction I was tilting it.

'The acquisition of these skills was necessary before I could go on to object recognition. It must be noted here that I never acquired the ability to identify an object on the basis of my tactile experience of the world, so when an object was first introduced I always had to be told what it was. Once I had "viewed" an object on TVSS and it had been named for me I was almost always able to recognize it on subsequent presentations. At first I had to scan an object in its entirety before I could tell what it was. Later I learned to pick out a distinctive feature which I used as a cue for identification.

'*Hand-held camera.* The changeover to the hand-held camera with its zoom lens proved to be both a help and a hindrance to object recognition. It enabled me to pick out identifying features that I previously could not "see", but it also upset my notions of familiar size. With the first camera, objects were always displayed at a constant distance, and always, therefore, appeared to be in a constant size. The zoom lens and the variable magnification it possessed changed that feature. In essence, I had to learn which zoom setting corresponded with the size of the object as seen with the spectacle-mounted camera—a task much less formidable than I thought it would be.

'*Comparing distances of objects.* Initially, during the object recognition phase, only one object at a time was displayed. The next phase of training consisted of comparing the distances of two or more objects. I was asked to tell which of the two objects was farther away from me. I was never asked to judge how far away a single object was from me, nor was I asked to judge the metric distance separating two objects. In performing the task of judging distance, I never thought of the distance as distance, but rather as being a function of the monocular cues for depth which the System was capable of showing. At this point, familiar size, inter-position, and apparent elevation in the visual field were the most important cues.

'Subsequently, I learned to recognize familiar objects in their various possible orientations, although I always had some difficulty in doing so. Up to this point, objects had always been presented to me in one particular orientation. But now, an object was rotated around its axis. A pair of synchronized turntables made it possible for me to rotate an object on display by remote control. This ability greatly aided me in recognizing an object in whatever orientation it happened to be.

'A large part of the last week of this first training period was devoted to illustrating some visual concepts with the aid of a plane mirror. After the mirror was introduced, I was able to observe some of the relationships that exist between an object and its virtual image. Also, the mirror enabled me to "see" the front and back of something simultaneously, a concept I found rather startling.

'*Camera–hand coordination.* The last major skill which I acquired was the rudiments of camera–hand coordination. One of the things I did to acquire this skill was to position the camera so that I could "see" an area to the left of my left shoulder. I could reach into this area with my left hand and "see" it move. I could "see" the separation between thumb and fingers, but not the individual fingers themselves. I could reach for and grasp the hand of my assistant when it was placed within my field of view. I could also duplicate some of her hand movements—waving and so forth. In addition, in order to sharpen this skill, I was taught how to draw. Shapes and figures were drawn and I had to shade them in; that is, I had to stay within the lines of the particular figure. One of the things that added to the difficulty of this task was the fact that I was again using the spectacle-mounted camera. I had difficulty in aiming it at what I wanted to "look" at, apparently because I thought of the camera as being located on or near my midline. I never really adjusted to the change in cameras in that regard. I have been told that this transition occurs with adequate practice and that my few hours of training were not sufficient to expect mastery of this skill.

'At the end of this initial period, I was pleased with my progress and had acquired many of the concepts that would be elaborated and refined in my second training period. A second training period was deemed essential because the equipment used during the first period had various limitations and because three weeks were not sufficient to permit accomplishment of all of our goals.

'*Second training period.* When I returned to San Francisco in February 1975, I was able to obtain some measure of mobility experience with the TVSS. I spend much time learning about such visual phenomena as perspective, foreshortening, and shadowing in a stationary setting prior to the mobile situation so that I would be able to make sense out of rooms, corridors, doors, windows, and the like. However, before I could begin working with complex visual concepts, I had to reacquire my facility in using the System. I repeated much of what I had done during the earlier part of the first training program. I again did such things as line orientation, discrimination, object recognition, and determining whether or not two lines intersected or just approached each other rather closely. I was surprised at how rapidly my ability to scan returned. This skill was the most important I had to reacquire because without it I could not recognize anything.

'During the second training period I worked with two different tactile display systems. One consisted of a matrix mounted inside the back of a wheelchair and a miniature camera mounted on spectacle frames. The other consisted of a matrix of tactors which was placed against the abdomen. The electronics for the second system were housed in a suitcase. With this system we used another miniature camera that had two interchangeable lenses. One lens, similar to that used with the wheelchair TVSS, was mounted on spectacle frames. The second was a zoom lens that could either be hand-held or placed on a pivot mount. The zoom lens was idea for work requiring "seeing" much detail or for viewing the objects close to the camera. Unless it is relevant, I will not mention in the following discussion which system we were using.

'*Relationship of moving object to stationary object.* One principle I learned concerned the apparent change in relationship of two objects when one is moving. This principle was demonstrated by viewing an object against a background consisting of a horizontal line. As the object is moved closer to the observer, the line appears to move higher and higher on the object. I was shown this phenomenon with the system and also had the optical principles behind it explained to me.

'I was also introduced to the concept of foreshortening. In order to illustrate this concept, we used a cone, which was placed in various orientations by either tilting the cone or rotating it onto its side. Foreshortening was one of the few concepts with which I had difficulty: I always found it somewhat confusing. Again, the limited practice time with each concept may have contributed to my difficulty.

'*Two-point perspective.* Another major concept I learned concerned two-point perspective and the artistic convention of the two vanishing points. I have always been fascinated by the idea of being able to draw three-dimensional objects on two-dimensional sheets of paper, and I found this experience one of the most exciting parts of this training period.

'A metal board and magnetic strips of tape were used to construct line drawings of cubes and other simple shapes. I "looked" at them with the System and examined them tactually. I was ultimately able to interpret a drawing of an inside corner of a room with a door in one of the walls. Once I had mastered the concept, it was no longer necessary for me to feel the drawings. I was also able to draw what I had seen, and add features not present in a particular display.

'*Simulated room.* Following the making of line drawings of a room, we began "looking" at a simulated room. We constructed this room by taking a cardboard box and cutting off one of its sides. Thus, I was presented with an inside corner, a ceiling and floor, and two intersecting walls. The inside of the box had to be covered with special paper to provide the high contrast necessary for the TVSS.

'For the work I did with the simulated room I used the suitcase system with its hand-held camera. I was interested in "seeing" how the room looked from various positions within it. I found it to be rather awkward to lean back into the tactile display matrix and attempt to hold the camera absolutely straight and level at the same time. In order to solve this problem, I had a pivot mount constructed for this camera and zoom lens. The mount held the camera at any desired height and allowed it to be rotated so as to give the effect of looking up towards the ceiling or down to the floor. The camera could also be locked in any desired position. When "looking" at the simulated room, the zoom lens became extremely valuable. Without this lens, the simulated table and rug that we placed in the room would not have been visible at all.

'*Convergence of parallel lines.* When I reached the point of being able to describe my position in the "room" by means of the angles formed by the intersecting walls, ceiling, and floor, we stopped working with the "room" and began working with the apparent convergence of parallel lines. During the first training period I had been shown how parallel lines appear to converge when they are located below the observer's gaze line. I had no difficulty in recognizing this when it was again presented to me. Here again, we used the metal board and magnetic strips to make line drawings. I did have enormous difficulty with the phenomenon of looking up at a pair of parallel lines and "seeing" how they appear to converge as I "looked" toward the horizon. My assistant and I, and the other members of the staff to whom we mentioned the fact, were surprised, but no one was really sure why I had such difficulty. We tried to clear up the problem by examining a ceiling which had acoustical tiles and feeling the parallel lines made by their edges. Again to our surprise, these experiences really did not help very much. Further experience with such displays was apparently needed before I fully understood this phenomenon.

'*Direction of shadows.* A concept with which I expected to have great difficulty, but which I did not, was that of shadowing. We took a sphere and illuminated it from various positions. At one point we simulated something approximating the phases of the moon. To give me a better understanding of what was occurring, my assistant would cut from paper the various segments of the sphere which would appear when the light was in different positions. I was also shown the difference between a partially shadowed sphere and a partially shadowed circle. With some practice and with increased independent mobility permitting the use of parallax (viewing the display from various angles), I am sure I would have been able to tell the difference between the two-dimensional and three-dimensional objects.

'*Mobile system*. I began the second week of this training program by attaching a 100-foot-long extension cord to the wheelchair System. By being wheeled around the corridors of the research building, I received my first mobile experience with the TVSS. I could not distinguish much in the way of doors, windows, and other things in the corridors. The most important part of this particular experiment was that I was finally able to "see" and understand how parallel lines appear to converge when the observer is looking up at them from below. This concept was made clear because I was now able to view from four to six fluorescent ceiling lights at a time. Viewed from the wheelchair, they appeared to me to be horizontal bars. These "bars" looked shorter and shorter the farther away from me they were. If I imagined the ends of the "bars" as being connected by straight lines, then I would be "seeing" a perfect illustration of the convergence of parallel lines when they are "seen" from below.

'Inasmuch as the wheelchair system did not pick up enough detail and did not provide proprioceptive information through walking, we improvised a mobile system using the suitcase model. Straps were put through the handles of two matrices, one of which acted as a counterweight and hung down my back, and the other rested against my abdomen and provided the vibratory display. We placed the suitcase on a cart which was wheeled along behind me. A spectacle-frame model camera was attached to this system. I could then walk as far as my 100-foot extension cord would allow. With this system, too, I could not "see" much except the ceiling lights and patches of glare.

'A major problem was the lack of sufficient illumination in the corridors. We partially solved this problem by plugging a spotlight into the power source on the cart. As I walked around I could point it at whatever I wished to illuminate. The spotlight was only partially successful because it emitted a large amount of infrared which rapidly saturated the solid-state camera. (A heat filter placed in front of the lens reduced the infrared reaching the camera to some degree, but did not improve the camera's effectiveness sufficiently.)

'The modified mobile arrangement worked reasonably well when we put the System on black–white reversal, i.e., dark regions were displayed as vibration and lighted areas were silent. I could then "see" doors, part of a drinking fountain, and people as they walked by. The most interesting part of this experiment for me was to be able to focus the camera on a particular ceiling light and "watch" the changes in shape it underwent as I approached it. In my opinion I was able to distinguish so little at this time because I did not have the time to do the exercises which would have been necessary to develop this skill sufficiently.

'The experiments involving the mobile suitcase which I have just described took up most of the second week of this training period.

'*Optical illusions.* I spent one morning viewing some simple optical illusions. I shall describe them and state my responses to them. We did not engage in any sort of psychophysical tasks to measure my responses to them. It should be borne in mind that the camera possesses a narrow field of view and that only a part of most objects can be seen without having to move it. This means that if the figures presented were too large or contained too much detail, it would be impossible to "look" at them in a short enough time for it to feel like a simultaneous display.

'We tried several illusions, but I had difficulty interpeting them; before I could respond to an illusion, I had to be able to "see" it clearly and know in what part of it the illusion lay.

'One of the illusions I viewed consisted of a vertical and a horizontal line intersecting at right angles. The horizontal line was below the vertical and the lines were actually of equal length. The vertical line appeared to me to be much longer than the horizontal line. Another illusion I viewed consisted of a square; inside it were a set of parallel lines which were parallel to two of its sides. When the square was positioned so that the set of parallel lines within it was vertical, the square appeared to be taller than it was wide—that is, it appeared to be rectangular; but when it was oriented so that the parallel lines within it were horizontal, it looked more like a square.

'The last illusion that I would like to describe consisted of a group of five vertical stripes that were uniformly spaced and rather close together. To the right of this group was a single vertical stripe. In actuality, the space between this sixth or right-most stripe and the group of five equaled the area encompassed by the group of five stripes. It appeared to me, however, as if the space or area covered by the group "looked" larger than the space between the group and the single stripe.

'*Viewing corner of an actual room.* I began the third week of my training program by moving the apparatus into a conference room and observing a corner of an actual room. In one corner we placed tape to make distinct divisions between the floor, walls and ceiling. I could "see" the line made by the intersection of the two walls, also the lines made by the intersection of the walls with the floor and ceiling. They looked much as they did in the simulated room, but since they were longer they would run into areas of shadow. I could walk around freely in this corner and orient myself in relation to the walls; I could determine which wall was closer to me. I had some initial difficulty in learning the head movements necessary to look up at the ceiling, but I soon became used to doing it. I found it even more difficult to learn to look down at the floor. I could not get used to having to tip my head so far down. I had a tendency to bend my knees and torso.

'As was the case when I "looked" at the simulated room, I "saw" the corner of the actual room as if it were a drawing with a vanishing point on either side and my height determining the horizon line. One of the most interesting experiences I had while working in the corner of the room occurred when I sat on the floor and "looked" up at the ceiling. It struck me as being incredibly high. The other exciting experience was simply that of being able to "watch" the angle of the intersecting lines change shape as I moved about. I was ultimately able to use this information to move about and guide myself to a target.'

Theoretical Aspects of the TVSS Studies

One of the major goals of the TVSS project was to study brain plasticity, the capacity of the brain to reorganize following injury and to restore function. Thus, our principal work was with congenitally blind persons: these were considered to be 'natural' experiments, in whom the major source of afferent information had been eliminated before they had the opportunity to develop the mechanisms for the analysis of visual information. A discussion of brain plasticity is beyond the scope of this chapter. It has been extensively discussed elsewhere (Bach-y-Rita, 1967; 1971; 1972; 1975a, b; 1976a, b; 1980b).

Practical Applications of Vision Substitution Devices

A number of factors must be considered in the development of a practical sensory substitution system. In the first place, it is necessary for the device to have a sound physiological basis. This sometimes occurs, either by chance or by appropriate interaction with physiologists and other members of a development team. Often, however, the devices have no sound physiological basis and, although a great amount of money is expended, no practical device can be developed. Even when a physiologically sound device is developed, the chances of it ever becoming practical are limited. Some factors involved include: per unit cost, cost of developing a product from the successful prototype, limited potential market, availability of other approaches to the problem that may be well established or less costly, maintenance and reliability problems and cosmetic and acceptability problems (Bach-y-Rita, 1979). The enthusiasm of the research team is thus rarely crowned by the success of a product that is actually *used* by handicapped persons.

I. THE TVSS

Our TVSS system is an example of a rehabilitation instrumentation development project that has not yet been translated into practice. We were certain that this crude prototype would quickly lead to the development of practical visual substitution systems for the blind, for school, vocational, mobility and general adaptation. Furthermore, it seemed feasible to apply the same principles to other sensory losses (our tactile auditory substitution system and our touch prosthesis for leprosy patients without tactile sensations in their hands both proved feasible, and successful prototypes were developed). We seemed to be in a particularly favourable environment for substitution system development, and our research team included psychologists and consumers to complement our professional qualifications.

The five years following the appearance of the first prototype were full of theoretical and instrumentation development successes (summarized in Bach-y-Rita, 1972). However, the *practical* device eluded us.

The technical problems are enormous, since normal sight is such a highly complex function and is so difficult to reproduce with present-day machines. The interface between machine and man is another major problem. Developing devices that are physiologically acceptable, that take advantage of receptor and transmission capacities of the substitute sensory system (e.g. the skin of the abdomen and its receptors and pathways, or the cochlea and the highly sequential nature of the auditory system), is a major challenge. Experimental subjects for the development projects have generally been highly intelligent, well-adapted blind persons; in other words, unusual persons who may not reflect the capabilities of the great majority of the blind. The technical problems of developing research prototypes are great, but those of developing a useful product from a successful prototype are even greater and at least ten times as costly. If a successful system were developed, future problems would include: unit cost and distribution, maintenance and reliability, cosmesis and acceptability. And on top of all of these problems, the psychological factors involved in the transition from a blind person to one who had acquired some degree of 'sight' would have to be carefully considered.

One limitation is the result of differing properties of the individual sensory systems. For example, the visual system is able to receive a great deal of information simultaneously: a brief flash (or tachistoscopic presentation) is sufficient to recognize a face. However, it is very poor at resolving high frequencies. The ear, on the contrary, has a very high frequency response; it is excellent for resolving sequential information, but poor at simultaneous information. The skin is in between: it resolves more simultaneous information than the ear, but less than the eye, and higher frequencies than the eye, but less than the ear. Thus, blind subjects using the TVSS do not perceive objects instantaneously. They scan the object, which consumes considerable time. Furthermore, receptor density and two-point discrimination are important factors (although less so than could have been predicted). The nervous system extracts information from dynamic patterns of stimulation more than from static unpatterned stimuli, such as the two-point discrimination studies (discussed in Bach-y-Rita, 1972); however, one of the limitations of a sensory substitution system is that the receptors and pathways of the substitute normal system may not be capable of adequately carrying the information required to provide a practical sensory substitute.

At present, no blind or deaf person is using our tactile sensory substitution devices on a regular basis. The studies have demonstrated that the brain is a highly plastic organ and that the perceptual mechanisms are sufficiently malleable to enable a congenitally blind person to interpret the information from a tactile sensory substitution system in visual terms. Furthermore, the development of a mobility device is being actively pursued and the auditory tactile substitution system has a very good chance of becoming a practical system for deaf persons. A teaching device for blind children is feasible, especially in the classroom setting, where portability is not a concern, where focal length and lighting can be easily controlled, and where specific training can take place: for example, to teach geometry and graphical material, to train the blind children in the three-dimensional world, to allow them to observe moving animals, to teach microscopic information (such as the structure of a fly wing or of a red blood cell). Yet,

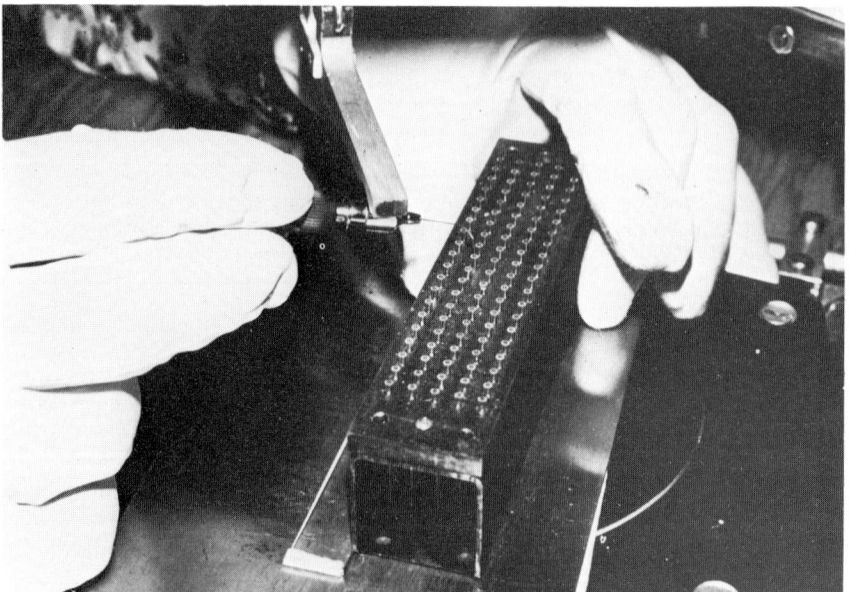

Fig. 13.2. A blind worker on an assembly line for diode construction in an electronics firm. The metal frame ('boat') contains 100 glass cylinders. The blind assembler is in the process of filling one of the cylinders, which he found to be empty by moving the boat into his 'field of view' under a television camera. (Photo courtesy of Al Alden)

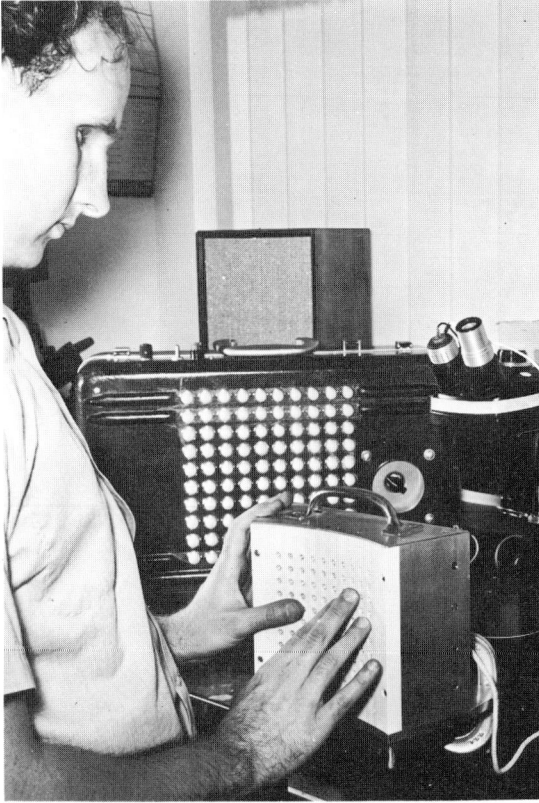

Fig. 13.3. A blind subject is shown examining a laboratory version of the system used in Fig. 13.2. The array of vibratory stimulators is clipped to the workbench (the subject has his right hand on the array). A TV camera is shown in a microscope, substituting for an ocular. The array of lights (middle background) provides a visual display corresponding point-for-point to the tactile display, thus allowing the instructor to monitor the blind subject's activities.

even such a relatively simple form of the tactile vision substitution system is a long way from being practicable.

A vocational test of the TVSS revealed its potential application to jobs presently reserved for sighted workers. A person totally blind since two months from birth spent three months on the miniature diode assembly line of an electronic manufacturer. During the assembly process, he received a frame containing 100 small glass cylinders with attached wires as the frame emerged from an automatic filling machine that filled the cylinders with a small piece of solder (lead [Figs. 13.2 and 13.3]). The automatic process was 95% efficient, and so approximately 5% of the cylinders remained unfilled. His first task after receiving each frame was to inspect each of the cylinders and to fill by hand those

(5%) that remained unfilled. This was accomplished with a small TV camera under which the blind person passed the frame containing the cylinders. The information from the TV camera was passed through an electronic commutator in order to transform it into a tactile image and delivered to the skin of the abdomen of the blind worker by means of 100 small vibrating rods in an array clipped to the workbench. In order to receive the image, the worker had only to lean his abdomen against the array (without removing his shirt). The blind worker did not wear any special apparatus and his hands were left free to perform the assembly task under the microscope. He filled the empty cylinders by means of a modified injection needle attached to a vacuum: he placed the needle into a dish filled with small pieces of solder. The needle picked up only one piece, since the suction was blocked when the tip of the needle was covered by a piece of solder. He then brought the needle with the piece of solder into the 'visual' field under the microscope and by hand–'eye' coordination placed the needle in an empty cylinder. When the needle was in the cylinder, he released the vacuum, allowing the piece of solder to fall into the cylinder.

The blind worker repeated the process for each of the empty cylinders encountered. When all 100 were filled, the frame passed to another loading machine where it was automatically filled with the diode wafers. Again, the task was to identify the unfilled cylinders (5%) and to fill them by hand as described above. However, this stage offered two extra problems: the wafers were very thin and light and they did not always fall flat into the cylinders. Sometimes they landed on edge. Furthermore, the wafers were gold on one side and silver on the other, and they had to be correctly orientated: the worker had the additional task of turning over the 50% of wafers that were incorrectly orientated. This task was accomplished by identifying the colour (silver or gold) on the basis of light reflectance, since the silver reflected more light.

The blind worker was able to come into the criterion established for the sighted workers in regard to velocity of performing the assembly task, and in regard to errors. Thus, the feasibility of the vocational device was established. However, with the prototype device used for this task the blind worker became fatigued from the effort of concentration more often and required more frequent rests. The assembly line manager, although satisfied that the task had been performed to the pre-established requirements, was unwilling to consider employing a blind worker. His objections to this included unwillingness to provide the small extra space occupied by the device, fear that the blind worker might not be able to perform the task if it had to be modified, and fear that it would be difficult to terminate the blind worker's employment, should this become necessary.

Thus, although the feasibility of the vocational device was demonstrated, it is not being used. This is a common fate of many potentially successful devices developed for the handicapped.

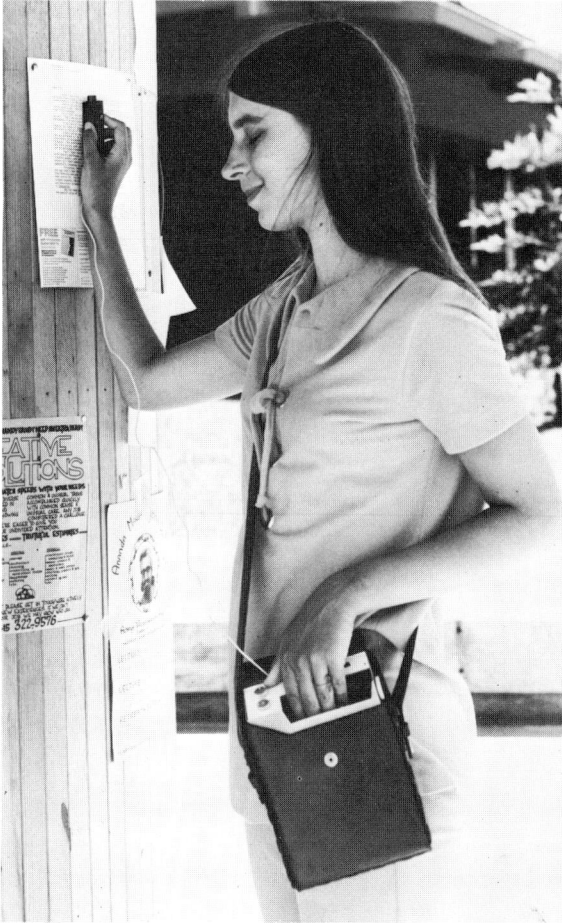

Fig. 13.4. A blind subject is shown using an Optacon. The right hand holds a television camera picking up the letters as it is passed across a line of print. The left hand is held on a vibrating tactile display of the letters. (Photo courtesy of Dr James Bliss)

The Optacon

Some sensory substitution devices do become practical. The Linvill–Bliss research team (Bliss, 1971) at Stanford University was able to develop a practical sensory substitution system* that enables a blind person to read ordinary print by passing a small television camera over a line of print, while receiving a tactile image of each letter on a finger placed over a matrix of 144 vibrating stimulators

* Optacon—Telesensory Systems, Palo Alto, California, USA.

(Fig. 13.4). This is one of the very few devices that have become products available to the public.

II. ELECTROMYOGRAPHIC SENSORY SUBSTITUTION

A sensory substitution technique that is now in common use is the substitution of head, trunk or limb position and muscle contraction information normally supplied by proprioceptors, by artificial receptors (electromyographic (EMG) needles or surface electrodes) that convert the proprioceptive information into visual and/or auditory displays.

A number of research and clinical groups (e.g. Brudny *et al.*, 1976; Basmajian, 1978) have been studying the application of EMG feedback (sometimes called 'biofeedback') to patients with various manifestations of disturbed neuromotor control. Brudny *et al.* (1976) have applied these techniques to patients with various such diseases, including hemiparesis, torticollis and dystonia, with favourable results in the majority of their 114 patients. They displayed the integrated EMG on an oscilloscope in the form of a continuous trace that reflects, instantaneously, the degree and rate of muscle contraction. They also used an auditory display that reflects, instantaneously, the change in the integrated EMG activity either by proportional changes in click rate or tone intensities.

Prior to treatment, the deficient motor activity of each patient was evaluated, and therapeutic goals defined, e.g. reaching, grasping and pulling, in the evaluation of upper extremities in hemiplegics. The degree of involuntary spasmodic activity was evaluated in patients with spasmodic torticollis.

The desired functional goals were analysed in terms of simple tasks performed by the primary movers (agonists). For example, in treating a hemiplegic non-functional upper extremity, the therapeutic effort was directed toward learning volitional control of muscles, starting proximally and progressing distally. The main goals were decrease of spasticity during movement or stretch and increase of contraction and strength of paretic or atrophied muscles. Other muscles (synergists, antagonists) were then treated in a similar manner. In patients with spasmodic torticollis the goals were decrease of involuntary spasmodic activity during rest and movement and strengthening of contralateral muscles if they were atrophied. A brief demonstration was usually carried out on a normal muscle preceding the treatment, allowing the patients to understand the relationship between muscle contraction and relaxation and the corresponding changes in the auditory and visual displays. Initially, the patient's efforts were directed toward minimal volitional changes of the audiovisual displays of integrated EMG activity derived from a functionally deficient muscle. Such changes were accomplished by maintaining a sustained state of voluntary contraction or voluntary relaxation of the muscle for 10–20 seconds. In the next stage of training, emphasis was placed on alternating the voluntary contraction and the voluntary relaxation of the trained muscle in increasingly shorter time periods.

Following this, the actual motor task (e.g. extension of the forearm) was attempted in a step-by-step manner, using the shaping technique described below.

The simultaneous use of auditory and visual displays allows for therapeutic shaping of the patient's response. Shaping is modification of the behaviour (in this case, motor) by defining a desired response, and reinforcing closer and closer approximations to this pattern. Patients were made aware of success of their performance by auditory signals (tones) delivered upon successful completion of the spatial and temporal components of the electromyographic task.

The voltage display representing patient's volitional muscle performance was matched against an arbitrary voltage line, representing the therapeutic goals and subject to gradual changes by the therapist in the desired direction, over a number of sessions. When the patient repeatedly responded with closer approximations of the muscle activity to the optimal therapeutic goals, the visual feedback was withdrawn. Further functional return was facilitated by continuing auditory feedback with concomitant direct visual observation of the limb displacement or by mirror viewing of the neck position. Feedback from the activity of two muscles at the same time (one auditory and one visual, or both visual with one additionally auditory) provided a means for inhibiting and/or suppressing the undesired involuntary activity in the antagonist muscles. As the return of functional components of a desired task occurred, and the speed and accuracy of performance improved, all feedback was gradually withdrawn. If functional movement was carried out adequately and repeatedly under the therapist's guidance without any feedback, the sessions were spaced farther apart and gradually discontinued.

The authors believe that,

'... during sensory feedback therapy, the audiovisual signals reflecting muscle activity have matching or resonance characteristics with the neural coding of the information on the intensity and rate of muscle contraction. Normally, this information, derived from the proprioceptive (kinesthetic) system, is processed in many CNS centers interconnected by a neural network of feedback loops, with eventual relay to the sensorimotor cortex and to the descending pathways of the brainstem reticular system. Thus, disruption of a closed-loop type of servosystem of patterned movements may occur as a result of an insult to various areas of the CNS. In the case of the hemiparetic syndrome, the insult may involve numerous cortical and subcortical structures, while in the dystonic syndrome it is generally believed that it is the basal ganglia which are primarily involved. Either form of neuropathology disrupts the ultimate voluntary motor function. The audiovisual sensory feedback from integrated EMG, when considered as a substitute for the proprioceptive internal feedback loops, forms an external feedback loop in the disrupted system. This external loop thus augments or restores the sensorimotor interaction of the closed loop system, of voluntary patterned movements' (Brudny *et al.*, 1976).

III. LIMB SENSORY SUBSTITUTION

A major problem in the rehabilitation of upper-extremity amputees is the paucity of sensory information in the artificial limb. This is not as great a problem for lower-extremity amputees since the control required for the prosthesis is less fine, and since the contact with the ground during gait produces a stimulus to the skin and deeper receptors of the stump.

The paucity of sensory information from the prosthetic upper extremity is undoubtedly an important reason for not using a non-motorized prosthetic upper extremity, but even these do provide some sensory information through contact of the hook with objects: some stimulation of the stump does occur and this information is useful. A greater problem appears to occur with motor-driven upper-extremity prosthesis since the artificial (motor-driven) joint is insufficiently linked to accurate sensory receptors. Our sensory substitution studies have confirmed the necessity of motor-sensory linkage for accurate perception of self-induced movement and the integration of that movement information with other proprioceptive information in the accurate self-localization in space (discussed in Bach-y-Rita, 1972). A comparable problem occurs in hemiplegics, primarily left hemiplegics, with absent or distorted perception of proprioception on the affected side.

Cutaneous Sensory Substitution in Leprosy Patients

A preliminary study of sensory substitution of touch, pressure and temperature in leprosy patients with absence of these sensations has provided valuable information for the development of a sensory substitution system for amputees. Fig. 13.5 shows a leprosy patient with absent cutaneous sensation in the hands wearing a glove containing strain gauges providing information on touch and pressure. The skin stimulation site was the forehead, since his sensation there was intact. Within a few hours he could accurately locate the sensations to his fingers, and could gain pleasure from perceiving textures.

Sensory Substitution in Limb Prosthesis

With most upper-extremity prostheses, the position of the shoulders provides some kinaesthetic feedback, but the eyes must provide most of the information on forearm position. Thus an amputee rarely uses his prosthesis outside his field of view. Normally he cannot carry on a conversation while he uses the prosthesis to eat, since controlling the prosthesis requires his full attention. Indeed, Alles (1968) has pointed out that if the amputee who wears a prosthesis with multiple degree of freedom 'is to feel that it is an extension of his body and not that he is just the operator of a remote manipulator, he must receive kinesthetic information through a sensory channel in addition to his eyes. Otherwise he will operate it like a steam shovel, one joint at a time' (Alles, 1968).

Kinaesthetic feedback systems for amputees have been designed by several groups of investigators. Among these Alles (1968) has designed a feedback system for an artificial elbow joint utilizing two stimulators located approximately four inches apart on the upper arm. His system is based on the von Bekesy phantom sensation principle: the relative amplitude of stimulation at each stimulator is altered as the amputee flexes his elbow, and the sensation travels up his arm between the two stimulators.

Several possible approaches to tactile kinaesthetic sensory substitution (TKSS) have been discussed previously (Bach-y-Rita & Collins, 1970). The ultimate aim of the amputee, using a TKSS, would be to have the information processed automatically and subconsciously. Only in this way would he be able to manipulate his prosthesis to achieve a goal, such as picking up an object, without consciously thinking of degrees of flexion at each joint. An amputee, using a prosthesis that included a high resolution tactile display delivered to a suitable area of skin (upper arm, torso), should learn to respond to the stimulation as if it originated in the appropriate part of the prosthesis. Thus the ultimate result could be that the prosthesis would become functionally a part of his body. One example may suffice to indicate why we feel that the amputee

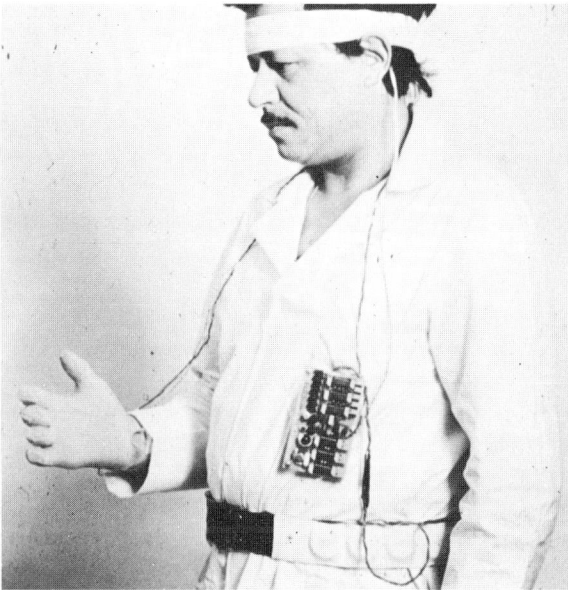

Fig. 13.5. A leprosy patient is shown wearing a glove fitted with strain gauges. The signals are converted to tactile stimuli by the commutator clipped to his shirt pocket, and delivered to the skin of his forehead. He is wearing a belt containing batteries.

may achieve this ultimate goal. When one is learning to use a typewriter by the touch system, one must concentrate on the relative position of each letter on the keyboard, and on the relative positions of all the fingers. Yet once the learning process is complete, full attention can be given to the meaning of the words being typed; the fingers do the actual typing without conscious direction.

IV. TACTILE AUDITORY SUBSTITUTION SYSTEM

For the last few years a group in our laboratory have been developing a tactile auditory substitution system (TASS). It is comparable to the TVSS discussed in Section I, but is simpler in conception and construction. The aid presents sound information as flowing, dynamic patterns on the skin, which is learned like a new language.

The deaf subject wears a 'belt' contining 32 stimulators in contact with the skin. The frequency response of the TASS described by Saunders *et al.* (1978) covers the range of normal hearing, from 30 to 16 000 Hz, with a frequency discrimination threshold of 1/12 octave.

Speech and environmental sounds are analysed according to frequency and are displayed on the belt of tactile stimulators, worn around the abdomen. Each stimulator is sensitive to a specific frequency, and its output represents the amount of energy present within its specific bandwith. The frequency bands are displayed linearly, from low to high; a 'siren' produces a sensation which moves back and forth across the belt.

The resonances which characterize different vowel sounds are perceived as a characteristic pattern of two or three simultaneous sensations. Diphthongs combine these patterns in a moving sequence.

Unvoiced stop consonants (*p*, *t*, *k*) are perceived as a brief burst of energy at a single place on the belt, whose position is dependent upon the place of articulation. Voiced stops (*b*, *d*, *g*) provide, in addition, a sensation in the frequency range of vocal cord activity. Fricative consonants such as *s* and *sh* are perceived as longer in duration and broader in bandwidth than the stop consonants, and the presence or absence of voicing may be similarly distinguished.

The sensory aid provides information both about the frequency content of the signal and also about the time-varying envelope properties known as prosodic or suprasegmental features. These features include duration (rhythmic) patterns, intensity stress patterns, and changes in inflection. A wearable, 20-channel prototype of the teletactor is shown in Fig. 13.6.

Previously reported experiments have indicated that untrained subjects can learn to discriminate the basic phonemic features of the English language via the tactile display alone, eliminating all acoustic and lipreading cues, within ten hours of training. Vocabularies of common words, consisting of a few dozen items presented in isolation, can be learned in a comparable period of time. With

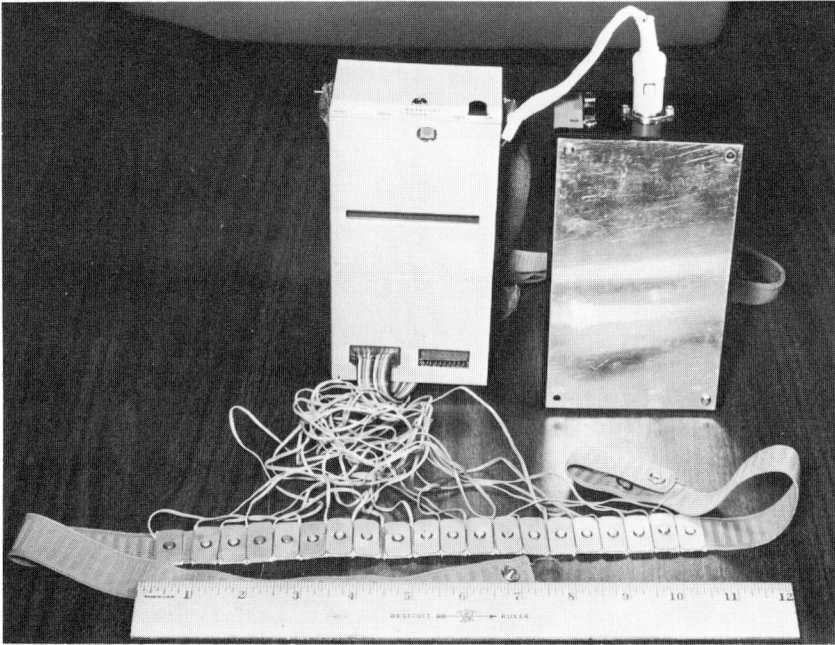

Fig. 13.6. A 20-channel model of the tactile auditory substitution system is shown. In the foreground is a linear array of electrodes worn on the abdomen as a belt. In the background are the microphone to pick up the words and environmental sounds, the electronic apparatus with batteries, and a linear array of lights (in the slit in the device on the left) to enable the instructor to monitor visually the tactile stimulation received by the deaf subject. (Photo courtesy of Dr Frank Saunders)

further training, words learned in isolation can be discriminated when presented within sentence frames, in connected discourse.

It is clear, however, that the task of learning and discriminating individual words is radically different from the fluent comprehension of ongoing speech. The discrimination of syllables and phonemic features is only a beginning; the learner must also develop the ability to utilize more complex, partially redundant cues such as the prosodic, syntactic and semantic structure of each utterance. In other words, the process is equivalent to the learning of a new language. For this reason, young children are the most appropriate candidates for this type of training, since they are still within their primary language acquisition age, and studies are in progress with profoundly deaf children (Saunders *et al.*, 1978). The child must respond by touching the display; a correct response is rewarded, while hints and other instructional pointers are given for incorrect responses.

V. DISCUSSION AND CONCLUSIONS

Evidence from our laboratories and others has shown that sensory substitution devices can, at least in the laboratory, provide information that the brain can learn to integrate with information from intact sensory systems.

The most extensively studied sensory substitution devices have been for vision substitution. However, this is the most difficult sense to substitute. Although reading devices are now practical, it is unlikely that a vision substitution system allowing perception of the three-dimensional world will be practical in the foreseeable future. On the other hand, EMG sensory substitution is already in practical use, and auditory and limb sensory substitution devices show promise of becoming practical in the foreseeable future. A sensory substitution device must be extremely reliable and easy to repair if it is to become widely used. A person using such a device would depend on it for mobility, employment and recreation, and unless it were as dependable as a pair of glasses, a cardiac pacemaker or a long cane (for blind mobility), it could not be widely used. Thus, technical difficulties and expense will continue to be major barriers to common usage of these devices even if they do become available.

REFERENCES

ALLES D.S. (1968) Kinesthetic feedback system for amputees via the tactile sense. Ph.D. Thesis, Massachusetts Institute of Technology, Cambridge, Mass.

BACH-Y-RITA P. (1967) Sensory plasticity: applications to a vision substitution system. *Acta Neurologica Scandinavica*, **43**, 417–26.

BACH-Y-RITA P. (1971) Neural substrates of sensory substitution. In *Zeichenerkennung durch biologische und technische Systeme—Pattern Recognition in the Biological and Technical Systems* (Eds. Klinke R. & Grüsser O.J.), pp. 130–42. Springer-Verlag, Berlin.

BACH-Y-RITA P. (1972) *Brain Mechanisms in Sensory Substitution*, 192 pp. Academic Press, New York.

BACH-Y-RITA P. (1975a) Plastic brain mechanisms in sensory substitution. In *Cerebral Localization* (Eds. Zülch K.J., Creutzfeldt O. & Galbraith G.C.), pp. 203–16. Springer-Verlag, Berlin.

BACH-Y-RITA P. (1975b) Plasticity of the nervous system. In *Cerebral Localization* (Eds. Zülch K.J., Creutzfeldt O. & Galbraith G.C.), pp. 313–27. Springer-Verlag, Berlin.

BACH-Y-RITA P. (1976a) Brain plasticity demonstrated by sensory substitution and stroke studies. In *Contemporary Aspects of Cerebrovascular Disease* (Ed. Austin G.M.), pp. 87–93. Professional Information Library, Dallas.

BACH-Y-RITA P. (1976b) Comments on central nervous system plasticity. In *Proceedings of the Second World Congress of the International Rehabilitation Medicine Association*, pp. 761–76. Mexico.

BACH-Y-RITA P. (1979) The practicality of sensory aids. *International Rehabilitation Medicine*, **1**, 87–89.

BACH-Y-RITA P. (1980a) Outlook. In *Rehabilitation of the Visually Handicapped and the Blind* (Ed. Gloor B.), pp. 136–43. H. Huber, Bern, Switzerland.

BACH-Y-RITA P. (1980b) Brain plasticity as a basis for therapeutic procedures. In *Recovery of Function: Theoretical Considerations for Brain Injury Rehabilitation* (Ed. Bach-y-Rita P.), pp. 225–63. H. Huber, Bern, Switzerland.

BACH-Y-RITA P. & COLLINS C.C. (1970) Sensory substitution and limb prosthesis. In *Advances in External Control of Human Extremities* (Eds. Gavrilovic M.M. & Wilson A.B. Jr), pp. 9–21. Etan, Dubrovnik.

BACH-Y-RITA P., COLLINS C.C., SAUNDERS F., WHITE B. & SCADDEN L. (1969) Vision substitution by tactile image projection. *Nature, London*, **221**, 963–4.

BASMAJIAN J.V. (1978) Biofeedback in therapeutic exercise. In *Therapeutic Exercise* (Ed. Basmajian J.V.), 3e, pp. 220–7. Williams and Wilkins, Baltimore.

BLISS J.C. (1971) A reading machine with tactile display. In *Visual Prosthesis: The Interdisciplinary Dialogue* (Eds. Sterling T.D. *et al.*), pp. 259–63. Academic Press, New York.

BRUDNY J., KOREIN, J., GRYNBAUM B.B., FRIEDMAN L.W., WEINSTEIN S., SACHS-FRANKEL G. & BELANDRES P.V. (1976) EMG feedback therapy: review of treatment of 114 patients. *Archives of Physical Medicine and Rehabilitation*, **57**, 55–61.

COLLINS C.C. & BACH-Y-RITA P. (1973) Transmission of pictorial information through the skin. *Advances in Biological and Medical Physics*, **14**, 285–315.

GUARNIERO G. (1974) Experience of tactile vision. *Perception*, **3**, 101–4.

GUARNIERO G. (1977) Tactile vision: a personal view. *Viz. Impairment and Blindness*, March, pp. 125–30.

SAUNDERS F.A., HILL W.A. & EASLEY T. (1978) Development of a Plato-based curriculum for tactile speech recognition. *Journal of Educational Technology Systems*, **7**, 19–27.

SCADDEN L.A. (1974) The tactile vision substitution system: applications in education and employment. *New Outlook for the Blind* (American Federation of the Blind, New York), **68**, 394–7.

WHITE B.W., SAUNDERS F.A., SCADDEN L., BACH-Y-RITA P. & COLLINS C.C. (1970) Seeing with the skin. *Perception and Psychophysics*, **7**, 23–7.

Chapter 14

Stimulation Procedures

The earliest accounts of the use of electricity or electrical stimulation in the treatment of disease date back to the first century. The ancient, and indeed some of the more modern, descriptions are of historical interest and are sometimes of great entertainment value, such as the enthusiastic experiments of the Abbé Nolet who discharged a Leyden jar through 180 of the King's guards at Versailles and repeated this performance with great panache on the entire membership of a Carthusian monastery. Unfortunately the techniques were of little or no therapeutic value. However, physiologists and neurologists used electrical stimulation techniques to good effect in the investigation of the central nervous system. Beginning with Fritsch and Hitzig's demonstration of the electrical excitability of the motor cortex in 1870 and culminating in Sherrington's (1906) exposition of the integrated action of the nervous system, electrical methods of stimulation resulted in the accumulation of a vast body of knowledge about the responses of nervous tissue to electrical currents. More recent advances in electronics have brought reliability, miniaturization and economy of power consumption.

EXPERIMENTAL STUDIES

Experimental studies of the long-term effect of repetitive stimulation on the morphology and function of the central nervous system are relatively few. Most of such studies, particularly those involving physiological experiments, have been related directly or indirectly to learning theory. The two major theories involve either reverberatory neural networks; or the possibility of repetitive stimulation of synapses producing some long-lasting change in structure with a resultant increase in efficiency and an easier transmission of subsequent impulses along previously used pathways. These two theories are not mutually exclusive.

It should be emphasized that although there is good evidence for environmental changes producing a demonstrable alteration in neural structure and response to stimulation, the precise part this alteration plays in neurological function remains unclear.

Morphological changes following repetitive stimulation have been reported in terms of synaptic size, synaptic vesicle change and changes in dendrite branching.

384

This brief review is confined to vertebrates and, unless otherwise stated, to mammals. The term *synapse* refers to the site of chemical transmission in the central nervous system, but is sometimes used in this sense in peripheral ganglia and at neuromuscular junctions. The swollen or dilated ends of axon terminals where they make contact with other nerve cells have various terms, such as *end-feet, terminal knobs, boutons terminaux,* etc. The term synapse includes the terminal swelling of an afferent axon, containing mitochondria, synaptic vesicles and, in most sites, neurofibrils; and the specialized ultra-structural thickenings at the junction of the swollen terminal and the post-synaptic cell. The synaptic vesicles are minute structures containing the chemical transmitter.

De Robertis and Ferreira (1957) stimulated the splanchnic nerve and looked at the endings of this nerve in the adrenal medulla. They demonstrated an increase in synaptic vesicles. However, faster rates of stimulation (over 400/s) led to a decrease in synaptic vesicles. Similar results were found by Feher *et al.* (1972) who found an increase in vesicles in reticulo-cortical endings with auditory stimulation, but with a concomitant decrease in the endings of thalamo-cortical pathways. Rats reared in an 'enriched environment', when compared to litter-mates, showed an expansion of visual cortex, probably due to an increase in dendritic branching, an increase in glia, an increase in cholinesterase and a possible increase in blood supply (Diamond *et al.,* 1964). Bazanova *et al.* (1965) found that peripheral nerve stimulation in the frog produced enlargement of synapses which persisted for hours after stimulation and with an increase in the uptake of silver stains. This enlargement of synapses with repetitive stimulation was confirmed by Illis (1969) in the spinal cord of adult cats following repetitive stimulation of a single posterior root. Synapses showed a shift towards larger sizes and with an increased staining with silver stains. The size and the morphology of the synapses were similar to the normal 'giant' synapses found on Clarke's column cells. In the synaptic zones of Clarke's column there is normally a system by which synaptic transmission is much more readily accomplished than at the anterior horn cells (Lloyd & McIntyre, 1950). Perhaps the enlarged synapses seen after repetitive stimulation could be responsible for the changes of post-tetanic potentiation. Jorgensen and Bolwig (1979) investigated the effect of electroconvulsive stimulation in rats using protein markers of various components of the synapse and synapse organelles. They found changes which indicated an increase in synaptic vesicles and also synaptic remodelling.

It appears that the number of synaptic vesicles (which contain the chemical neurotransmitters) in central synapses, as well as peripheral endings, may increase or decrease as a result of repetitive stimulation. The rise or fall appears to depend on the functional state, the rate of stimulation and the metabolic climate.

Rats exposed to daylight only after weaning differ significantly from litter-mates reared totally in the dark (Cragg, 1967). In the superficial half of the visual cortex the synapses are larger while in the deeper half of the cortex the distribution of synaptic profiles is towards the smaller sizes compared with the dark-reared rat. Experiments which involve comparing animals subjected to an enriched environment or reared in the light as opposed to reared in the dark are perhaps more 'physiological' than those involving isolation and preparation of individual nerves or nerve roots and repetitively stimulating with an artificial impulse. Tetanus toxin poisoning is an interesting example of a natural experiment. Tetanus toxin produces a progressive depression of inhibition and the most likely explanation is that the toxin acts on inhibitory synapses (Eccles, 1965). The clinical and experimental changes seen are those of increased excitation, for example repeated convulsions. Clinical follow-up of survivors from tetanus indicates an increase in irritability, sleep disturbance, myoclonus, epileptic fits and electroencephalographic abnormalities (Illis & Taylor, 1971). Clinically therefore one may look at tetanus poisoning as a type of central nervous system stimulation experiment. Experimentally tetanus toxin produces an increase in synaptic vesicles (Yates & Yates, 1966) and an enlargement of boutons terminaux with no evidence of degeneration (Illis & Mitchell, 1970).

Physiological experiments of disuse indicate a depression of monosynaptic reflexes compared to the control side (Eccles & McIntyre, 1953). Another way of reducing afferent impulses is by tenotomy (see Eccles, 1964), but surprisingly this results in more powerful monosynaptic action than on the control side. This has been explained as due to an actual increase of afferent impulse in tenotomized muscle; unfortunately this increase is in the small afferent nerves and not the muscle spindle afferents which make monosynaptic connections, or by increased supraspinal activation of gamma motoneurons with a consequent increase in group 1a (the appropriate fibres) discharge. A further way of producing long-term change in synaptic activity is by denervating all the muscles but one of the synergic group (Eccles *et al.*, 1962). Both the tenotomy and the denervation of muscle experiments demonstrate an increase in synaptic potency, but they do not definitely indicate that it is a consequence of excessive use. There is a further complication in that synapses at different functional levels of the central nervous system have quantitative differences. For example, frequency potentiation is powerful in cortical cells but is very poorly developed in interneurons of the spinal cord. Experiments designed to look at the effect of excess use or repetitive stimulation in higher centres such as the cortex are subject to technical difficulties, but Morrell (1961) has shown that prolonged activity in a cortical area produces hyperexcitability which continues in the homologous area of the other hemisphere long after its isolation from the original focus. The two areas are, of course, connected by a commissural pathway.

While frequency potentiation has been observed in many sites in the nervous system, it is not ubiquitous. Recent work has concentrated on the hippocampus where synaptic transmission is greatly enhanced by stimulation of afferents at rates above 0.2 Hz. Potentiation by a factor of 4 and with the total duration lasting many hours or even days has been observed (Anderson, 1978; Bliss & Gardner-Medwin, 1973). The interest in the hippocampus and its afferents lies partly in its anatomical arrangement which makes specific biochemical and pharmacological experiments possible and partly because of its proposed role in memory processes. A number of biochemical changes have been noted in association with frequency potentiation and at present potentiation is explained by an enhanced release of transmitter substance at the synaptic terminal rather than by any change in excitability of the post-synaptic neuron. It is of interest that the greatest potentiation is seen at stimulus rates of 10–20 Hz which are physiological rates of impulse firing. Higher and lower rates produce less potentiation. There has been no demonstration of frequency potentiation in man, but few would doubt that it occurs. It is just possible that the enhanced cervical somatosensory evoked potential seen in multiple sclerosis patients undergoing spinal cord stimulation is a reflection of frequency potentiation (Sedgwick *et al.*, 1980).

The first important clinical use of electronic technology was that of cardiac pacing in the 1960s with the advent of therapeutically useful, reliable and eventually implantable stimulators. In neurology, the clinical therapeutic application of electrical stimulation began with Melzack and Wall's (1965) illuminating theory of gate control of pain. Melzack and Wall summarized the established physiological, psychological and clinical facts and theories concerning pain, and put forward the suggestion of a gate which opens and shuts according to the balance of activity between small and large afferent fibres, with large fibre activity tending to close the gate to nociceptive impulses. It was well known that large nerve fibres are easily stimulated by electrical current without stimulating small fibres and once the suggestion had been made it was easy to see the application of electrical stimulation for the relief of pain. Electrical stimulation can be applied by electrodes on the skin (transcutaneous stimulation—TNS), directly to the nerve (peripheral nerve stimulation—PNS), implanted in the central nervous system, usually over the dorsal column of the spinal cord (spinal cord stimulation—SCS), or in other places in the central nervous system. Stimulator devices were first used by Shealy *et al.* (1967), and since that time peripheral nerves, phrenic nerves, spinal cord, cerebellum, midbrain, thalamus and cerebrum have been subjected to stimulation to reduce pain, to improve diaphragmatic function, bladder function, reduce neurological deficit, alter peripheral blood flow, aid the blind and the deaf, and treat intractable epilepsy. Some more careful studies which have been published show clear evidence of both clinical improvement and objective physiological change. Clinical improvement has occurred in chronic untreatable conditions and has produced alteration in function surpassing that achieved by any previous techniques or methods of treatment. In addition, the use of stimulation techniques has opened a new phase in the understanding of how the nervous system reacts to disease or injury and how this may be modified in order to improve function.

SPINAL CORD STIMULATION IN
NEUROLOGICAL DISEASE

Until Cook's report in 1973 (Cook & Weinstein, 1973) spinal cord stimulation was used exclusively in the treatment of chronic pain. Any changes in neurological function with spinal cord stimulation had been interpreted as complications or untoward effects. Unrelated experimental work on the effects of partial lesions on the central nervous system and the subsequent processes of reorganization and regeneration, together with studies of the effects of repetitive stimulation on synaptic boutons, had suggested that patients with chronic neurological deficit may respond to attempts to influence the intact nervous system by 'active re-education' (Illis, 1973). Cook and Weinstein reported that repetitive stimulation of the spinal cord in patients with multiple sclerosis produced marked improvement in neurological function. The original patient had multiple sclerosis and was stimulated to relieve pain and her neurological state improved. Instead of disregarding these changes as untoward effects, Cook and Weinstein carefully treated other patients with multiple sclerosis and demonstrated remarkable improvements related to the procedure of spinal cord stimulation. In 1976 the first cases of spinal cord stimulation in multiple sclerosis outside the USA were reported and the first objective neurophysiological data which ruled out any possibility of the so-called placebo effect were demonstrated (Illis *et al.*, 1976). The effect of spinal cord stimulation in improving neurological function in patients with multiple sclerosis was further reported from Cook's group (Abbate *et al.*, 1977) who showed that in 40 patients with multiple sclerosis and urinary symptoms, there was a 77% subjective improvement in sphincter control and a 42% objective improvement as shown by cystometry and sphincter electromyography. Improvement in peripheral blood flow has been reported (Cook *et al.*, 1976; Dooley & Kasprak, 1976). Improvement in neurological function has been observed in spinal injury and Friedreich's ataxia (Dooley, 1977; Richardson & McLone, 1978; Campos *et al.*, 1978).

Method of Stimulation

The usual procedure is carried out with normal sterile techniques with the patient prone on an X-ray table. Local anaesthesia is infiltrated around the interspinous ligament in the lower thoracic area. Under X-ray control, an epidural needle is introduced in the interspinous space to reach the epidural space in the midline. The stylet of the needle is removed and it is ascertained that there is no leakage of cerebrospinal fluid. An electrode is then passed through the needle pointing rostrally and advanced under X-ray control to the mid or high thoracic levels and positioned in the midline in the epidural space. The needle is removed and a second electrode is introduced in the same way so that the two electrodes are positioned in the midline about one to three vertebral bodies apart. The stimulator is connected and, if necessary, the electrodes moved until a bilateral tingling sensation is felt. The electrodes are fixed to the skin either with sutures or with Steri-strips, and antero–posterior and lateral X-rays are obtained to document the position of the electrodes. The loop antenna from the stimulator is placed over the receiver and a sterile dressing applied to secure the electrodes and the receiver.

In a trial of spinal cord stimulation carried out in Southampton, patients were not told precisely what type of sensation they would feel and eventually the patients were grouped into those who had had stimulation symmetrically into the legs and those who had had other kinds of sensation. It was quite clear that for clinical improvement to occur, patients must receive symmetrical sensation (Illis *et al.*, 1980).

Stimulation is carried out at about 33 Hz with 200 μs width pulses at a voltage adjusted by the patient to give a pleasant warm tingling sensation. In our centre we carry out ten days of stimulation, and if a good response is obtained clinically and physiologically then the electrodes are implanted subcutaneously to a subcutaneous receiver.

Spinal Cord Stimulation in Multiple Sclerosis

Since the original observations by Cook and Weinstein in 1973, many centres now carry out spinal cord stimulation for multiple sclerosis. Six centres reported their results at the Sixth International Symposium on External Control of Human Extremities in 1978 and all demonstrated improvement in patients with spinal cord stimulation. The selection of patients and the method of assessment vary from centre to centre but, in general, it appears that something like 50% of patients have a worthwhile improvement with spinal cord stimulation. The improvement is most marked, in terms of numbers and the degree of improvement, in those patients with severe bladder disturbance. Improvement in mobility is less consistent and the overall number of patients who show improvement in mobility is smaller. At the Wessex Neurological Centre, 28 patients with multiple sclerosis have had 43 studies of spinal cord stimulation. All the patients had had periods of clinical stability for 6–12 months before spinal cord stimulation and many of the patients had two periods of spinal cord stimulation separated by a period of 3–6 months. The mean follow-up at the time of writing is 18 months and the longest follow-up is 36 months of permanent stimulation; 25% of the patients showed improved mobility and 75% showed improvement in bladder function. There were associated changes in neurophysiological measurements (Illis *et al.*, 1980; Sedgwick *et al.*, 1980). With two exceptions the bladder improvement was maintained, but mobility improvement was maintained in only two patients. The bladder improvement is often quite marked and easily quantifiable. For example, patients who are permanently catheterized may regain normal bladder function within a few days. The degree of improvement in mobility is less easy to measure. A very mild degree of improvement from the observer's point of view may mean a significant change in the patient's way of life and the degree of dependency upon other people. For example, an improvement sufficient to enable the patient to stand unaided may appear to be quite insignificant, but from the patient's viewpoint this means that he may be able to transfer unaided from a bed to a wheelchair and to a toilet. If, in addition, spinal cord stimulation has produced an alteration in bladder function in terms of a diminished urgency, then this improvement would mean that the patient is no longer incontinent of urine and is no longer dependent upon others. It should be emphasized that the type of improvement described occurred in patients who were neurologically stable before spinal cord stimulation and in patients who had had standard methods of treatment, including courses of physiotherapy and ACTH injections, with no response. Similar results were obtained by Read *et al.* (1980) who treated 16 patients with static or progressive multiple sclerosis and demonstrated bladder improvement and reduction in spasticity.

Two groups have reported failure of SCS to produce any benefit in patients with MS (Rosen & Barsoum, 1979; Young & Goodman, 1979). On the other hand, Hawkes *et al.* (1978) reported improvement but did not ascribe it to spinal cord stimulation. The reason for failure of SCS is not apparent, but the most likely cause is in electrode placement. Centres such as New York, Southampton and Houston have emphasized the need not only for careful electrode placement but also for the necessity of continuous monitoring of stimulator sensation and manipulation of electrodes if indicated. It may be necessary to adjust the electrodes daily until a good stimulator sensation and clinical response are achieved.

Hawkes *et al.* (1978) ascribed improvement in their patients to motivation and training. However, in a later paper (Hawkes *et al.*, 1980) they reported 19 cases in more detail with an improvement in bladder function in 75% and supported this with objective bladder function tests showing improved urinary flow and reduced external sphincter pressure as judged from urethral pressure profiles. These changes were attributed to SCS. Concurrent changes such as an increase in walking speed in 50%, relief of chronic central pain, development of erections in three patients who had been impotent for several years and improvement in posture and balance were also noted but not attributed to SCS and were regarded as insignificant.

Read *et al.* (1980) carried out temporary SCS in 16 patients with MS and recorded improvement of bladder function in 10. Reduction of lower limb spasticity was obtained in 8. This careful study included detailed and repeated clinical, electrophysiological and urodynamic assessments.

Cook (1979) has also emphasized the need for careful selection of patients and treatment of intercurrent illnesses. That there is an objective response in SCS in patients with MS seems beyond question in view of the neurophysiological findings, changes in urodynamics and changes seen in peripheral blood flow (Tallis, Illis & Sedgwick, in preparation).

Placebo Effect

It has been suggested that the results produced with spinal cord stimulation in multiple sclerosis could be the result of a placebo response and that to demonstrate otherwise would require a double-blind trial. A double-blind trial, controlled and randomized, is a sound statistical method of testing the safety and efficiency of a new drug. The process involves the administration of the test drug to some patients while giving placebo to the rest. The patients are chosen at random and neither the physician nor the patient knows who receives the test drug or the placebo and it is therefore presumed that the same care would be received by all patients in the study. Unfortunately this type of trial, though easy to perform in drug assessment, is impossible to administer in spinal cord stimulation for the simple reason that the patients being stimulated experience a subjective sensation. One half of the double-blind is therefore invalid. Similarly, the adjustment of voltage, pulse rate and pulse width, and the changing of batteries depend on the patients reporting sensation to the physician, who also, therefore, is aware of which patient is undergoing stimulation. The other half of the double-blind is also invalid.

There are three main reasons for carrying out a randomized double-blind trial in clinical medicine:

1. To determine which of two apparently equal methods of treatment is the better. (This does not apply since there are no methods of treating multiple sclerosis in the chronic stationary phase.)

2. To compare an untested method of treatment with standard care. However, where the patient's previous course is known, and where the disease has been stationary for 6-12 months, there is no reason why the patient should not act as his own control, particularly if periods of treatment (SCS) are compared to periods of non-treatment (i.e. without SCS) with objective physiological measurements. The primary purpose of studying SCS is to determine effectiveness of one treatment rather than comparison of two types of treatment.

3. To determine toxic effects or unknown side-effects. SCS has been used for years in the treatment of pain and the incidence and nature of unwanted effects are well known.

There are strong ethical reasons for not placing electrodes in the epidural space of patients unless they are to receive stimulation. A trial which is sound sense in drug testing is inapplicable in this kind of study.

The double-blind trial is not a suitable method for studying stimulation just as it is not suitable for studying surgical procedures. It is mandatory, however, to design a study with an adequate control group and with reference to the possibility of placebo reactions. The trial of Illis *et al.* (1980) used patients as their own controls and made a number of observations pertinent to the placebo phenomenon.

Improvement did not *precede* SCS as might be expected if hospitalization and

motivation were the causes of improvement. The patients had been neurologically stable for at least nine months prior to SCS so any spontaneous
improvement would be unlikely to coincide with SCS in one patient, let alone in
10 out of 19. It is even less likely that a further episode of improvement would
coincide with the second period of stimulation unless the improvement and the
stimulation were causally related (in the Wessex Neurological Centre trial most
patients had at least two periods of stimulation separated by three to six months
without stimulation). Patients with severely disturbed bladder function, in 75%
of cases, showed marked improvement and this is considerably more than any
reported placebo effect as well as being greater than any reported improvement
with other therapy.

Two patients were 'stimulated' without batteries and three had surface
stimulation. None of these showed any improvement, though they received the
same treatment as the patients undergoing epidural stimulation. When SCS was
begun they all responded. Nine patients in the Wessex Neurological Centre
study had stimulation producing sensation in the chest, shoulder or into one leg
only. There was no clinical change in these patients. Sixteen patients had symmetrical sensation into both legs and 11 showed clinical response. Some of the
patients who had shown no clinical response with unilateral stimulation responded to symmetrical stimulation. This indicates that it is not the *fact* of
stimulation which produced improvement but the *type* of stimulation—namely
that which produced bilateral sensation into the legs. A further example of the
importance of the type of stimulation was shown in one of our patients who
responded well and had a permanent implant but began to deteriorate after four
months. This coincided with an alteration in stimulator sensation. Radiology
showed that one electrode had moved 5 mm from the midline. After this electrode
was replaced he again improved (Fig. 14.1). There were also objective neurophysiological changes associated with SCS which cannot be attributed to a
placebo effect (Sedgwick *et al.*, 1980). The neurophysiological responses, with
the exception of the contingent negative variation, are not under voluntary
control and it is difficult to see how they could be placebo mediated. The
contingent negative variation (CNV) is a cortical evoked response which *can* be
altered by the patient's motivation, but the CNV in our patients were not altered
by SCS (Sedgwick *et al.*, 1980).

In the Wessex Neurological Centre trial the patients' stimulation requirements
were carefully monitored (Jobling *et al.*, 1980). The current requirements of
patients who showed a good clinical response tended to lie in the range 6–12 mA
for a pulse duration of 0.2 ms. Some of the 'unsuccessful' patients had a very
much higher current requirement. Although not all patients choosing a current
in the 6–12 mA range were successful, all of those consistently choosing a higher
current have been unsuccessful. The lower current requirement was frequently
associated with a satisfactory bilateral sensation down the legs, but patients
choosing a higher current usually only experience the tight and unpleasant
sensation in the chest. Presumably the choice of current and response is depen-

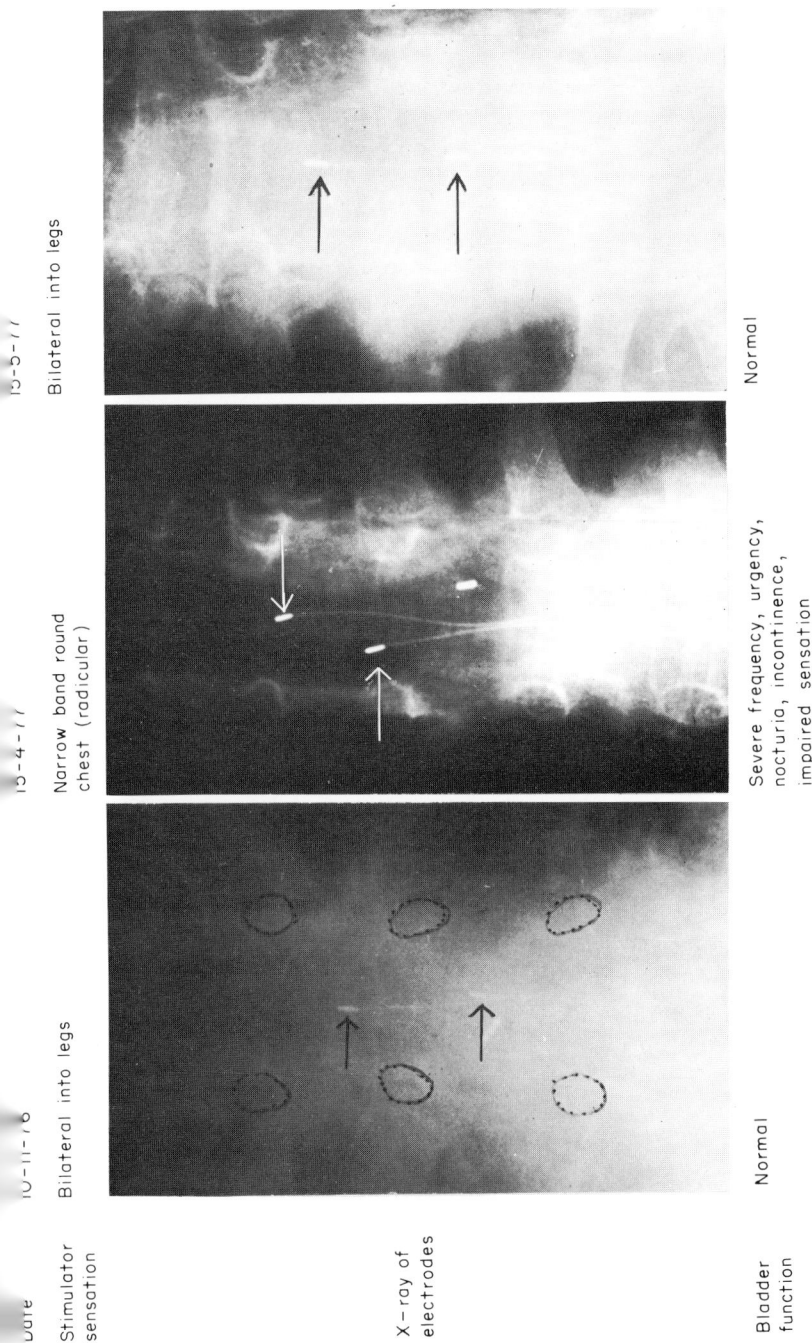

Fig. 14.1 A series of three radiographs showing the position of a pair of epidural electrodes. 10.11.76—Original position with bilateral stimulator sensation in the legs and a good clinical result. 15.4.77—At a time of clinical deterioration with a change in stimulator sensation. The lower electrode has shifted 5 mm to the right of the midline. 15.5.77—Electrode replaced now giving bilateral sensation in the legs and a clinical improvement in bladder function.

dent upon stimulation of the dorsal columns themselves. When the dorsal columns are refractory to stimulation, possibly because of extensive damage or badly sited electrodes, the patient would continue increasing the stimulus amplitude until the spinal roots were stimulated with resultant discomfort in a local distribution. Such patients did not respond well to SCS. The findings can be summarized as follows: a good stimulator sensation and a low current requirement implied a successful stimulation of the dorsal columns and the probability of a good response; a low current requirement accompanied by a bad sensation suggests that the electrodes were badly sited so that dorsal roots were stimulated instead of the dorsal columns; a high current requirement accompanied by a bad sensation is probably associated with damaged dorsal columns and a good response was most unlikely.

Spinal Cord Injury

Conventional treatment is limited to maintenance of skin nutrition and integrity, the prevention and treatment of renal complications arising from loss of bladder sensation and function, and the management of spasticity and spasms with drugs such as Diazepam and Baclofen. These measures, together with psychological counselling, are, in many cases, life-saving, but nevertheless the morbidity and mortality are high. No treatment has hitherto improved the neuro-logical function of the spinal cord. Matinian (1976) has reported functional recovery following spinal cord trauma, using enzyme therapy: elastase, trypsin, hyaluronidase. However, these results have not been confirmed.

Spinal cord stimulation has been used in patients with spinal cord trauma (Dooley, 1977; Richardson & McLone, 1978; Campos *et al.*, 1978; Waltz & Pani, 1978; Meglio *et al.*, 1980). Many of the reports are incomplete and the total number of patients is still small, but there appears to be a definite neuro-logical and functional improvement in patients with partial lesions of the spinal cord. The improvement is seen in spasticity, pain, mobility, sphincter function and autonomic hyper-reflexia. The improvement in bladder function is parti-cularly important since urinary tract and renal complications represent the greatest threat to life. Many patients appreciate the increased sense of alertness and freedom from drowsiness which follows reduction or cessation of anti-spastic medication.

Spasmodic Torticollis

Medical and surgical treatment of this condition is unsatisfactory. Medical treatment includes the use of Levodopa, Bromocriptine (Dopamine recep-tor agonist), Haloperidol (Dopamine receptor blocker) and Tetrabenazine (Dopamine depleting agent). Psychotherapy and biofeedback methods have been used. Surgical treatment includes antero-cervical rhizotomy with section of the spinal accessory nerve and bilateral stereotactic thalamotomy. For the majority of sufferers, the condition is intractable.

Gildenberg (1978) reported the use of spinal cord stimulation in 20 patients with torticollis and 2 patients with dystonia musculorum deformans. Twelve of these patients were rejected after a trial of transcutaneous stimulation and percutaneous dorsal column stimulation (either because of poor response or patient refusal). Of the remainder, there was one 'excellent' and one 'good' result. The stimulating electrode was placed inconsistently in front or behind the spinal cord at C5/6 level. Waltz (Waltz & Pani, 1978) carried out spinal cord stimulation in 17 patients with spasmodic torticollis with an age range of 30–61 years and with a duration of symptoms from 8 months to 11 years (mean ±4.2 years). The follow-up was from 6 months to 3 years. Twenty-nine per cent showed no effect during a period of trial stimulation of 7–10 days. These cases were stimulated at multiple levels and with varying stimulation parameters. Of the remaining 12 cases, satisfactory response was achieved with initial stimulation: 5 showed marked improvement, 4 showed moderate improvement and 1 case showed mild improvement. The best results were obtained in those patients who were stimulated in the C2/3 area. The best improvement was obtained in young female patients. In addition, Waltz carried out spinal cord stimulation in 25 patients with dystonia musculorum deformans. The overall result in these dystonic cases was disappointing, except in those cases where the primary problem or the major manifestation of dystonia was torticollis.

Standard medical and surgical techniques are unsatisfactory. If there is no response to medical treatment, spinal cord stimulation should be considered as a percutaneous procedure. The morbidity is considerably less than the therapeutically unsatisfactory surgical techniques.

Cerebral Palsy

Standard treatment of patients with cerebral palsy consists entirely of supportive or symptomatic treatment. Such treatment, at best, may improve spasticity, behavioural problems or the patient's morale and often results in considerable improvement in well-being. In no sense, however, is there improvement in neuronal functioning or neurological deficit.

Waltz and Pani (1978) have used SCS in 38 patients with cerebral palsy with an age range of 7–42 years. These cases included spastic diplegia and spastic quadriparesis with and without athetosis. The patients with spastic quadriparesis with marked athetosis showed no response. Of the other patients some degree of improvement was reported in 75% and 30% showed marked improvement. Improvement was seen in spasticity, improved articulation with smoother speech delivery, balance, hand function, spasms, walking, swallowing with decrease in drooling and improved bladder control. The authors noted that the best results were seen with SCS at C2, 3, 4 in patients aged 11–20 years with spastic diplegia and, to a less extent, with spastic quadriparesis without athetosis.

Further studies, particularly regarding the long-term effect of SCS, are needed, but these results indicate an encouraging approach to an otherwise intractable condition. No serious complications were reported. Another technique which seems promising in cerebral palsy patients is cerebellar stimulation (pages 399–401), but this again is a technique which at the present time remains under investigation and is recommended only as a research procedure to be undertaken at centres with appropriate staff and techniques.

Spinal Cord Stimulation in Homeostasis

The use of spinal cord stimulation in patients with disordered homeostatic mechanisms as a result of disease, in particular autonomic dysreflexia, hypertension and disorders of peripheral blood flow, is a matter of anecdote rather than carefully designed study. The reported features are, however, of great interest since they concern conditions where standard treatment is either unsatisfactory or mutilating (amputation of limbs).

Bayliss, in 1901, described hindlimb vasodilator nerves in the cat. In 1933 Foerster demonstrated that stimulation of dorsal roots in humans could produce vasodilatation of the skin in the appropriate dermatome. Foerster suggested that this was due to stimulation of efferent fibres from the spinal cord and was not due to anti-dromic stimulation of afferent fibres.

In our experience, at the Wessex Neurological Centre, patients receiving spinal cord stimulation frequently describe a sensation of warmth in the feet. The limbs feel warmer to the touch and the sensation of warmth is not associated with pain or relief of pain, and it is postulated, therefore, that the sensation is not due to spinothalamic stimulation. In addition, those patients with discoloration of the feet, due to stagnant anoxia associated with poor peripheral circulation, show improvement in the colour. One of our patients with arteriographically demonstrated peripheral vascular insufficiency and severe claudication was receiving spinal cord stimulation for multiple sclerosis. Claudication ceased to be a problem although his mobility increased as a consequence of spinal cord stimulation. He also noted regrowth of distal hair and accelerated toe-nail growth. Another patient, with severe peripheral vascular disease and an indolent ulcer, constant rest pain and night pain, and a claudication distance of 50 yards, showed marked improvement with spinal cord stimulation: complete relief of pain, healing of the previous indolent ulcer, and an increased claudication distance of 350 yards. In 1974 Friedman *et al.* reported an increase in skin temperature in the region of analgesia during spinal cord stimulation for pain. Cook *et al.* (1976) described eight patients with arterial disease 'unresponsive to sympathectomy or by-pass' who developed increased temperature and blood flow with spinal cord stimulation. In addition, these patients showed healing of ulcers which broke down again when stimulation was stopped.

Dooley and Kasprak in 1976 reported increased peripheral blood flow as measured by pulse plethysmography with epidural stimulation. Ebershold *et al.* (1977) found no change in skin temperature on transcutaneous nerve stimulation and no alteration in skin impedance. However, Owens *et al.* (1979), using infra-red thermography in healthy volunteers, demonstrated an increase in skin temperature with TNS which they interpreted as indicating indirect evidence of decreased sympathetic tone.

One of the severe complications of high spinal cord injury is the autonomic abnormality known as autonomic hyper-reflexia or dysreflexia. This produces an acute hypertension with severe throbbing headache. There is sweating above the level of the lesion with peripheral vasoconstriction below, dilatation of the pupils, bradycardia and syncope. Factors which may precipitate the rise in blood pressure and associated features include bladder distension (outlet obstruction or catheter obstruction); pelvic and rectal manipulation; painful stimuli in the perineal area; and distension of any hollow viscus. This syndrome occurs most frequently in patients with a lesion above T6 and the mechanism is probably due to an exaggerated reflex sympathetic activity in the isolated spinal cord. Standard treatment includes the use of ganglion blocking agents, carotid artery compression, as well as treatment of the precipitating cause. Prophylactic therapy is frequently disappointing. Richardson *et al.* (1979) reported the use of percutaneous epidural stimulation in five patients with autonomic dysreflexia secondary to spinal cord injury. In four of the patients no further episodes of autonomic dysreflexia occurred during the period of spinal cord stimulation. In the fifth patient the changes of dysreflexia occurred when the voltage was rapidly reduced.

STIMULATION AND BLADDER FUNCTION

In 1864, Budge used direct spinal cord stimulation with resulting bladder contraction to map out efferent bladder pathways. The first use of clinical stimulation of the bladder was in 1940 by Dees but was of no practical application (see Dees, 1965). Since that time several techniques have been used but with limited success. These techniques have involved direct stimulation of the bladder wall and of sacral nerve roots; they often resulted in voiding, but the clinical improvement was inconsistent. This was possibly related to the technique or to anatomical structural differences in the two sexes, or spread of current into adjacent pelvic and sphincter musculature with inappropriate contractions, pain and interference with sphincter relaxation. The most promising techniques of electrical stimulation involve stimulation of the spinal cord. Thoracic spinal cord stimulation and the resulting improvement in bladder function is described on pages 389–90. Sacral spinal cord stimulation with implantation of the spinal neuroprosthesis offers the possibility of good control of bladder function in patients with traumatic paraplegia.

Sacral Cord Stimulation

Friedman *et al.* (1972) implanted a spinal neuroprosthesis over the sacral cord at various levels but usually at S2. The electrode tips were located within the intermedio-lateral column of the central grey matter of the sacral cord—the so-called 'sacral micturition centre'. Experiments were carried out on normal and paraplegic animals and they obtained good results in terms of an increased bladder pressure and an increased volume expelled. After most stimulation episodes there was no residual urine in the bladder and the authors emphasize the importance of a sterile bladder. During the periods of bladder infection the volume voided decreased, but with treatment the volume of urine voided increased. In 1972, Nashold *et al.* reported the use of this type of stimulation in four paraplegic patients and further cases were reported in 1975 (Grimes *et al.*, 1975). The authors emphasize careful screening and selection of patients. Those patients with marked reflux or with trabeculated and rigid bladders are excluded as are those in whom intermittent catheterization or external sphincterotomy would be sufficient to keep them free from infection. It is essential that the conus and cauda equina are undamaged and that the patients have been clinically stationary for a period of at least 12 months since the traumatic paraplegia occurred. Patients with neuropathic bladders, as in multiple sclerosis, are probably not candidates for this kind of procedure. The authors use a psychological screening test to rule out any serious psychiatric disturbances. The patients have a careful neurological examination as well as the normal physical examination and urinary function and urine culture are performed. The lower urinary tract is evaluated with cystometrography and endoscopy. Myelography was carried out to evaluate the exact level of the spinal cord lesion. Percutaneous flexible electrodes, placed through a spinal needle, were used to evaluate the bladder response to sacral cord stimulation. Following this, the patients were subjected to a laminectomy and bipolar electrodes were used to determine the cord level producing the highest bladder pressure. The depth electrodes were then positioned at this level and held in place with a Dacron mesh strip and metallic clips. Electrode leads were tunnelled subcutaneously to an implanted receiver in the same way as for spinal cord stimulation in multiple sclerosis. Optimal bladder emptying occurred with stimuli of 200 μs at about 15–20 Hz using 10–15 volts for 20–30 seconds.

Most of the patients who have had this procedure carried out void with the stimulation and maintain a low residual urine and reduced incidence of infection. If the urine does become infected the residual urine (usually less than 10 ml with stimulation) rises promptly until the infection is treated. There appear to be two types of response: either sphincter relaxation with detrusor contraction and voiding; or the sphincter and bladder neck contract with the onset of stimulation, but as soon as the stimulus is stopped the vesical neck and urethra open and the patient voids. Associated or autonomic responses of piloerection occur and increased skin temperature. Occasionally penile erection is a problem. Adductor spasm and diffuse pelvic pain may also occur.

Ventral Root Stimulation

A technique for stimulating sacral ventral roots (S3, 4) to effect bladder emptying has been developed by Brindley (1977) and used chronically in baboons. Stimulation caused contraction of the detrusor and the external sphincter and pelvic striated muscles, but emptying occurred during two second gaps in the stimulus train when the striated muscle relaxed abruptly but the slowly responding smooth detrusor muscle maintained tension, thus forcing urine through the urethra. The author did not mention the possibility of ureteric reflux which could lead to hydronephrosis and could preclude the use of ventral root stimulation in humans. Successful use has been reported but the stimulus is painful in those with partial cord lesions.

Torrens and Fenely (Chapter 8) refer to stimulation of perineal structures to inhibit bladder spasms which lead to incontinence.

Patients with impaired bladder control should probably receive a trial of percutaneous spinal cord stimulation. Those patients with complete spinal cord injury, or in whom there is no response to thoracic spinal cord stimulation, would probably benefit from a trial of sacral stimulation. The use of an electronic spinal neuroprosthesis in man remains experimental at the present time, and requires further evaluation before it can be recommended for general use. However, the initial observations are encouraging.

CEREBELLAR STIMULATION

Since the demonstration by Sherrington and by Horsley that cerebellar stimulation in decerebrate animals reduces extensor tone, the evidence over the past 70 years or so has suggested that the cerebellum has a regulatory effect on muscle activity.

Cerebellar stimulation in man was first introduced by Irving Cooper in 1972 as a method of treating spasticity (see Cooper, 1978). The stimulation procedure involves silicone mesh plates bearing platinum electrodes which are placed over the anterior and posterior lobes of the cerebellum on both sides. The electrodes are stimulated by a subcutaneously implanted receiver which is activated by a radio-frequency signal from a power pack carried by the patient. The optimum number of electrodes, the optimum position, the exact electrode configuration and the best type of pulse to use are still unresolved problems. Anterior lobe cerebellar stimulation produces ipsilateral inhibition of spinal cord reflexes whereas stimulation of the posterior lobe inhibits the contralateral cerebral cortex. Chronic cerebellar stimulation has been used mainly in the treatment or modification of epilepsy and cerebral palsy. In addition, there have been changes reported in so-called behavioural aspects.

Epilepsy

The largest number of cases have been studied by Cooper and his colleagues; 18 out of 32 patients with intractable epilepsy have shown a good clinical response, i.e. with at least a 50% reduction of seizures, and in some the improvement was even more marked; for example seizure reduction from 25 per day to 4 per day. Other benefits included a return to employment, reduction or cessation of drugs, a sensation of increased alertness, increased concentration and reduction in aggression. Nine patients were therapeutic failures, but none were made worse as a result of the procedure. One patient died from post-operative extradural haematoma (cerebellar stimulation not actually carried out), and 4 patients died subsequently during sleep: 6 weeks, 17 months, 26 months and 28 months after cerebellar stimulation. These deaths were not attributable to stimulation.

   Nine of the patients were studied physiologically with visual evoked responses, H-reflex and other spinal reflexes and cortical somatosensory evoked responses. Cerebellar stimulation produced inhibition of all responses except the visual evoked response.

Cerebral Palsy

Cooper's group have used cerebellar stimulation in cerebral palsy for the past five years or so and have studied over 140 patients. Most of these had a history of birth trauma and more than a third had epilepsy. Overall improvement was seen in about 46% (moderate to marked), and 39% showed mild improvement. However, 73% showed benefit in spasticity overall, and 61% showed benefit in athetosis. In 9 patients studied neurophysiologically, there was evidence of inhibition of spinal reflexes and somatosensory evoked potentials, and there was a reduction of the variability of responses and of clinical deficit producing a 'smoothing' effect.

Conclusion

In view of the clinical results produced by Cooper and his colleagues, it would seem that the time is long overdue for a careful trial of cerebellar stimulation in other centres. Ablative surgery for epilepsy should be delayed until cerebellar stimulation has been tried, following observation with continuous EEG monitoring and repeated determination of anticonvulsant blood levels. In cerebral palsy it would appear that cerebellar stimulation, or spinal cord stimulation, is the only therapy that offers real promise, but the techniques still require further evaluation.

FUNCTIONAL NEUROMUSCULAR STIMULATION

Since the early 1960s there has been a considerable amount of work directed towards the activation of paralysed muscles by electrical stimulation. Initially all neural prostheses were devices or techniques which were used to supplement or replace lost or impaired function in people with neurological deficit. More recently, it has been realized that many methods of electrical stimulation do not simply supplement or replace lost function but, in some way, favourably modify the remaining structurally intact nervous system. When functional electrical stimulation is restricted to stimulation of nerves and muscles it is referred to as functional neuromuscular stimulation (FNS) or functional electrical stimulation (FES), or, when the stimulator is over the peroneal nerve, functional peroneal stimulation.

Peroneal Nerve Stimulation

Where a lower motoneuron lesion has occurred and the neurons innervating the muscles are irreversibly damaged, atrophy cannot be reversed by functional stimulation. However, if the muscle paralysis is due to an upper motoneuron lesion, electrical stimulation may reverse the muscle atrophy and produce functional muscle contractions. The stimulation in this case can be applied directly to a peripheral nerve, as for example in phrenic nerve stimulation for control of respiration, or by means of electrodes placed on or in the muscle. One of the first applications of FNS was for the correction of foot drop in patients suffering from stroke. Stimulating electrodes were placed over the peroneal nerve with resultant contraction of the tibialis muscle during the swing phase of gait (Liberson *et al.*, 1961). Since that time the technique has been developed and it has been estimated that more than 2000 patients with stroke, head injury, multiple sclerosis and cerebral palsy have been treated (Gracanin, 1978). Implantable systems, with the electrodes placed directly on the peroneal nerve, have been used as well as surface stimulation with the electrodes held in place over the skin by some type of knee bandage. Similar techniques have been used to stimulate the femoral nerve in patients with quadriceps muscle weakness, and multi-channel systems in patients with paraplegia. Devices aimed at restoring functional use of the hand in patients with high-level spinal cord injuries have been rather less successful and many single and multi-channel stimulators have been used with varying effects (Hambrecht & Reswick, 1977).

If repetitive stimulation is applied too slowly, the muscle responds in a series of coarse twitches. As the stimulation frequency is raised the response becomes smooth. However, stimulation can also excite sensory nerves as well as motor nerves and this may produce reflex activation of muscles and, in certain circumstances, pain may be felt. The techniques of electrical stimulation cannot, as yet, select and control individual motor units, so that when FNS is carried out the first muscle fibre groups activated are those with fast-contracting, high-output and rapidly fatiguing fibres, and those with slow low output and relatively resistant to fatigue are only excited with higher stimulus strengths. This may result in a marked variability in response, particularly during periods of sustained muscular contraction. This, however, does not detract from the use of FNS and could, if necessary, be partly overcome by proportional feedback control of the stimulator (Chandler & Sedgwick, 1973). Proportional feedback also goes some way to overcome movement of the stimulating electrodes with respect to the nerve.

Functional neuromuscular stimulation when applied to the leg for foot drop (one of the commonest uses) requires control by the patient. Control signals which have been used include position, pressure, electromyographic and electroencephalic signals, as well as single unit activity of individual brain cells. The most useful controls have been a pressure switch for use in peroneal stimulation and a position transducer for control of the hand. One of the major complaints of patients who have used these systems is the lack of information about the position of the limb and the force exerted. Ideally sensory feedback signals with a stable closed loop need to be provided.

Stimulation for the Treatment of Scoliosis

The usual treatment for progressive mild or moderate scoliosis is the application of an external device such as the Milwaukee brace. Many patients are reluctant to wear this kind of device because of psychological, cosmetic and restrictive problems, and as a result the curvature may increase to a point where surgical correction is the only feasible solution. An alternative to using such a brace is the use of electrical stimulation to paraspinal muscles. Stimulation, using surface electrodes or by cork-screw electrodes inserted into the paraspinal musculature, has now been used. More recently stimulating electrodes have been used not in the paraspinal musculature but to the more lateral trunk muscles. Stimulation is applied at night-time only, using a portable stimulator with surface electrodes. The results are encouraging and at the present time a multi-centre clinical investigation is being carried out (see Axelgaard *et al.*, 1978).

Phrenic Nerve Stimulation

Apnoeic quadriparesis and Ondine's curse* are the two indications for phrenic nerve stimulation. Glenn *et al.* (1976) reviewed respiratory pacing by phrenic nerve stimulation in 37 quadriplegics, and he and others with experience point out that to switch from positive pressure ventilation to phrenic nerve stimulation takes many weeks and requires a skilled and dedicated multi-disciplinary team of workers. The benefit to an otherwise totally paralysed patient may seem marginal at first sight, but this is not so; even small reductions in the dependency of these more seriously disabled patients can make a great difference to their lives and morale. This is one stimulation procedure which is life-preserving and even the most successfully stimulated patient must never be without an alarm and back-up system in case of failure.

In the case of spinal trauma at C4 or higher, phrenic stimulation should not be considered until at least three months after injury, and then only if other rehabilitation problems, such as the bladder, are under control and there has been no improvement in respiratory function despite appropriate physiotherapy. Respiratory function can recover significantly during the first three to four months after trauma. The patients should be trained in positive pressure respiration or whatever system is to be used as a back-up. Before implanting the phrenic nerve stimulator investigations should establish the functional integrity of both phrenic nerves by percutaneous or needle electrode stimulation with fluoroscopic observation of the diaphragm and measurement of the vital capacity.

Each side is usually implanted separately with a two-week interval. Current thresholds and current for maximum effect should be measured at the time of implantation. Muscle relaxants should not be used at surgery. After recovery a long period of rehabilitation of the diaphragm is begun with a programme of gradually increasing periods of stimulation and checks on blood gases. In Glenn's series, 13 of 37 patients were satisfactorily paced for 100% of the time and a further 10 for 50% of the time. Phrenic nerve damage, when it occurred, was probably sustained at the time of surgery and did not happen as a result of chronic stimulation. Glen *et al.* (1976) make the remarkable claim that, after successful pacing has been achieved, the incidence of chest infection is no more than in the general population. This and the normalization of haemodynamics by restoring a negative intrathoracic pressure must be in itself sufficient justification for the procedure.

---

* A Germanic mythological water-nymph, Ondine, deprived her deserting husband of all automatic function so that he had to remember to breathe. When he finally fell asleep he died. The term Ondine's curse has been applied to any patient whose respiratory centre has lost its responsiveness to CO_2.

ONDINE'S CURSE

Loss of responsiveness of the respiratory control system to hypercapnia can arise from different pathological processes and sometimes a permanent state of unresponsiveness develops. Ventilation is usually adequate when the subject is awake and alert, but during rest and sleep ventilation falls and CO_2 accumulates in the blood. Glenn *et al.* (1973) showed phrenic nerve stimulation during sleep prevented deterioration of, or improved the blood gas levels. Oxygen could be administered safely as the danger of reduced hypoxic drive to ventilation was obviated. The authors state that phrenic nerve stimulation is contra-indicated in respiratory failure due to pulmonary or muscle disease.

CONCLUSION

Functional neuromuscular stimulation is a useful mode of treatment in the management of some central nervous system disorders. The technique may be used to strengthen paralysed muscles, to produce active movement at joints which are operated by paralysed muscles in order to prevent spastic deformities, to serve as a permanent means of producing functional use in place of static devices, and to facilitate recovery. The use of these devices, for example the functional peroneal brace in patients with foot drop following stroke, is best carried out in a department where the devices are in constant use. It is necessary to select patients who are motivated to use the device and where proper follow-up facilities are available.

Although most patients within hospital have little trouble in using functional neuromuscular stimulation equipment, there are many problems when they return home. Most of these problems are not physiological, but the patients tend to take poor care of the equipment with resultant breakage and there is often inadequate motivation by the patients to use the external apparatus when they are at home. The patient requires a fair amount of tolerance to external gadgets, and unless the equipment is reliable and easily serviceable and economic to buy, it is unlikely that the patient will continue to use the equipment. As with all rehabilitation techniques, the requirements of the patient must be the primary concern and it is necessary to ask the question, for each individual patient, as to whether functional neuromuscular stimulation can do more for the patient than any other currently available technique or device.

SAFETY OF ELECTRICAL STIMULATION OF NERVOUS TISSSUE

The aim of electrical stimulation is to excite reliably the appropriate neural tissue without causing damage or other adverse effect.

Materials used for the electrode are usually platinum with small amounts of iridium or rhodium. Tests in artificial serum or CSF show these materials can carry appropriate electrical currents for many years without corrosion, but corrosion over durations longer than a decade or so remains uninvestigated. A new type of electrode made from tantalum pentoxide is being studied and may prove superior to platinum as it does not pass electrons across the electrode-tissue interface and oxidation–reduction reactions are said not to occur (Donaldson, 1974; Guyton & Hambrecht, 1974).

Electrochemical reaction at the metal–tissue interface is a constant problem (*IEEE Transactions*, 1976). All stimulators should be capacitance coupled and some workers use only alternating phase stimulators. This means making one electrode the anode for one pulse and the cathode for the next so that the algebraic sum of current flow is zero. These techniques reduce but do not eliminate the risks of electrochemical reaction. Further safety is offered by constant current stimulators and a short duration pulse which is not permitted to reach a constant voltage (Bergveld, 1976). In some situations the electrochemical reaction products, if produced, could be satisfactorily removed by dilution, but with depth electrodes and electrodes pressed on to the surface of the brain there is minimal 'mixing' and toxic concentrations could quickly build up.

Biological changes due to the passage of current through the tissues are well known to occur. In the extreme there is heat generated by passing a current through a resistance (nervous tissue), but this would take much greater currents than are employed for neurostimulation.

The stimulus strength or current passed is reported in different ways in the literature. The experimental studies of Pudenz (1977) indicate that the critical stimulation parameters are charge and charge density per pulse, which is more correctly called the electric flux density per pulse. Charge is expressed in coulombs (C) and electric flux density as coulombs per square metre (Cm^{-2}). For stimulation purposes a flux density expressed in μCmm^{-2} appears a more sensible scale, but the numerical value is the same. Workers in the field of cerebellar stimulation now consider $0.4\,Cm^{-2}$ a safe electric flux density per phase when using alternating phase stimulators. If the electrodes are of unequal size then tissue damage will occur first beneath the smaller. The rate of pulses (within the physiological range of rates up to 200/s) does not seem to relate to damage, but safety is increased by a factor up to 10 by using pulses of alternating polarities. Pulse width does not relate directly to damage, but neurologically effective stimuli need to be 0.1–0.4 ms in duration. Longer or shorter pulses are less effective and long pulses obviously increase the charge passed (Girvin, 1978; Jobling *et al.*, 1980).

The first evidence of damage is said to be breakdown of the blood–brain barrier which can be reversible. Charges of $>0.45\,\mu C$/phase were needed to produce damage to the cerebral cortex of cats (Mortimer *et al.*, 1970; Pudenz *et al.*, 1975).

Morphological changes in stimulated cortex are the accumulation of glycogen and astrocytosis. Dendrites appear to be most sensitive, but oligodendrocytes are resistant to high currents (Brown *et al.*, 1977; Girvin, 1978).

Early and alarming reports of damage caused by cerebellar stimulation in monkeys (Gilman *et al.*, 1975) have not been substantiated by later work. There are few autopsy observations of patients undergoing cerebellar stimulation; in one case a very local change involving loss of Purkinje cells beneath the electrodes was seen, but this was attributed to pressure rather than electrical current. Another case showed no lesion while others have shown slight and localized changes which appear to relate more to physical effects of the implant rather than to the passage of current. Many of the patients receiving cerebellar stimulation for epilepsy have pre-existing pathological change in the cerebellum (Cooper, 1978).

It is clear that stimulation can be accomplished without causing significant neuronal damage, but one must be vigilant and take every opportunity to study the stimulus parameters used and to check on changes seen at autopsy should material become available.

Pulse parameters used for stimulation should be quoted in full, including duration, current, frequency, whether monophasic or alternating, etc. Electrode geometry must be considered, as possibly only a fraction of the current actually passes through nervous tissue. The current passed is frequently known only approximately as the radio-frequency coupling to implanted devices is dependent upon the distance between the antenna and receiver and their spatial relationship. Some form of calibration is necessary and can be done directly if the electrodes are led out through the skin, implantation being delayed until after the clinical effectiveness of stimulation has been confirmed. Spinal cord stimulation produces a sensation which becomes unpleasant at high stimulus strengths, but cerebellar stimulation gives no sensation until current spread excites nerves of the dura or neighbouring brain-stem structures such as the trigeminal nerve. In these situations it is easy for excessively high or low currents to be used inadvertently. Devices could be modified to limit their outputs, but none of those presently available have a current-limiting circuit which could be pre-set by the physician. Low currents due to poor coupling between transmitter and receiver also occur. Both these problems could be partially solved by feedback control from the receiver to the transmitter so that constant strength stimuli would be delivered to the electrode tips. Some warning device could be incorporated to warn if too high or too low a stimulus was being induced.

HARDWARE COMPLICATIONS

The most troublesome complication is electrode slippage. Periodic radiological checks should be carried out, though slippage is more frequent in the initial two weeks. At later times the electrodes can break or lose their insulation and re-implantation is required. Diagnosis of a broken lead is aided by mapping the distribution of amplitude of the stimulus potential at the skin surface soon after implantation. Any change on re-mapping, particularly a high amplitude poten-tial appearing along the course of the lead, indicates a breakage.

We have not seen a failure of an implanted receiver, but the transmitter and antennae fail due to wear and tear. There is a built-in test to check the function of stimulators and their antennae, but further checks can be accomplished simply by replacing the battery and listening for the pulse on a radio placed next to the device.

Nothing is known of possible harmful effects during pregnancy. The placing of electrodes involves radiology and therefore stimulation cannot be recom-mended during pregnancy. Stimulation procedures of any sort cannot be used in patients with cardiac pacemakers. The 'on demand' pacemakers can interpret the stimulation field as of cardiac origin and will not deliver a pulse. Pulsed radio-frequency fields are a potential source of unintentional stimulation. Such fields can occur in the vicinity of radar transmitters, badly serviced electric motors and poorly screened microwave ovens.

SURGICAL COMPLICATIONS

Patients are exposed to the usual surgical risks, but those specific to stimulation are nervous tissue damage at the time of implantation, CSF leak when the dura has been opened, and infection. Infection has been rare but, especially when leads are left passing through the skin, constant vigilance is essential. Our practice has been to remove the implant if a superficial infection proves resistant to one course of antibiotics. CSF leaks are common but frequently self-limiting.

It is said that surgical procedures can trigger a relapse in multiple sclerosis. The evidence seems to be anecdotal and we have not observed such an occur-rence. Allergy to implanted silastic has been reported but is very rare.

REFERENCES

ABBATE A.D., COOK A.W. & ATTALAH N. (1977) The effect of electrical stimulation of the thoracic spinal cord on function of the bladder in multiple sclerosis. *Journal of Urology*, **117**, 285–8.

ANDERSEN P. (1978) Long-lasting facilitation of synaptic transmission in functions of the septo-hippocampal system. Ciba Foundation Symposium No. 58. Elsevier, Amsterdam.

AXELGAARD J., McNEAL D.R. & BROWN J.C. (1978) Lateral electrical surface stimulation for the treatment of progressive scoliosis. *Sixth International Symposium on External Control of Human Extremities, Dubrovnik*, pp. 63–70. Yugoslav Committee for Electronics and Automation, Bel-grade.

BAYLISS W. (1901) On the origin from the spinal cord of the vasodilator fibres of the hind limbs and the origin of these fibres. *Journal of Physiology*, **26**, 173–209.

BAZANOVA I.S., EVDOKIMOV S.A., MAIOROV V.N., MERKULOVA O.S. & CHERNIGOVSKII V.N. (1965) Morphological and electrical changes in interneuronal synapses during passage of rhythmic impulses. *Fiziolgicheskii Zhurnal SSSR*, **51**, 457. In *Federation Proceedings*, 1966, **25**, T187–90.

BERGVELD P. (1976) Simple test for electrophysiologically tolerable parameters of artificial stimulation. *Medical and Biological Engineering*, **14**, 479–82.

BLISS J.V.P. & GARDNER-MEDWIN A.R. (1973) Long-lasting potentiation of synaptic transmission in the dentate area of the unanaesthetized rabbit following stimulation of the perforant path. *Journal of Physiology*, **232**, 357–74.

BRINDLEY G.S. (1977) An implant to empty the bladder or close the urethra. *Journal of Neurology, Neurosurgery and Psychiatry*, **40**, 358–69.

BROWN W.J., BABB T.L., SLOPER H.V., LIEB J.P., OTTINO C.A. & CRANDALL P.H. (1977) Tissue reaction to long-term electrical stimulation of the cerebellum in monkeys. *Journal of Neurosurgery*, **47**, 336–76.

BUDGE J. (1864) Über den Einfluss des Nervensystems auf die Bewegung der Blase. *Zeitschrift rationelle Medizin*, **21**, 1.

CAMPOS R.J., DIMITRIJEVIC M.M. & SHARKEY P.C. (1978) Clinical evaluation of the effects of spinal stimulation on motor performance in patients with upper motor neurone lesions. *Sixth International Symposium on External Control of Human Extremities, Dubrovnik*, pp. 569–74. Yugoslav Committee for Electronics and Automation, Belgrade.

CHANDLER S.A.G. & SEDGWICK E.M. (1973) A proportional stimulator for the treatment of the disabled. In *Advances in External Control of Human Extremities*. Proceedings of the 4th International Symposium, Belgrade (Eds. Gravrilovic M.M. & Wilson A.B.), pp. 547–53.

COOK A.W. (1979) Comment on Young and Goodman (1979). *Neurosurgery*, **5**, 225–8.

COOK A.W., OYGAR A., BAGGENSTOS P., PACHECO S. & KLERIGA E. (1976) Vascular diseases of the extremities. Electrical stimulation of spinal cord and posterior roots. *New York State Journal of Medicine*, **76**, 366–8.

COOK A.W. & WEINSTEIN S. (1973) Chronic dorsal column stimulation in multiple sclerosis. *New York State Journal of Medicine*, **73**, 2868–72.

COOPER I.S. (1978) *Cerebellar Stimulation in Man*. Raven Press, New York.

CRAGG B.G. (1967) Changes in visual cortex on first exposure of rats to light. *Nature, London*, **215**, 251–3.

DEES J. (1965) Contraction of the urinary bladder produced by electric stimulation. *Investigations in Urology*, **2**, 539–47.

DE ROBERTIS E. & FERREIRA A.V. (1957) Submicroscopic changes of the nerve endings in the adrenal medulla after stimulation of the splanchnic nerve. *Journal of Biophysiology, Biochemistry and Cytology*, **3**, 611–14.

DIAMOND M.C., KRECH D. & ROSENZWEIG M.R. (1964) The effects of an enriched environment on the histology of the rat cerebral cortex. *Journal of Comparative Neurology*, **123**, 111–20.

DONALDSON P.E.K. (1974) The stability of tantalum-pentoxide films *in vivo*. *Medical and Biological Engineering*, **12**, 131–5.

DOOLEY D.M. (1977) Demyelinating, degenerative and vascular disease. *Neurosurgery*, **1**, 220–4.

DOOLEY D.M. & KASPRAK M. (1976) Modification of blood flow to the extremities by electrical stimulation of the nervous system. *Southern Medical Journal*, **69**, 1309–11.

EBERSHOLD M.J., LAWS E.R.J. & ALBERS J.W. (1977) Measurements of autonomic function before, during and after transcutaneous stimulation in subjects with chronic pain and in control subjects. *Mayo Clinic Proceedings*, **52**, 228–32.

ECCLES J.C. (1964) *The Physiology of Synapses*. Springer-Verlag, Berlin.

ECCLES J.C. (1965) Pharmacology of central inhibitory synapses. *British Medical Bulletin*, **21**, 19–25.

ECCLES J.C. & MCINTYRE A.K. (1953) The effects of disuse and of activity on mammalian spinal reflexes. *Journal of Physiology, London*, **121**, 492–516.

ECCLES R.M., KOZAK W. & WESTERMAN R.A. (1962) Enhancement of spinal monosynaptic reflex responses after denervation of synergic hind-limb muscles. *Experimental Neurology*, **6**, 451–64.

FÉHER O., JOO F. & HALÁSZ N. (1972) Effect of stimulation on the number of synaptic vesicles in nerve fibres and terminals of the cerebral cortex in the cat. *Brain Research*, **47**, 37–48.

FOERSTER O. (1933) The dermatomes in man. *Brain*, **56**, 1–39.

FRIEDMAN H., NASHOLD B.S. & SENECHAL P. (1972) Spinal cord stimulation and bladder function in normal and paraplegic animals. *Journal of Neurosurgery*, **36**, 430–7.

FRIEDMAN H., NASHOLD B.S. & SOMGEN G. (1974) Physiological effects of dorsal column stimulation. *Advances in Neurology*, **4**, 764–73.

FRITSCH G. & HITZIG E. (1870) Über die electrische Erregbarkeit des Grosshims. *Archives of Anatomy and Physiology*, **37**, 300–32. Translation by Bonin G. von. In *The Cerebral Cortex*, pp. 73–96. C. C. Thomas, Springfield, Illinois.

GILDENBERG P.L. (1978) Treatment of spasmodic torticollis by dorsal column stimulation. *Applied Neurophysiology*, **41**, 113–21.

GILMAN S., DAUTH G.W., TENNYSON V.W. & KREMZNER L.T. (1975) Chronic cerebellar stimulation in the monkey. *Archives of Neurology*, **32**, 474–7.

GIRVIN J.P. (1978) A review of basic aspects concerning chronic cerebral stimulation. In *Cerebellar Stimulation in Man* (Ed. Cooper I.S.), pp. 1–12. Raven Press, New York.

GLENN W.W.C., HOLCOMB W.G., HOGAN J.F., METANO I., GEE J.B.C., MOTOYAMA E.K., KIM C.S., POVRIER R.S. & FORBES G. (1973) Diaphragm pacing by radiofrequency transmission in the treatment of chronic ventilatory insufficiency. *Journal of Thoracic and Cardiovascular Surgery*, **66**, 505–20.

GLENN W.W.C., HOLCOMB W.G., SHAW R.K., HOGAN J.F. & HOLSCHUK K.R. (1976) Long term ventilatory support by diaphragm pacing in quadriplegia. *Annals of Surgery*, **183**, 566–77.

GRACANIN F. (1978) Functional electrical stimulation in control of motor output and movements. In *Contemporary Clinical Neurophysiology* (Ed. Cobb W.A. and Duijn H. von (EEG Suppl. No. 34), pp. 355–68.

GRIMES J.H., NASHOLD B.S. & ANDERSON E.E. (1975) Clinical application of electronic bladder stimulation in paraplegics. *Journal of Urology*, **113**, 338–40.

GUYTON D.L. & HAMBRECHT T.F. (1974) Theory and design of capacitor electrodes for chronic stimulation. *Medical and Biological Engineering*, **12**, 613–20.

HAMBRECHT F.T. & RESWICK J.B. (1977) *Functional Electrical Stimulation: Applications in Neural Prostheses.* Marcel Dekker Inc., New York.

HAWKES C.H., WYKE M., DESMOND A., BULTITUDE M., SMALL D., JONES S. & ROBINSON K. (1978) Epidural stimulation in 21 patients with multiple sclerosis. *Proceedings of the Sixth International Symposium on External Control of Human Extremities*, pp. 603–607. Yugoslav Committee for Electronics and Automation, Belgrade.

HAWKES C.H., WYKE M., DESMOND A., BULTITUDE M.I. & KANEGAONKAR G.S. (1980) Stimulation of dorsal column in multiple sclerosis. *British Medical Journal*, **280**, 889–91.

IEEE Transactions on Biomedical Engineering (1976) Special issue on neurological signals, current application and electrode design. **23**, No. 4, 273–356.

ILLIS L.S. (1969) Enlargement of spinal cord synapses after repetitive stimulation of a single posterior root. *Nature, London*, **223**, 76–7.

ILLIS L.S. & MITCHELL J. (1970) The effect of tetanus toxin on boutons terminaux. *Brain Research*, **18**, 283–95.

ILLIS L.S. (1973) Regeneration in the central nervous system. *Lancet*, **i**, 1035–7.

ILLIS L.S., SEDGWICK E.M., OYGAR A.E. & AWADALLA M.A.S. (1976) Dorsal column stimulation in the rehabilitation of patients with multiple sclerosis, *Lancet*, **i**, 1383–6.

ILLIS L.S., SEDGWICK E.M. & TALLIS R.C. (1980) Spinal cord stimulation in multiple sclerosis: clinical results. *Journal of Neurology, Neurosurgery and Psychiatry*, **43**, 1–14.

ILLIS L.S. & TAYLOR F.M. (1971) Neurological and electroencephalographic sequelae of tetanus. *Lancet*, **i**, 826–30.

JOBLING D.T., TALLIS R.C., SEDGWICK E.M. & ILLIS, L.S. (1980) Electronic aspects of spinal cord stimulation in multiple sclerosis. *Medical and Biological Engineering and Computing*, **18**, 48–56.

JORGENSEN O.S. & BOLWIG T.G. (1979) Synaptic proteins after electro-convulsive stimulation. *Science*, **205**, 705–7.

LIBERSON W.T., HALMQUEST H.J., SCOTT D. & DOW M. (1961) Functional electrotherapy:

stimulation of the peroneal nerve synchronized with the swing phase of the gait of hemiplegic patients. *Archives of Physical Medicine*, **42**, 101–5.

LLOYD D.P.C. & MCINTYRE A.K. (1950) Dorsal column conduction of Group 1 muscle afferent impulses and their relay through Clarke's column. *Journal of Neurophysiology*, **13**, 39–54.

MATINIAN L.A. (1976) Enzyme therapy in organic lesions of the spinal cord. Presented at National Paraplegia Foundation 4th Biennial International Neuroscientific Conference. Hollywood, Florida.

MEGLIO M., CIONI B., D'AMICO E., RONZONI G. & ROSSI G.F. (1980) Epidural spinal cord stimulation for the treatment of neurogenic bladder. *Acta Neurochirurgica*, **54**, 191–9.

MELZACK R. & WALL P.D. (1965) Pain mechanisms: a new theory. *Science, New York*, **150**, 971–9.

MORRELL F. (1961) Lasting changes in synaptic organisation produced by continuous neuronal bombardment. In *Brain Mechanisms and Learning* (Ed. Delafresnaye J.F.), pp. 375–92. Blackwell Scientific Publications, Oxford.

MORTIMER J.T., SHEALY C.N. & WHEELER C. (1970) Experimental non-destructive electrical stimulation of the brain and spinal cord. *Journal of Neurosurgery*, **32**, 553–9.

NASHOLD B.S., FRIEDMAN H., GLENN J.H., GRIMES J.H., BARRY W.F. & AVERY R. (1972) Electromicturition in paraplegia. *Archives of Surgery*, **104**, 195–202.

OWENS S., ATKINSON E.R. & LEES D.E. (1979) Thermographic evidence of reduced sympathetic tone with transcutaneous nerve stimulation. *Anaesthesiology*, **50**, 62–5.

PUDENZ R.H. (1977) Adverse effects of electrical energy applied to the nervous system. In *Symposium on the Safety and Clinical Efficacy of Implanted Neuro-augmentive Devices* (Eds. Burton C.V., Ray C.D. & Nashold B.S.). *Neurosurgery*, **1**, 186–232.

PUDENZ R.H., BULLARA L.A., DRU D. & TALALLA A. (1975) Electrical stimulation of the brain. II. Effects on the blood–brain barrier. *Surgical Neurology*, **4**, 37–42.

READ D.J., MATTHEWS W.B. & HIGSON R.H. (1980) The effect of spinal cord stimulation on patients with multiple sclerosis. *Brain*, **103**, 803–33.

RICHARDSON R.R., CERULLO L.J. & MEYER P.R. (1979) Autonomic hyper-reflexia modulated by percutaneous epidural neurostimulation: a preliminary report. *Neurosurgery*, **4**, 517–20.

RICHARDSON R.R. & MCLONE G. (1978) Percutaneous epidural neuro-stimulation for paraplegic spasticity. *Surgical Neurology*, **9**, 153–5.

ROSEN J.A. & BARSOUM A.H. (1979) Failure of chronic dorsal column stimulation in M.S. *Annals of Neurology*, **6**, 66–7.

SEDGWICK E.M., ILLIS L.S., TALLIS R.C., THORNTON A.R.D., ABRAHAM P., EL-NEGAMY E., DOCHERTY T.B., SOAR J.S., SPENCER S.C. & TAYLOR F.M. (1980) Evoked potentials and contingent negative variation during treatment of multiple sclerosis with spinal cord stimulation. *Journal of Neurology, Neurosurgery and Psychiatry*, **43**, 15–24.

SHEALY C.N., TASLITZ N., MORTIMER J.T. & BECKER D.P. (1967) Electrical inhibition of pain: experimental evaluation. *Anaesthesia and Analgesia—Current Research*, **46**, 299–304.

SHERRINGTON C.S. (1906) *The Integrative Action of the Nervous System*. Cambridge University Press (1947), 2e.

TALLIS R.C., ILLIS L.S. & SEDGWICK E.M. (1982) Spinal cord stimulation in peripheral vascular disease. Third International Meeting on Spinal Cord Stimulation. (In preparation.)

WALTZ J.M. & PANI K.C. (1978) Spinal cord stimulation in disorders of the motor system. *Sixth International Symposium on External Control of Human Extremities, Dubrovnik*, pp. 546–56. Yugoslav Committee for Electronics and Automation, Belgrade.

YATES J.C. & YATES R.D. (1966) An electronmicroscope study of the effects of tetanus toxin on motoneurones of the cat spinal cord. *Journal of Ultrastructure Reasearch*, **16**, 382–94.

YOUNG R.F. & GOODMAN S.J. (1979) Dorsal spinal cord stimulation in the treatment of multiple sclerosis. *Neutosurgery*, **5**, 225–8.

Index

411